T0386060

HISTORIES OF THE TRANSGENDER CHILD

Histories of the Transgender Child

. . . .

Julian Gill-Peterson

University of Minnesota Press
Minneapolis
London

Portions of chapter 1 were previously published as
"Implanting Plasticity into Sex and Trans/Gender: Animal and
Child Metaphors in the History of Endocrinology," *Angelaki:
Journal of the Theoretical Humanities* 22, no. 2 (2017): 47–60,
www.tandfonline.com.

Published by the University of Minnesota Press
111 Third Avenue South, Suite 290
Minneapolis, MN 55401-2520
http://www.upress.umn.edu

Printed on acid-free paper

The University of Minnesota is an equal-opportunity educator and employer.

Library of Congress Cataloging-in-Publication Data
Names: Gill-Peterson, Julian, author.
Title: Histories of the transgender child / Julian Gill-Peterson.
Description: Minneapolis : University of Minnesota Press, [2018]. | Includes
   bibliographical references and index. |
Identifiers: LCCN 2018008947 (print) | ISBN 978-1-5179-0466-1 (hc) | ISBN 978-1-5179-0467-8 (pb)
Subjects: LCSH: Transgender children—United States—History. | Gender
   nonconformity—United States—History.
Classification: LCC HQ77.95.U6 G55 2018 (print) | DDC 306.76/80835—dc23
LC record available at https://lccn.loc.gov/2018008947

UMP LSI

Contents

Contents

Preface

We fear the children we would protect.

—Kathryn Bond Stockton, *The Queer Child*

A LIBEL PLACED ON THE VERY EXISTENCE of trans children, a vicious question mark snaked around being, is what passes for a rational object of "debate" among adults every day in the media, online, in schools and clinics, and in the social milieu in which trans children must find a way, despite all the odds, to survive, to grow, and to endure. Subject to radical skepticism and verification in the best instances and to being dismissed as unreal or brainwashed in the worst, trans children's consistent experience in this country is to be excluded from having a voice, from having a say in the public battle over whether they should find themselves allowed *to be*, as if such determinations are not procedurally genocidal in their holding open the door to a world where trans life would be violently extinguished from growing in the first place. We have not even yet begun to ask what it would mean to let trans children name their own desires and be recognized as entitled to direct their own affairs. Adults, whether anti-trans hate groups, trans exclusionary feminists, conservative activists, parents, so-called interested observers, or even allies and advocates, tarry within the dangerously limiting circumstances of a system that continues to assay the value of trans children's being in terms not of their humanity and personhood but via questions absurd in their abstraction for how they ask us instead to wonder if trans children "prove something" about the biological basis of sex and gender or how identity politics have so injured a cis, white, heteronormative imaginary that cannot fathom the obvious fragility of its claims to universalism in the face of a defiant *no*. While anti-trans forces mobilize and collude to enforce binary childhoods in schools, in gender-segregated organizations, in the normative family, and in public accommodations that make trans childhood a life-threatening place to be every day, trans-inclusive and trans-affirmative voices struggle to find a way to protect trans children that does not imagine them as deserving of protection because they are, finally, the *property* of adults, not people with the right to gender self-determination. In the midst of this false fight, the real demographic majority of trans children, who do not have access to medicine, who do not fit the white, middle-class, desexualized image trafficked in the media, and whose lives go on and grow in spite of the many denials of being thrown at them, have no viable status in which to be recognized or welcomed. Trans children have been reduced to figures for what they are so clearly not, abstract ciphers of this or that etiology of gender, this or that political platform. Trans childhood, under such circumstances, has yet to visit us. Yet trans children already exist, left to fend for themselves in a culture that suffers from being unable to imagine children with a richly expressive sense of who they are.

If childhood is already a very dangerous time and space for children in the United States, trans childhoods—and, so much more specifically and insistently, *black* trans and *trans of color* childhoods, *nonbinary* trans childhoods, *low-income* trans childhoods, *disabled* trans childhoods, and *undocumented* trans childhoods—have been evacuated of formal meaning and abandoned by adults as less-than-human precincts, caustic reminders of the effects of a culture in which the delusional adoration of the rosy figure of the Child abuts the most heinous quotidian modes of violence in the lives of real children. We make children vulnerable by the force of law, the deprivation of their economic earnings, and the infantilization of their personalities, only to raid their bodies, minds, and souls to enrich an order of things that cannot stomach their savvy and enviable divergences from normativity.

This book works slowly and at length, over diachronic and synchronic modes of historiography, to visit as much destruction as possible upon one central libel that limits the livelihood of trans children: that they have no history, that they are fundamentally new and, somehow, therefore deserving of less than human recognition. Throughout, my point of departure is that trans children's right to be is not up for debate. Instead, the affirmation of that right directs my thinking. Such a project of historiography requires a certain way of writing and engaging with the grain of the incredible twentieth-century archive of trans childhood, race, and medicine. But before entering that mode, which necessitates giving up others, let me speak a little differently, to say that the urgency of giving up our foolish attachment to an *adult* innocence about trans childhood also motivates me in the pages that follow (and not, say, a retrospective desire for a trans childhood that I or anyone else might have had). The truth is, we don't know trans children because we have inherited, reinforced, and perpetuated a cultural system of gender and childhood in which they are unknowable and, what's worst of all, unable to be cared for except through forms of harm. The staggering, nauseating arithmetic of trans youth suicide and the truth that we have just witnessed again, in 2017 *more than in any year on record before it,* of the murder of black and brown trans women, are two real costs of that innocence and its normative delusions about childhood, gender, and race.

In writing this book, I have become possessed by the haunting insistence of the many trans children who populate it, archived under circumstances of simultaneous violence and remarkable flourishing that inspire in me—and, I hope, you—a profound *responsibility* to understand that our relation to trans children is not given but must be thoughtfully and carefully negotiated. Throughout the text, I use "*[sic]*" to mark instances in which quoted materials contradict the pronouns used by the person being discussed. In underlining my disagreement with discourses that have refused to honor trans people's pronouns, I hope that these trans children from the past are far from contained by it. On the contrary, they might erupt out of history and into the present, finding company alongside the countless trans children, today and tomorrow, whose vulnerabilities are not really by reason of age but actually engineered by adults and who call upon us each to account for our complicity with the violent arithmetic of bullying, suicide, murder, and life deprived of safety and collective or self-determination. I find myself confronted at the end of writing this book with the certain knowledge that we are not worthy of the care of trans children we have accorded ourselves. Until we see that, and from such a realization work toward a radical reckoning with the ways that the concept of childhood, binary gender, medicine, racism, and capitalism have transacted unbelievable degrees of harm in the name of care, guardianship, development, and pedagogy, we will find ourselves ever lacking in the company, comfort, rich knowledge, inspiring worlds, and tenacity of the trans children who, despite adults, call this world home. We scarcely yet know what it would mean to care for trans children, and in that way, they are *not* ours.

India Monroe
Mesha Caldwell

Jamie Lee Wounded Arrow
Jojo Striker
Jaquarrias Holland
Tiara Richmond
Chyna Gibson
Ciara McElveen
Alphonza Watson
Kenne McFadden
Chay "Juicy" Reed
Mx. Bostick
Sherrell Faulkner
Imer Alvarado
Kendra Adams
Ebony Morgan
TeeTee Dangerfield
Gwynevere River Song
Kiwi Herring
Anthony "Bubbles" Torres
Derricka Banner
Ally Lee Steinfeld
Stephanie Montez
Candace Towns

—JULIAN GILL-PETERSON
   November 20, 2017
   (Transgender Day of Remembrance)

Toward a Trans of Color
Critique of Medicine

AMID THE ACCELERATING AND CONTESTED PUBLIC VISIBILITY
that trans life has accrued in the United States in recent years, certain
figures have become oversaturated. Made to carry starkly different narratives for mass consumption, while simultaneously offering very narrow
windows to contest the terms of their representation, images of black trans
women and trans women of color on the one hand and transgender children on the other circulate seemingly without end. These very different
figures are, somehow, meant to signify and embody the so-called newness
and now-ness of trans life. As Laverne Cox and Janet Mock speak out from
their perspective as black trans women or CeCe McDonald writes letters
from prison, Jazz Jennings stars in a reality television show about entering
high school as a trans girl and Gavin Grimm pursues a legal case against the
school board of Gloucester County, Virginia, over its transphobic bathroom policy.[1] While there may be a growing awareness of the rising and
unmatched violence black trans women and trans women of color face, a
seemingly never-ending stream of documentaries, independent films, journalistic profiles, novels, and digital platforms simultaneously circulates
images and narratives about a "new" generation of children growing up as
transgender *during* their childhoods.[2] The public figurations of black trans
women, trans women of color, and trans children have become pervasive
but markedly distinct, with profoundly different significance and impact.

The contrast is instructive about the fault lines of the seismic shifts
underway in U.S. trans visibility but also incredibly misleading. The pub-
licness of black trans women and trans women of color is registered,
paradoxically, through ongoing forms of social death that reduce their personhood to the barest zero degree, hiding it from view and converting
their images and names more often into objects of necropolitical value.[3]
As scholars in black trans studies, including Treva Ellison, Kai M. Green,
Matt Richardson, C. Riley Snorton, Elías Cosenza Krell, Syrus Marcus

Ware, and Erin Durban-Albrecht, have argued, this visibility is specifically predicated on antiblack modes of subjection whereby the surveillance and exposure of being visible elicits the extreme and paradoxical charge of nonexistence.[4] Trans children, meanwhile, are presented as powerful emblems of futurity. Sanitized, innocent, and always highly medicalized, they are domesticated figures, either reassuring that the so-called trans tipping point heralds a new generation of liberal progress and acceptance or, to the transphobic agitators involved in political campaigns focusing on bathrooms and schools, acting as proof that trans life deserves to be repressed in its incipient forms for the threat to the social order that its future would represent. Children, by design deprived of civil rights and infantilized, are easy targets for political violence—just as easily, it turns out, as concerned adults can claim them for protection.

The problem with this figural contrast, of course, is that it arbitrarily separates black trans and trans of color life from trans childhood. The dominant figure of the trans child trafficked in the public sphere today underwrites, as the child has long done in the United States, a potent "racial innocence" that empties trans childhood of its content, including race, rendering it conceptually white while simultaneously libeling the existence of black trans and trans of color childhood.[5] There is tremendous damage in the figurative separation of racialized trans negativity and white trans childhood futurity.[6] And the part played by the figure of the child in this process has received very little, if any, attention. Despite the overwhelming material vulnerability of actual trans children, most of whom live at a great distance from the imagined world represented in dominant media narratives, the figure of the trans child as emblem of a new and futuristic generation is part of a larger strategy that continues to disavow and naturalize the reduction of black trans women and trans women of color's personhood to nothingness, what Eva Hayward calls "an attack on ontology, on beingness, because beingness cannot be secured."[7]

Yet an even more fundamental assumption about trans children that floats this contrast has yet to be challenged: that they are, in fact, new and future-bound. The narrative that we are in the midst of the *first* generation of trans children is so omnipresent as to be ambient. It is repeated ad nauseam in the media, online, by doctors, and by parents.[8] Trans children, these various gatekeepers say in unison, have no history at all. Trans children are unprecedented and must be treated as such, with caution or awe. What happens if this consensus turns out to be baseless? The bleached and medicalized image of the trans child circulating as unprecedented in the twenty-first century is actually prefaced by an entire century of trans children, including black trans children and trans children of color. And trans children played a decisive role in the medicalization of sex and gender, rather than being its newest objects. These are two of the key ruptures that *Histories of the Transgender Child* uncovers. If the contrasting effect of contemporary figurations of black trans and trans of color life, placed next to trans childhood, is so damaging in its staging of an antinomy between negativity and futurity, this book argues that the twentieth century provides a surprising archive of trans childhood that undoes them from the inside.

Histories of the Transgender Child rewrites the historical and political basis for the supposed newness of today's generation of trans kids by uncovering more than a century of what came before them. From the 1910s, children with "ambiguous" sex were medicalized and experimented upon by doctors who sought in their unfinished, developing bodies a material foothold for altering and, eventually, changing human sex as it grew. In the 1930s, some of the first trans people to seek out American doctors connected their requests for medical support to reports that "sex changes" on children were being regularly performed at certain hospitals. In the 1940s and 1950s, five decades of experimental alteration of children's sex directly led to the invention of the category gender, setting the stage for the emergence of a new field of transsexual medicine and the postwar model of binary transition. And in the 1960s and 1970s, as that field of medicine became institutionalized, many children took hormones, changed their names, attended school recognized in their gender identities, and even underwent gender confirmation surgeries. Trans children not only were present but also were an integral part of the transgender twentieth century *and* the broader twentieth-century history of sex, gender, and race in medicine.

If there are so many trans children hiding in plain sight in the past, how have we failed to see them? I argue that trans children were central to the medicalization of sex and gender during the twentieth century in a very specific way, made valuable through a racialized discourse of plasticity. Examining the history of trans children through the shifting terrain of that plasticity helps to explain, precisely, *why* trans children have so easily gone unnoticed or been ignored. By limiting trans children's value to an abstract biological force through which medicine aimed to alter sex and gender as phenotypes, those children became living laboratories, proxies for working

out broader questions about human sex and gender that had little investment in their personhood. Children were by the design of medical discourse meant to recede into the background of the alteration of sex and
gender by being reduced to reservoirs of plasticity, the raw material of phenotype. Children became the incarnation and etiology of sex's plasticity
as an abstract form of whiteness, the capacity to take on new form and be
transformed by medical scientific intervention early on in life. And the
twentieth-century discourse of child development naturalized this function in the medical clinic.

   In the early part of the century this resulted in reading trans (and intersex, as we shall see) children's "abnormal" or "mixed" sexual development
through eugenic and evolutionist paradigms that sorted sexual morphology through racial typology. By the 1960s, it allowed the inaugural gatekeepers of transsexual medicine to imagine an etiology of transsexuality in
the indeterminacy of childhood gender acquisition, opening the door to
the genocidal fantasy of eradicating trans life altogether in its developing
forms, even as children also successfully transitioned and secured access to
gender confirmation surgery. Far from being a progressive vector of malleability or change, the racial plasticity of sex and gender was a decidedly
disenfranchising object of governance from the perspective of trans children. At its institutional best, it granted access to a rigid medical model
premised on binary normalization. At its institutional worst, it allowed gatekeeping clinicians to reject black and trans of color children as *not plastic
enough* for the category of transsexuality, dismissing their self-knowledge
of gender as delusion or homosexuality. The value of plasticity came to
stand in for the value of trans children's personhood, enabling their continual instrumentalization in the service of medical science over and above
any recognition of their embodied self-knowledge or desire. This book's
uncovering of a century of untold stories is therefore not a recuperative
or reparative project. I instead underline a massively overlooked way that
children's bodies, because of their unfinishedness and plastic potential to
be changed as they grow, have been key sites of the modernizing violence
of medicine. Trans children have been forced to pay one of the heaviest
prices for the sex and gender binary, silenced *as* the raw material of its
medical foundation.

   At the same time, however, framing trans children through a discourse
of plasticity was a risky wager for medical science, as embodied plasticity itself, despite being ostensibly domesticated through its racialization as

whiteness, retained a demonstrable *autonomy* that threatens normalizing models of the sex and gender binary, along with medical technique, to this day. In key moments throughout the twentieth century, trans children's plasticity enacted forms of partial material refusal that threatened to cause a crisis for doctors in the categories sex and gender.[9] Plasticity, an invisible force in the trans child's body, seemed to always retain a certain material agency for itself, partly indifferent or oblivious to scientific rationality. Whether the strange forms of plastic growth that resulted from these moments, interrupting the orderly flow of medical reason, actually provided trans children any leverage is a complex problem that this book unfolds slowly, over a century's worth of clinical history. While I argue against the current romance with plasticity in the humanities and STEM fields, showing how the concept and its material referent encourage no particular form of political agency, the book's archive testifies to how difficult it is to imagine that trans children, already lacking patient rights, could have resisted its capture by medicine.[10]

Still, there are important and startling moments in the archive when some trans children's plasticity afforded them brief movements outward and away from the capture of modern medicine. While there is no clear-cut scene that rises to the pitch of resistance or even subversion, and there is otherwise a great deal of violence, both epistemic and material, there remains something vital to consider about the limits of plasticity in building different futures around childhood transition and pediatric medicine. To that end, this book does investigate the enigma of trans children's plasticity, not so much to affirm its value as to look *through* it for ways to undermine the rationality of medicine, challenge the racialization of sex and gender as phenotypes, and imagine different futures for trans children that do not instrumentalize their living bodies and dismiss their self-knowledge.

The Generational Trouble of Trans Children

Histories of the Transgender Child wades into a subject about which we have almost nothing in the way of reference points. There are no existing accounts of trans children's history in the United States, only speculation and retrospective theorizing from the point of view of the present. The myth that there were no trans children until recently is so widespread and unchallenged that it is present even in the small but rich and growing scholarship on the trans child, most of which focuses on the twenty-first-century pediatric endocrine clinic or media representation.[11] In "Child," a keyword entry in the inaugural issue of *Transgender Studies Quarterly*, Tey Meadow observes that, "A relatively new social form, we see no references to transgender children prior to the mid-1990s."[12] Although in a strict sense this is correct, because the term "transgender" did not come into widespread use until the 1990s and would have been unavailable to attach itself to children before then, the second dimension of Meadow's claim—that adults are confronted with a "new social form" in trans children—is an important clue as to why their history has been forgotten or erased. Much of the celebration and controversy over trans children today departs from the fact that they express self-knowledge about something as profound as their gender, flouting social, medical, and parental gender assignment. This initial focus frequently travels to fixate on medical therapies to pause puberty and pursue childhood transition as either a biologically "reversible" or "irreversible" process.[13] The ostensible concern is that the effects of these "new" hormonal technologies are in some important way unknown or that children are too young to undergo hormonal therapy or even make the decision to alter their bodies—as if sex and gender were otherwise natural, unmodified forms in cisgender bodies.[14] This narrative also grants immense authority to medicine in making the trans child an ontological possibility, as if trans children were unthinkable, nonexistent even, prior to puberty suppression therapy.[15] The novelty of today's medical technique is deeply questioned by this book, which traces an entire century of medicalizing trans children and their biological development, while also stressing the many ways in which trans children had no need for medicine to live trans lives. Even if medical technologies do not play a causal role in the production of new social forms, however, the social meaning invested in them does seem to be very important for many *adults* today.

In "Trans*—Gender Transitivity and New Configurations of Body, History, Memory and Kinship," Jack Halberstam seizes on a speculation in Meadow's work to dramatize this point. Halberstam's interest is in a perceived "disjunction in transgender histories" between today's trans children, who are growing up in an environment where the trans child is a distinct and partially recognized social and medical category, and older trans and gender-variant adults who came of age in a different political, cultural, and medical milieu during the second half of the twentieth century.[16] The issue boils down to a generational split. If today's trans children can have a recognizable trans childhood, with options to transition, Meadow proposes that "this new generation may have wider latitude to disidentify with transgender history and those who came before them."[17] That "is quite a mind-blowing statement," Halberstam interjects, developing Meadow's speculation further:

> Unlike other social justice formations where young people might acknowledge and even thank the adults who came before them and made the world a more hospitable place, Meadow proposes that the support that many trans children now enjoy from their families and communities affords them a radically different experience of childhood than that of trans people even a decade older. While transgender individuals of my generation, now in their forties and fifties, who often could not transition until they were adults, lacked a complex language for their gender variance and had to live large parts of their lives in relations to gender identities with which they were at odds, today's gender nonconforming children, Meadow reminds us, with parental support, may grow up trans rather than struggling through long periods of enforced gender normativity. While that is a cause for some amount of celebration, it also, Meadow hints, puts them at odds with the history that produced the conditions for their smooth(er) passage from trans childhood to adulthood.[18]

While I agree that a potentially difficult generation gap is growing in the twenty-first century between trans children and adults, and I do not wish to interrogate Halberstam's generational experience, this book puts significant pressure on the historical premises upon which this reflection rests. Setting aside for a moment the problem of *which* trans children Halberstam is calling upon, given how highly racialized and class-stratified access to competent medical care is in the United States, I would point out that the apparent disidentification of today's trans children with the trans past may in large part be premised on a fundamental misrecognition of that past.[19] We do not know trans children's history because we have assumed they do not, generationally, belong in the trans past. The fact that trans children have been forced in the twenty-first century to fare without a history may itself *be* a major cause of the generational tension that Halberstam identifies.[20] How different would this passage look in light of several key points that this book works to unfold? Today's trans children are *not* the first generation to identify and live openly as trans during child-hood. They are not even close to the first generation to transition or to be medicalized during childhood and grow up as publicly trans. In fact, trans children outright precede the category "transsexuality" and the contemporary medical model. Trans children have a documentable past stretching the *entirety* of the twentieth century, long before today's trans and gender-variant adults were even born.

With a distinctly different take on Meadow and Halberstam's reflections, then, *Histories of the Transgender Child* departs by considering the extent to which the twenty-first-century framing of trans children as new and lacking historicity is actually *complicit* with their ongoing political infantilization, particularly by medicine. Investing in the idea that today's trans children either are new or represent a major break with the past may actually be a significant obstacle to forming cross-generational relationships between trans adults and children that do not do the latter harm or continue to render their actions and embodied self-knowledge unintelligible. And, particularly of concern in this book, the myth that trans children have no history has significantly reinforced the rationality of medicine by allowing the twentieth and twenty-first centuries to be defined by the limiting parameters of transsexuality and puberty suppression therapy, discourses that rely on children being the nearly invisible, plastic bedrock of medical technique or an etiology for gender in general.

This presumes, of course, that there is a meaningful "transgender child" in the past, rather than another projection of contemporary categories backward. I deploy an array of terms in a careful way to explore how we have arrived at a moment where it is possible to claim trans children are somehow new. But before focusing on the historiographical problems of the period that this book covers, it is worth laying out exactly what I mean conceptually both by "transgender" and "child" in this book. "Trans" is invoked throughout in an expansive sense, as it has been theorized in transgender studies, sometimes as a prefix and sometimes with an asterisk, to mark a *political* distinction from medical or pathological meanings that have accrued to the term "transgender" in recent years, many of which have been borrowed from the earlier term "transsexual."[21] While it is technically anachronistic to name a child in 1930 "trans," I do so precisely to make an intervention, as Susan Stryker puts it so well: to "[tell] a story about the political history of gender variance that is not limited to one experience."[22]

The terms "transvestism" and "transvestite" also appear in this book, as they had both medical and lay connotations in the first half of the twentieth century, as well as relatively uneven adoption in the United States compared to Europe. I use them in precise historical contexts, largely before "transsexuality" and "transsexual" came into use. Similarly, I use the terms "hermaphrodite," "intersex," "sexual inversion," and "homosexuality" when their appearance in archival documents matters. In many instances these terms bleed over into trans domains, making their overlap important. Finally, I name "transsexuality" to explicitly mark a *medical* discourse and biopolitical apparatus, a colonial form of knowledge with racializing and disenfranchising effects. Transsexuality arrogantly pretends to know and seize trans life as an object, making it a difficult concept to write with and against, as Sandy Stone first theorized through the concept of the "posttranssexual."[23] More than some of the other terms used in this book, "transsexuality" is an artifact of a dominant knowledge system to be constantly questioned and undermined from the inside. Transgender studies has excelled at the critical use of terminology to make sense of *and* challenge scientific and medical authority, but perhaps my attention to now obsolete categories or now politically incorrect terms may, at times, strike readers as awkward. What's more, it is likely that the categorical landscape will continue to change in the future, at some point rendering the language of this book anachronistic, something that I embrace. Here I follow Leslie Feinberg's lead in *Transgender Warriors*: "Since I am writing this book as a contribution to the demand for transgender liberation, the language I'm using in this book is not aimed at *defining* but at *defending* the diverse communities that are coalescing."[24]

If it seems odd, by contrast, to take the time to define what a child is, there is good reason to be equally critical and careful. Rather than taking for granted the existence of children as a demographic group defined somehow by age, this book takes a fairly simple approach to defining who is a trans child. Anyone under the medical age of consent during the twentieth century—typically twenty-one, but sometimes eighteen—is a child in the pages that follows. I draw on the medical age of consent not because it refers to a meaningful distinction but precisely because its arbitrariness and obvious construction illuminate how the figure of "the child" and actual living "children" are entangled products of historical processes of Western subjectification, rather than representing a natural category of human life. While there are infants, toddlers, five-year-olds, teenagers, and even twenty-year-olds throughout this book, I refer to all of them as children because they were subject to a specifically *infantilizing* form of governance (this is also why the category "adolescent" did not meaningfully come into play in trans medicine during this period). The medical age of consent, which deprived children of the ability to make medical decisions for themselves, proved to be a deciding factor in shaping their experiences and limiting their ability to act. Drawing on Paul Amar's critical reading of the field of childhood studies, I agree that the child is a dehumanized social form, the product of historical and political processes of infantilization "designed to control various populations" through sexual and racial difference, rather than to index meaningful age differences.[25] As Amar points out, one of the most pernicious effects of the production of children through infantilization is "a failure to recognize children as agents," to render their lives politically *informal*—effectively unintelligible to adults.[26] The Western form of the child and childhood is a powerful obstacle to seeing "the mechanism and practices by which social actors branded as children challenge the regime of infantilization," whether through collective organization or individual itineraries that stray from developmentalism.[27] For that reason, this book names the trans *child* not as a distinct subgroup within the trans community but as a politically disenfranchised person subject to a regime of racially and gender normative governance by medicine and other social institutions, including the family.

While the children who populate this book, particularly those in the early twentieth century, may not look recognizably trans by today's dominant definition, this is precisely because the signature effect of medicalization over the past century has been to restrict trans life to a singular definition *while simultaneously placing an etiological question mark upon trans people,* and children especially, forcing them to constantly prove and account for their embodied self-knowledge instead of taking their transness seriously. The social reality of trans children across the twentieth century in this book begins to suggest some of the many ways that children whose lives differed from the normative patterns for the sex and gender they were assigned at birth actually multiply the meanings of "trans," moving it in many different directions. In so doing, I stress that the being of trans children—the content of their "transness," as such—is *not* the place to ground the meaning of trans childhood, for that etiological discourse is precisely the one in whose name medicine has inflicted incredible harm. The trans child represents a further case of what Kathryn Bond Stockton has described as the ghostliness of certain "impossible" children during the twentieth century.[28] Not meant to exist at all in the present tense of their childhoods, the ghostliness of trans children over the past one hundred years takes unique residence in the medical archive, hiding in plain sight, invisible to the inverse degree of being pervasively present, yet always slightly out of reach even as they come into discourse. To pursue the trans twentieth century *through* the perspective of trans children, as this book does, shows how Halberstam's assumed "history that produced the conditions for their smooth(er) passage from trans childhood to adulthood" is really not at all what we adults have come to imagine.

The Trans (and Intersex) Twentieth Century

This book begins at the turn of the twentieth century, when sex was brought under the jurisdiction of a modernizing project of medicine that sought to alter its form, and traces the medicalization of trans children until 1980, the year in which the publication of a new edition of the *Diagnostic and Statistical Manual* with an entry on "Gender Identity Disorder of Childhood" inaugurated the medical matrix in which we still live today. By beginning in the early twentieth century, the moment in which sex was redefined through the concept of plasticity by fields like endocrinology and urology, I read the medical archive to *contest* the historiography of the trans past monopolized by the parameters of transsexuality. While this book is first and foremost an account of trans children's past, its broader historiographical intervention within transgender studies has four specific ends: to continue the work of displacing the 1950s as a default starting point for trans history; to undermine the rationality of medical science from its inside by reading trans people as complex participants in the production of scientific knowledge, rather than its objects; to highlight the overlooked entanglement of intersex and trans bodies during the first half of the twentieth century; and to uncover the vital but unexamined role of the child's body in the medicalization of sex and gender as racially plastic, alterable phenotypes. These four characteristics of the trans twentieth century played decisive roles in shaping the lives of trans children, and vice versa.

The 1950s have been granted too much weight in transgender studies and popular accounts as the reference point for the twentieth century, overrepresenting the advent of transsexual medicine and Christine Jorgensen's

celebrity.[29] The shadow cast by the midcentury also comes in the form
of historical argumentation, like Paul B. Preciado's in *Testo Junkie*, which
imagines something especially distinct about the postwar era that enabled
the emergence of transsexuality and its correlate medical techniques.[30]
This thinking runs perilously close to reproducing the kind of technodeterminism that characterizes Bernice Hausman's reading of the history
of trans medicine in *Changing Sex*, which has been roundly critiqued from
Jay Prosser on for what he terms the transphobic "conception of transsexuals as constructed in some more literal way than nontranssexuals."[31]
It is also historically inaccurate, as Joanne Meyerowitz points out, considering that medical procedures to change human sex long predated the willingness of American doctors to actually provide them to trans people, a shift
that this book reexamines.[32] In reality there was no revolutionary techno-
logical or medical shift in midcentury. Transsexuality is, rather, a medical
discourse that distracts from forms of knowledge and being that are disqualified by its rationality and its timescale, minimizing a half-century of
trans life and interaction with medicine that both precedes and informs it.

Since institutional medicine typically involves meticulous record keeping and voluminous discursive practices, and because it claims unrivaled
authority to know and govern trans life, it represents a significant source
of information on the trans past.[33] The distinct challenge of the early twentieth century, before transsexuality, is that we still do not know very much
about trans life *or* actual medical practice in this era. While there is an
established sense that in some places in Europe, particularly Germany, trans
people had access to various forms of medical support and built vibrant
social worlds in urban centers as early as the 1920s, their experiences in the
United States were not always comparable, as the second chapter of this
book explores. What we do know about the concept of "sex change" and
the hormonal theories of interwar endocrinology is framed in largely sche-
matic, discursive terms through published medical texts and journalistic
sources.[34] Meyerowitz argues on this basis that the entire concept of changing sex for trans people took root first in Germany, not the United States,
because of a "vocal campaign for sexual emancipation."[35] Yet there are no
clinical histories in the United States that examine what actually went on
in the hospitals and doctor's offices where sex was made plastic and alterable or what happened when trans people began to seek out those doctors
for assistance with their transitions. Nor do we have a concrete sense of
how trans people understood their relationship to medicine beyond their

interaction with popular-press accounts of dramatized "sex changes." In the face of this prevailing lack of evidence, one of the central contributions of *Histories of the Transgender Child* is to reconstruct clinical histories at key places around the country, including a long-term look at the Johns Hopkins Hospital from the 1910s to the 1960s. I show that trans people readily sought out American doctors in the absence of a category like transsexuality as early as the 1930s—but not because they needed a medical discourse to make sense of their lives—that there were trans social worlds in the same period that Berlin was renowned for its trans community, and that even in the early twentieth century a few trans childhoods made it into the medical archive.

Still, there is disagreement over the very viability of claiming early twentieth-century figures as trans, rather than lesbian and gay, because of the absence of a clear separation between categories.[36] Or rather, it would be more precise to say that our contemporary sense of categories that line up around separable phenomena of "sex," "gender," and "sexuality" did not exist until incredibly recently, coming into being perhaps only over the past forty years. This has resulted in a very slow recognition of obviously trans individuals who led public lives well before the availability of synthetic hormones or the concept of transsexuality, and several of them appear in the first few chapters of this book. And this problem has dogged the crossroads of queer theory and trans studies in particular. Take Ralph Werther, who went by the name Jennie June and whose peculiar 1919 text, *Autobiography of an Androgyne*, details her life as an "invert" and lower-class "fairie" in New York City from around the 1890s to the 1910s. In his introduction to a reissued edition, Scott Herring underlines the fascinating ways in which June's text at first glance serves a modernizing discourse of transatlantic sexology, adopting and commenting on Richard von Krafft-Ebing's typology of inversion from *Psychopathia Sexualis* and making frequent use of Latin to describe frank scenes of sex and cross-sex social life in the "underworld."[37] Perhaps to skirt obscenity censors, the *Autobiography* was published by a medical press, complete with an authorizing introduction by a well-respected physician, who framed the text as an account of "the congenital homosexualist" (11). Yet Herring also points out how June turns on the sexological premises of the narrative in key moments, authoring powerful critiques of the legal and social ostracism of the era, making the *Autobiography* "one of the inaugural acts of queer social theory in the United States" (xv).

Why *queer* social theory? Why not *trans* social theory? Although Herring is careful to point out that we know very little about the real person behind the nom de plume "Ralph Werther," he nonetheless claims June for the history of queer sexuality as a figure whose life writing undermines the sexological framing of modern *gay* American sexuality (xv, xxxi). Yet it is far less clear, within the text itself, why June's repeated professions to be "really a woman whom Nature disguised as a man" (25)—having wished to be a girl from early childhood (29), using the name "Jennie" from a young age (34), wearing women's clothing from childhood on, wishing to have her genitals recognized as a woman's (45), and eventually choosing to be medically castrated—would not invite a strongly *trans* reading. Alfred Herzog, the doctor who wrote the introduction to the original text, speculates about June's castration procedure that "he hated above all the testicles, those insignia of manhood, and had them removed to be more alike to that which he wished to be," a woman (14). Or, as June puts it herself: "were it not for certain masculine conformations of the body, I ought to go about in dresses as a woman, and always identify myself with the female sex" (13). In the retrospective frame of postwar American identity politics, where transgender has frequently been styled as a successor to gay and where trans studies has sometimes been cast as a successor to queer theory, June's account of inversion has inaccurately been routed through the same implicitly teleological model.

In *Transgender History*, Susan Stryker names Jennie June as a trans woman in her review of the era before transsexuality.[38] And there are compelling reasons to make that claim, not the least of which is that even June's definition of inversion reflects not quite proto-homosexuality as we would expect it from our contemporary vantage point but an entirely different epistemology of sex, one that is not well known anymore. June employs a scientific thesis on the natural bisexuality of the species that was very much in vogue at the time of the publication of the *Autobiography*, explaining that "there exists, in the human race, no sharp dividing line between the sexes."[39] Within that paradigm, June observes that "there are innumerable stages of transitional individuals" (21) between masculinity and femininity, including those described as inverts by sexology. June actually goes so far as to explain her life through a concept of sexual plasticity: a "protoplasm" theory of inversion, according to which "the presence in the male body of a particular kind of governing corpuscles or germs ordinarily found only in the protoplasm of females" (31) results, at birth, in a mixed body and person, somewhat male, somewhat female. While Herring reads this inversion as a harbinger of modern homosexuality, the very resistance to modernizing sexological narratives he identifies in the *Autobiography* also undermines the reading of June's life as gay instead of trans. The specifically trans quality of this life narrative is based in a lived epistemology of sex's *plasticity*, not a binary of homosexual and heterosexual personhood.

The point is not to decide for trans over gay in a categorical sense but to understand that the European sexological concept of "inversion" was a much more complex blend of what today is separated into sex or gender on the one hand and sexuality or sexual object choice on the other. What's more, as Emma Heaney explains in *The New Woman*, the discourse of sexology that produced inversion is premised on a staggering misrecognition and confinement of the rich social reality of trans feminine life and experience in this era. Quite unlike Herring, Heaney argues that "Jennie June bridges vernacular and medical understandings *of trans femininity*."[40] *Histories of the Transgender Child* follows Heaney's important historiographical intervention into the early twentieth century, that "the emergence of the trans feminine as a field distinct from both male homosexuality and cis womanhood is a weighty historical corollary to the emergence of homosexuality."[41] Heaney shows that the growth of sexological and medical paradigms at the turn of the century was not the teleological apprehension of trans life by science, as it has often been framed, but rather the emergence of a distinction between cis and trans femininity that did not previously exist socially in Europe and the United States. In this context, I argue for reading certain historical individuals as trans when the available evidence is clear, because otherwise we risk missing key evidence, such as June's reliance on a concept of plasticity to narrate her embodied trans feminine knowledge. More important than litigating any competition between queer and trans studies, as Peter Coviello argues about the consolidation of modern American sexuality, is that in an obsession over the emergence of discourses we have grown accustomed to overlooking what was simultaneously *curtailed* by modern forms of knowledge and being around sex. In undermining the inevitability of today's dominant discourses by looking at the transitional overlap between epistemes, Coviello directs attention to "any number of broken-off, uncreated futures, futures that would not come to be."[42] *Histories of the Transgender Child* takes a similar position from within transgender studies. Indeed, trans children's history is a

powerful case of a completely overlooked field of lived experience, knowledge, and embodiment that has been lost through the positivist mythologies
of twenty-first-century medical discourse, narratives of American identity
politics, and the partial biopolitical normalization of certain trans subjects.

Many early twentieth-century trans people, like June, also drew on the
language of intersex embodiment (then most often called "hermaphroditism") to describe themselves as sexually intermediate types, somewhere
between male and female. This was in addition to a growing medical discourse on hermaphroditism in the early twentieth century that was based
around experiments on infants and children born with ambiguous genitalia
and other morphological characteristics that could take on many nonbinary forms. For that reason alone, this book reads intersex children alongside trans children. Yet it turns out that it was precisely the same doctors
and psychiatrists who saw both groups of children, too. What's more,
experimental medicine practiced on intersex children, typically without
either their consent or even their knowledge, directly founded the modern
medical protocol for assigning a sex and then reassigning a child's body
to fit that sex, first surgically and, later, hormonally. The second chapter of
this book, which covers the 1910s to the 1940s, shows that the applicability
of intersex medical protocols and techniques to trans people was actually
proposed by trans lay persons, long before doctors were willing to consider the same. In this moment, trans people actually *anticipated* important
medical links that would not be institutionalized by doctors for more than
two decades. By seeing trans people as active participants in the construction and contestation of medical discourse in this way, rather than as passive objects of knowledge, I emphasize that at many key moments trans
people's embodied fluency in medical science far outpaced institutional
medical knowledge. The broader point is that trans life had no causal reliance upon medicine during the twentieth century and that the trans people
who did interact with doctors brought their own embodied knowledge
of the social realities of their transness with them to the clinic. What's
more, the medical model consisted of a strategy to deny the social reality
of trans life and confine it to a wrong body narrative by suggesting that
trans women and men were not already woman and men (as their lives
frequently testified) but that they somehow *aspired* to become women and
men.[43] For the first half of the century, trans people's embodied knowledge
borrowed heavily from intersex discourses to negotiate this growing power
of the doctor and the clinic.

The ongoing intersex-trans dialogue led in the 1950s to the invention of gender, a signal event with deep consequences for all human life. Scholars working at the crossroads of intersex and trans studies, including Jennifer Germon, Sharon E. Preves, David A. Rubin, and Jemima Repo, have reconstructed how the concept of gender was built out of clinical experimentation on intersex infants and children born with ambiguous genitalia or secondary sex characteristics.[44] Reassigning the sex of intersex infants led to a theory of gender that coordinated the development of the biological body with the psychological acquisition of an ineradicable identity, installing a new difference *between* sex and gender, a distinction that would have had very little intelligibility over the preceding fifty years.

The second and third chapters of this book, which reconstruct four decades of experimental medicalization of intersex children's plasticity at the Johns Hopkins Hospital, greatly expand our understanding of how intersex children informed the invention of gender by the psychologist John Money and his colleagues in the 1950s. Reconstructing such a detailed history of intersex medicine also serves to undermine Money's referential position—whether lauded or critiqued—as the ostensibly decisive factor in producing gender. I argue, instead, that Money only *interpreted* the results of many decades of complex surgical and hormonal experiments upon intersex children's plasticity at Hopkins, importantly smuggling the racialized sense of sex as phenotype into the postwar era, so that gender was designed to function as phenotype, too. In this book, Money emerges not as a singular historical force but more as a relay point between the pre- and postwar eras, joining discourses and practices of intersex and transsexual medicine by way of the invention of gender. The persistence of the entanglement of intersex and trans life in the bodies of children has been underappreciated; in fact, it endured well into the 1950s, if not later. It lasted nearly as long as we have had the discourse of transsexuality, and yet it has radically faded from contemporary conversations about the plasticity of sex and gender.

Overall, *Histories of the Transgender Child* contests and carefully rereads the normative medical archive by beginning in the early twentieth century and working to undermine the model provided by transsexuality for making trans life intelligible. The final chapter attends specifically to trans boys, in part to open up the problem of how a transsexual definition of surgery has become an implicit measure by which to judge the relative degree of reality of trans life in the past, producing a highly gendered asymmetry revolving around bottom surgery for trans women and girls, making trans men's and boys' transitions, which are more likely to revolve around top surgery, less legible—not to mention all who do not seek out surgery or do not have access to medicine.[45] This book militates against the implication, born of the discourse of transsexuality, that trans people *need* medical knowledge about themselves to name or understand their lives. Ironically, it is the medical archive itself that shows this to be untrue. The records of many trans people who interacted with American doctors contain their rich reminiscences of childhoods, adolescence, and years lived openly as trans, often with the acceptance of local communities, without searching for or even wondering about medical support or terminology. Very often medicine became important only *after* children and adults had lived significant trans lives. And medicine was transformed by its experience with their trans lives as much as the inverse was true.

These interventions into the trans twentieth century contribute to a broader movement in transgender studies that seeks to revisit the role played by trans people in scientific and medical research and to undermine the Western rationality and secularism too often reproduced by the field. Several key early figures in European and American trans medicine, after all, were trans men who became doctors and were in some cases able to experiment on themselves. In England Michael Dillon, likely the first trans man to undergo testosterone therapy in the 1940s, became a physician and penned what could be read as a major volume of trans knowledge before transsexuality, *Self: A Study in Endocrinology and Ethics*.[46] In the United States, Alan L. Hart, a physician, radiologist, and tuberculosis researcher, was one of the first trans men to transition with medical support, including surgeries, even earlier, in 1917 to 1918.[47] Other lay persons, such as Louise Lawrence, a major trans community leader in the San Francisco Bay Area and the head of a national network of trans correspondents, actively sought out and challenged medical experts and practicing clinicians, significantly shaping research on transsexuality at midcentury. "More and more I see the need (as Dr. [Alfred] Kinsey once told me about my appearance before the Staff at Langley Porter [Psychiatric Clinic in San Francisco])," she wrote in a letter in 1953, "to educate the doctors, to give them a thought to work on that doesn't come out of a text book."[48] Throughout this book are numerous trans people who decided, whether voluntarily or through exigent circumstances, to work with—and, almost as frequently, to antagonize—doctors. Some of them were trans children like "Vicki," who appears in chapter 4 and whose persistent letters to the endocrinologist Harry Benjamin in the 1960s interrogated his gatekeeping role from the perspective of a trans girl living in rural Ohio.[49]

Appreciating the active role played by trans people in twentieth-century medical science calls not just for an expanded sense of the medical archive but also for an interpretive practice that works against the rationality of the categories "transsexual" and "transgender." In their writing on the life of Reed Erickson, a wealthy businessman and trans man who founded the Erickson Educational Foundation (EEF) in 1964 after his own medical transition, Aaron Devor and Nicholas Matte have worked to shift thinking in this direction. By personally overseeing the dispensation of millions of dollars in philanthropic funding from the 1960s to 1980s, they argue, Erickson directly financed much of American transsexual medicine in the postwar era. His funding provided Harry Benjamin, often canonized as a founding figure, with the actual resources he needed for his clinical work; the EEF provided Hopkins with the money needed to open its Gender Identity Clinic in 1965; and the vital professional networks for researchers and doctors treating trans people in these decades were likewise financed by the foundation. Devor and Matte argue that the contemporary landscape of trans medicine and social services in the United States is in large part the result of Erickson's specific philanthropic vision, not only Benjamin's or Hopkins's approach. Rather than support a field of medical science with his money, Erickson took an active role in shaping it, meaning that his perspective on transition, transsexuality, and trans masculinity all played a role for too long underappreciated.[50]

Erickson's place in transgender studies, in particular, has remained marginal in comparison to the influence that Devor and Matte reclaim. In part, Abram J. Lewis argues, this is because of Erickson's many nonscientific and ostensibly irrational pursuits. As he got older, he funded a massive amount of New Age research into mystical, magical, and supernatural practices and knowledge. Erickson also became a chronic drug user, exploring psychedelic and transcendental practice before becoming a serious addict and, by the accounts of his contemporaries, descending into a period of paranoia and delusion toward the end of his life. Rather than reading Erickson's notorious "eccentricity" as evidence that these irrational matters were separate from or contaminated his work with medical science and represented a failure to live up to his empirical commitments to transsexual science, Lewis argues that Erickson's life instead precisely challenges the epistemological coherence of trans life as an object of knowledge. "Erickson's interest in psychedelia and para-psychology were not, as they have appeared in the historiography," he explains, "mere footnotes to his work on transsexualism."[51] Lewis asks how positivist connotations of the discourse of transsexuality might change if New Age mysticism, psychedelic drugs, and research into animal communication were understood as integral threads of the ostensible rationality of transsexuality rather than its convenient foil.

Reflecting on the experience of researching in the trans archive of the twentieth century, Lewis underlines an odd contrast between primary documents and the historiographical narratives in existing scholarship. "Possibly in an effort to resist popular notions of transgender people as at once insane, tragic, and absurd, this literature has seemed, if anything," he suggests, "to promote histories of agential and politicized communities—of subjects with sensible, self-interested aspirations." While that may be understandable in its context, "perhaps unsurprisingly, then," he adds, "much of the transgender archive is even more perplexing than secondary accounts suggest."[52] This tendency has both overvalued and overrepresented the authority of medical science, while underplaying the role of trans people who, like Erickson, may have had complex political agendas that in unexpected ways undercut medicine's rationality through ostensibly irrational or nonsecular commitments. As Lewis suggests, trans studies need irrational concepts, such as "trans animisms," to understand not only figures like Erickson but also trans activist efforts that took place outside the medical context, such as a 1970 protest against the police murder of gay and black trans people in Los Angeles, which involved an attempt to collectively "levitate" the Rampart Police Station in the hope that it might be made to disappear. Reina Gossett connects this manifestation to the present day as both a trenchant critique of "the normalized organizing tactics preferred by the Non Profit Industrial Complex" and a demonstration of being "accountable to the unborn, the dead and the living," a potential "shift in connection [that] would create more space in our movements to hold more people, more levity, more magic, less isolation, and less shame."[53]

Histories of the Transgender Child contributes to and extends Devor and Matte's, Lewis's, and Gossett's careful rereading of the archive, working to undermine medicine's self-appointed authority and self-referential rationality from within by emphasizing the ways that trans people were actively involved with the contested production of medical knowledge despite lacking, in most cases, expert education and, especially in the case of trans children, often producing theories of trans life that drew as much from magic or fantasy as from science. While the trans twentieth century uncovered here is drawn primarily from archival research in major medical institutions, including the Johns Hopkins Hospital, the University of California, Los Angeles Medical School, and Harry Benjamin's private practice in New York City, the depth and breadth of the archive's contents move well beyond these focal points. Trans children lived in every single region of the United States. The coasts were also far from the only locations in which trans children (or adults) encountered and interacted with medicine or one another. Indeed, it would be difficult to maintain any pretension to a trans "metronormativity" during the twentieth century, even if major urban centers such as San Francisco and New York City were important places for trans social life, community building, and activism.[54] In this book as much space is devoted to rural trans life and childhood in states like Ohio, Alabama, Missouri, and Wisconsin as to urban trans life and childhood in Los Angeles or Washington, D.C. What *does* typify the demography of the medical archive, however, is its overwhelming whiteness. To reckon with the implications of that pervasive whiteness in relation to trans of color life, this book draws on and contributes to trans of color studies.

Trans of Color Studies and Medicine

If the twentieth-century medical archive is compromised by the limited perspective of its rationality and by its overrepresentation of white, middle-class trans life, how can trans of color studies reckon with a reliance on that archive? Why not abandon the medical archive for alternative forms of knowledge? In reconstructing the history of trans children, this book could have begun, for instance, with Sylvia Rivera. Trans "street kids" are central to her political work and legacy. Rivera was also a trans street kid herself in the late 1960s. Running away from her grandmother's home on Long Island to New York City at the age of eleven, Rivera found her way to Greenwich Village, where she "was adopted by a few young (but older than I was) drag queens"[55] and soon thereafter joined a community of trans and queer street youth, including a teenage Marsha P. Johnson, as a sex worker on 42nd Street. Rivera lived openly and defiantly in her childhood, even wearing

makeup to elementary school. She was also held at the Bellevue psychiatric
ward after a suicide attempt and shortly before running away from home.[56]

Rivera's and Johnson's participation in the Stonewall riots, their affini-
ties with and critiques of gay liberation activism, and their trans of color
liberation activism at the turn of the 1970s present a rich tangle of categories, politics, and priorities that undermine the increasingly sanitized and
progressive narratives that collapse retrospectively into the U.S. "LGBT"
movement or the creation of "a generalized 'transgender' subject in the
narrative of Stonewall and the gay liberation movement," which, as Ehn
Nothing points out, "celebrate Sylvia Rivera's visibility as transgender,
conceal[ing] her status as a broke woman of color."[57] Rivera is also a difficult figure to reconcile with contemporary political taxonomies of sex,
gender, and sexuality. As a child, she recalled, "I was an effeminate gay boy.
I was becoming a beautiful drag queen, a beautiful drag queen child. Later
on, of course, I knew that Christine [Jorgensen] was already around, but
those things were still waiting on the backs of people's minds."[58] Donning
and contesting the *political* identity of "gay" in the early 1970s and referring
to herself here and there as a "drag queen" and a "transvestite" in the expansive idioms of the era, not adopting the term transgender until the 2000s,
Rivera remained mostly aloof from the medicalization of transsexuality.
In an interview about their work in Street Transvestite Action Revolutionaries (S.T.A.R.), Johnson asks Rivera about the difference between the
terms "drag queen" and "transvestite," and she responds:

> A drag queen is one that usually goes to a ball, and that's the only
> time she gets dressed up. Transvestites live in drag. A transsexual
> spends most of her life in drag. I never come out of drag to go
> anywhere. Everywhere I go I get all dressed up. A transvestite is
> still like a boy, very manly looking, a feminine boy. You wear drag
> here and there. Where you're a transsexual, you have hormone
> treatments and you're on your way to a sex change and you never
> come out of female clothes.[59]

When in response Johnson asks, "You'd be considered a pre-operative
transsexual then? You don't know when you'd be able to go through the sex
change?" Rivera responds, "Oh mostly likely this year. I'm planning to go
to Sweden. I'm working very hard to go." Johnson points out that surgery
in Sweden would be "cheaper" than at "Johns Hopkins," to which Rivera

agrees, "It's $300 for a change [in Sweden], but you've got to stay there for a year."[60] Yet some time later, in 1990, during an interview, the historian Martin Duberman asked Rivera about hormones. Duberman's notes record that Rivera said she "took them for a while but came to the conclusion that she did not want to be a woman. 'I like pretending, the whole world for me is a stage I like to dress up. I don't want to be a woman. I didn't think about the sex change, that's not what I want."[61]

Even if Rivera is a complex figure around whom to write a history of trans children, why are the street kids of major cities like New York not already recognized as proof that trans children have a past?[62] Why are they not brought up in present-day conversations about the "newness" of trans children? Their radical politics, which would hardly be compatible with the modernizing, progressive narrative of medicine and corporate political lobbying, is surely one reason. Rivera's and Johnson's work in S.T.A.R. undoes progress narratives of gender and sexuality. They prioritized a trenchant critique of the police, gay gender normativity, and institutional racism and pursued a celebration of Latinx and black trans life that led to their own marginalization within activist circles almost as soon as they began organizing.[63] Another reason, however, is that their lives are incredibly ephemeral—most "street kids" are anonymous as historical subjects, an unknowable diversity of experience hiding behind the collective noun. Even though Rivera and Johnson have generated perhaps the largest amount of archival documents and scholarly interest of any known street kids, even the account to which we have access is organized around a relatively sparse set of repetitive narratives that provides only small snapshots of what the lives of black trans and trans of color street kids were like in the 1960s and 1970s.[64]

S.T.A.R.'s work on behalf of trans children nevertheless offers an important set of contrasts to the clinical history that anchors this book. Formed in 1970 and led by Rivera and Johnson, S.T.A.R. "focused on survival, countered societal injustice, and asserted a revolutionary and unapologetic transvestite identity" in the face of an increasingly hostile and gender-normative gay liberation movement dominated by cisgender, white men.[65] S.T.A.R.'s efforts were guided, argues Jessi Gan, by Rivera's hope "of enacting a very grounded kind of social change: creating a home for 'the youngsters,' the underage street queens who, like her, had begun working on the streets at age ten, and who not long afterward ended up dead."[66] She and Johnson materialized this aim through the creation of a S.T.A.R. home, a place where street kids could live together, pool resources, and develop practices for addressing violence in the sex work industry, police brutal- ity, and overincarceration. In its first iteration, the S.T.A.R. home "was a parked trailer in an outdoor parking lot in Greenwich Village," where around two dozen street kids lived. When the trailer was suddenly driven away by a trucker, Rivera and Johnson "decided to get a building," hoping also "to get away from the Mafia's control of the bars." They found a place to rent in the East Village. Teaching themselves to make repairs and reno- vate the space, Leslie Feinberg explains, "they envisioned the top floor as a school to teach the youth, many of whom had been forced to leave home and live on the streets at a very early age, to read and write."[67] Johnson and Rivera worked to make sure that the children were fed and clothed. "We went out and hustled the streets. We paid the rent. We didn't want the kids out in the streets hustling."[68]

By prioritizing the lives of trans of color street kids and sex workers, S.T.A.R. had an extremely fractious relationship with the Gay Liberation Front and the Gay Activists Alliance, which culminated in Rivera's infa- mous exclusion from the 1973 Christopher Street Liberation Day rally, to which she responded by physically fighting her way on stage to deliver a scathing speech indicting gay men for ignoring the beating and rape of trans people in jail.[69] Because S.T.A.R. built itself through the situated knowledges of the arguably poorest marginal constituency of the trans community, it also did not address institutional medicine much during its short existence. Like Rivera, S.T.A.R. did not identify itself through the medical model of transsexuality, although it was certainly aware of it. What little work S.T.A.R. or its affiliates directed at medicine at the turn of the 1970s instead addressed access to other basic, life-sustaining health care. For instance, Bob Kohler, a gay activist and friend of Rivera and one of the only people who maintained a friendly relationship with the homeless and with the street kids of New York, worked with the Mattachine Society and the East Side Village Youth Project to bring a mobile medical trailer to serve the medical and psychotherapeutic needs of street kids in late 1969.[70] Rivera also focused some of her activist energy on psychiatric institutions, par- ticularly Bellevue Hospital, where family members or the state had many gay and trans people confined on spurious pretenses.

S.T.A.R.'s black trans and trans of color political organizing to provide livable worlds for street kids also took place at the end of the historical period that this book covers, making it too late to serve as a starting point for some of the interventions I make. Still, the many differences between this account of trans of color childhood and the accounts that are assembled across *Histories of the Transgender Child* are instructive in avoiding the reduction of black trans or trans of color life to singular narratives. S.T.A.R. and the ephemeral perspectives of trans street kids of color are also an important model for trans of color studies as it works to dismantle medical, state-sponsored systems of being and knowledge that continue to marginalize and extract necropolitical value from black trans and trans of color life and death, something with which transgender studies must continue to reckon as it becomes further institutionalized in the university.[71]

"Trans of color studies," of course, does not name a unified or even necessarily an extant field. It functions here instead as an invocation across several fields of a vital point of departure for this book, one that Rivera's and Johnson's lives reflect: race is not a new matter to *add* to transgender studies.[72] Multiple and differing racial formations, including blackness, coloniality, latinidad, indigeneity, and immigrant diasporas, are not *and should not be* new areas of inquiry for transgender studies to encounter or discover. In "We Got Issues: Towards a Black Trans*/Studies," Ellison, Green, Richardson, and Snorton argue instead for seeing black trans theory as an impetus to investigate "a series of questions about repressed genealogies that might come into view through a more sustained engagement with blackness, as an 'issue' that is both overseen and unknown."[73] Drawing on Édouard Glissant's work, they offer his concept of transversality "as *a collateral genealogy,* or an encounter with the past that also contains an ethical confrontation with the collateral damages involved in blackness as overseen and unknown."[74] The relation of blackness to trans life, as well as the relation of antiblackness to transsexuality and transgender, represents political problems of knowledge and being to be opened up through historical and politically engaged scholarship, rather than a frontier of new thinking to be discovered by more inclusive methodologies. Blackness problematizes the category trans—and vice versa.

Trans of color studies not only argues that race is integral to transgender studies, then, but also responds to a particular problem of black and trans of color hypervisibility with which the field is frequently complicit. In the introduction to *The Transgender Studies Reader 2*, Susan Stryker and Aren Z. Aizura observe that "current trans of color critique resists imperialist forms of knowledge production precisely by calling attention to which transgender bodies—and they are almost always the non-white ones—are made to represent the traumatic violences through which claims for rights are articulated."[75] In that volume, Snorton and Jin Haritaworn's essential essay "Trans Necropolitics" names as the "most urgent present task" of trans of color critique "explaining the simultaneous devaluation of trans of color lives and the nominal circulation in death of trans people of color." As they argue, "this circulation vitalizes trans theory and politics" precisely "through the value extracted from trans of color death."[76] This critique is particularly prescient in the wake of the ongoing biopolitical turn in transgender studies, which has been incredibly generative in identifying how trans life has been operationalized by normalizing and governmental techniques but also tends to follow Michel Foucault's lead in abstracting the category "race" out of its own historicity, abandoning the centrality of colonialism and transatlantic slavery to the racialized modernity of the human.[77]

Instead of taking Foucault's account of the modern biopolitical body for granted, scholars working toward decolonizing the field and the concept of transgender are increasingly looking to Sylvia Wynter's work on the overrepresentation of Western Man and the production of alternate genres of the human for scholarly coordinates that extend the work of trans studies in more productive directions.[78] Alongside growing conversations involving trans studies, Afro-pessimism, and indigenous studies is work that draws on a decolonial framework to think of transgender and transsexuality as imperial formations of knowledge that circulate transnationally, but unevenly, across the global north and the global south.[79] Joseli Maria Silva and Marcio Jose Ornat explain the "decolonialist approach" succinctly as "the opportunity to develop a strategy with which to overcome the notion of the primacy of scientific knowledge over those who suffer the effects of epistemic violence."[80] As the editors of *Transgender Studies Quarterly*'s special issue "Decolonizing the Transgender Imaginary" put it, "The term *transgender*—grounded as it is in conceptual underpinnings that assume a sex/gender distinction as well as an analytic segregation of sexual orientation and gender identity/expression . . . [is] simply foreign to most places and times."[81] *Histories of the Transgender Child* adds that one of those "places and times" might actually be the twentieth-century United States, if we read the medical archive through an interpretive practice aimed at its decolonization.

This book makes two arguments about the racialized genealogies of transsexuality and trans medicine on the one hand and the disqualification of trans of color life and knowledge from them on the other. First, its trans of color critique of medicine illuminates *how* the medicalization of trans life has always fundamentally racialized it, in more than one sense. Sex and gender were reconceived as plastic phenotypes during the twentieth century, which makes all human embodiment, including cisgender forms, a racial formation.[82] Second, because the concept of plasticity was abstractly racialized by medical science as a synonym for whiteness, in the clinic it had real demographic effects. The overwhelming majority of trans patients seen at institutions of medicine were white. Even in the most pathologizing and disenfranchising medical models, the abstract whiteness projected onto the white trans body justified the attention given by doctors. Black trans and trans of color patients were much rarer because they were by design not welcome within that discourse. The broader racialized and class disparities in access to American medicine were also particularly acute in trans medicine, making it far more difficult for trans people of color to find competent and caring professional attention, whether in 1920 or in 1975— or, for that matter, today. In this way, the medical model built during the twentieth century disavows its own racial knowledge and racial violence, a set of practices that, as C. Riley Snorton has shown, run much longer, into the eighteenth century at least, where "chattel slavery functioned as one cultural apparatus that brought sex and gender into arrangement."[83] The Johns Hopkins Hospital, which is a central focal point of this book, is emblematic of the disavowed racial genealogy of modern American medicine. Built in a historically black neighborhood in the late nineteenth century on the presumption of special access to black people's bodies for experimental research that was frequently nontherapeutic, practiced without consent, painful, and destructive, Hopkins produced many "modern" medical protocols out of experiments that were seen through a lens not of white plastic potential but of black fungibility. This held true for the Hopkins clinics involved in the production of protocols for altering human sex, where I show that black trans and black intersex life was framed in atavistic terms. This is a particularly pernicious racial effect of medicine in light of Snorton's rigorous detailing, in *Black on Both Sides*, of how "captive flesh figures a critical genealogy for modern transness, as chattel persons gave rise to an understanding of gender as mutable and as an amendable form of being."[84] The racial plasticity of sex and gender whose history this book locates in the twentieth century is very much part of the inheritance from that racial history.

A trans of color critique of medicine, then, insists on naming, following Susan Stryker, the "spectacular whiteness" of transsexuality as a colonial form of knowledge whose claims to jurisdiction over trans life must be contested.[85] Through a detailed historical investigation of the construction of trans medicalization from the opening of the twentieth century to the end of the 1970s, this book works from within the historicity of transsexuality and its predicates to demonstrate that medicine's reason is actually a highly impaired, partial perspective on trans life—and trans childhood especially—that can only masquerade as universal and objective through the constitutive violence that it disavows. Not only does the whiteness of medicine interfere with the intelligibility and livelihood of black, brown, indigenous, and other marginal trans people, but it substitutes for them a point of view rendered detached and transcendent through their exclusion. Trans children stand out as powerful examples of this process of producing objective vision out of the forced disappearance of the personhood of patients. Trans children became valuable to doctors for an abstract quality, plasticity, which they exceptionally incarnated in their growth from infancy to adulthood. Medicine made of children's living bodies proxies for the experimental alteration of racial plasticity and human sex, not by listening to children's desires or demands for gender self-determination but by making them into the raw material of medical techniques. The same plasticity of sex that was racialized as white, making white trans children valuable in the clinic, also silenced them, making their experimental treatment a means to other ends.

Marking the limited and partial perspective of medical science is a project whose roots I also find in feminist science studies and woman of color feminism. Donna Haraway argues for a concept of "situated knowledges" to both open up this problem in dominant Western forms of scientific knowledge and find a theory of feminist objectivity that can usurp its place without having to reject the practice of science altogether. For Haraway, the difference between a dominant form of objectivity and a feminist objectivity is that the latter is concerned with the ethical problem of *being held accountable for the production of a standpoint.* Unlike institutional science or medicine, in the production of situated knowledge "the scientific knower seeks the subject position not of identity, but of objectivity; that is, partial connection," which is quite distinct from the totalizing act of fully grasping an object of knowledge.[86] In other words, through a feminist practice of situated knowledge, which does not pretend to proceed from a transcendent, detached position or to split the observer and the object of knowledge, "we might become answerable for what we learn to see."[87]

Naming dominant epistemological practices and forms of scientific knowledge as situated, not universal or independent in their objectivity, is a powerful critique. Yet Haraway also offers the concept for building alternate forms of embodied knowledge, especially from the position of those whose lives have been long disqualified as unscientific, such as women, people of color, and colonized peoples. Still, Haraway is careful about not romanticizing the alternate production of knowledge from perspectives that have been subjugated:

> Many currents in feminism attempt to theorize grounds for trusting especially the vantage points of the subjugated; there is good reason to believe vision is better from below. . . . The positionings of the subjugated [however] are not exempt from critical re-examination, decoding, deconstruction, and interpretation. . . . The standpoints of the subjugated are not innocent positions. On the contrary, they are preferred because in principle they are least likely to allow denial of the critical and interpretive core of all knowledge. . . . Subjugated standpoints are preferred because they seem to promise more adequate, sustained, objective, transforming accounts of the world. But *how* to see from below is a problem requiring at least as much skill with bodies and language . . . as the 'highest' techno-scientific visualizations.[88]

This is a point that Chela Sandoval develops through a woman of color feminist lens in *Methodology of the Oppressed,* explaining that the production of situated knowledge from the perspective of the oppressed must be careful to avoid reducing that perspective to an identity. Sandoval cautions against this persistent problem, where minority forms of knowledge such as black feminist theory, queer of color critique, or indigenous epistemologies are misrecognized as correlate to a particular identitarian scope that reduces their sphere of applicability, rather than constituting "a theoretical and methodological approach in [their] own right."[89] For Sandoval, "These skills, born of de-colonial processes," would "insist on new kinds of human and social exchange that have the power to forge a dissident transnational coalitional consciousness."[90] A trans of color methodology of the oppressed might also be called a "science of the oppressed," a concept that micha cárdenas has adapted and developed in recent work connecting art, activism, poetics, and digital making.[91]

Trans of color studies grows out of these multiple genealogies, prioritizing as much as possible the "(De)Subjugated Knowledges" named in Susan Stryker's introduction to the first *Transgender Studies Reader*.[92] There is a rich and growing bibliography of work that problematizes transsexuality as an artifact of colonial forms of knowledge and governance, critiques the disqualification of trans of color life and knowledge as unscientific and unworthy of personhood, and authors situated knowledges from the perspective of trans of color lives that are never reducible to a single or transcendent position but instead implicate the researcher and the reader, asking them to confront their responsibility to trans of color subjects, *and* the varying "response-ability" of those trans of color subjects.[93] This book's trans of color framework is built not out of a unified voice or referent, then, but out of a generative and internally discordant bibliography drawn from trans of color scholarship, black feminist theory, black queer studies, woman of color feminism, queer of color studies, and decolonial studies. While I aim to cultivate responsibility to those fields, I also affirm the partially incompatible and contradictory elements involved in their mobilization together. There are distinct points of friction that I do not always try to resolve and that are the particular risk of the formulation "trans of color." I *do*, however, mean to avoid flattening the category "race," much as I aim to expand the meanings of "trans." In this book there are several distinct forms of racialization at hand whose historical entanglement is the object of inquiry. Naming modern sex and gender as racialized white though the medicalization of plasticity in children's bodies, for instance, implies an exclusionary and dehumanizing relation to the racialization of black trans life. The racial formations of blackness and indigeneity, in particular, are highly specific in the U.S. context and do not map onto Latinx or immigrant forms of race that have often been forced into competitive relationships by the state.

There are also important conceptual and political tensions within the theoretical perspectives mobilized in this book. Haraway and Sandoval's emphasis on situatedness, for instance, sits in tension with work in black studies on what Fred Moten calls "the refusal of standpoint" and the proposition "to think from no standpoint" in the case of blackness.[94] There is also an important tension in thinking about the relation of forms of symbolic or social death that have attached to black trans and trans of color life and the material lives of black trans and trans of color people. Admittedly, these larger and ongoing conversations across fields are mostly beyond the scope of this book. Still, they insist as an importantly recurring problem. The frequent absence of black trans and trans of color children in the clinic's archive, in particular, is not only a product of medical gatekeeping or the whiteness of transsexuality. It is also a product of a *distance* practiced by black trans and trans of color people from institutional medicine, which was well understood to be a dangerous and frequently violent apparatus. By the 1960s and 1970s, as formal gender clinics began to open in the United States, their overwhelmingly white clientele was contrasted with the continuing use of willfully faulty homosexuality and schizophrenia diagnoses to reject outright black trans children's personhood and to subject them to potentially infinite detention in psychiatric facilities, as well as more literal forms of incarceration.

The black trans children who appear in this book, particularly in the fourth and fifth chapters, occupy a difficult and risky position in its narrative, one magnified by the protocols of medical archival research, where the need to anonymize dilutes even the smallest details of black life whose traces are left behind. Black trans children are situated in these chapters in contrast to the white trans children whose lives are overrepresented in clinical archives. Although to preserve anonymity I do not use any real names from medical records in this book, it is worth pointing out that these black trans children frequently had no name recorded in those documents to begin with. They were also the least likely to have any pretense of their own voice recorded in interviews or to be discussed with even the most basic trappings of personhood. This is a dangerous situation to reconstruct out of the archive, for it risks reassigning a necropolitical value to black trans children, letting them vitalize the work of transgender studies without challenging their reduction to social death in the archive. To read contrary to the facticity of the archive and locate some form of escape or resistance is also exceedingly difficult because of the brevity and sheer misdirection of the medical discourse in those documents. To argue that their blackness therefore always sits in an irruptive position in relation to transsexuality, in certain instances threatening to puncture the racial order of things, also risks casting these black trans childhoods in a romanticized role as always-already outside the category transgender—not an easy position from which to find a livable life for a child.

Taking these risks on as part of the ethical project of cultivating responsibility toward the real lives behind historical discourses, I draw on Robert Reid-Pharr's "post-humanist archival practice."[95] Informed by rich thinking in black studies on how black social formations are forced to survive within the violent matrix of Western humanism's concept of "Man," how "the black operates in Western humanism as a nonsubject who gives meaning to the awkward and untenable concept of 'Man'" (8), for Reid-Pharr the historical archive of black sociality can reinforce the parameters of that humanism only if it is acquiesced to in advance. He argues convincingly that "though the conceits of humanism would have us believe that our ability to address human being must by necessity be a radically demarcated endeavor, the *lived* reality of black life demonstrates an unusually broad set of procedures that have challenged and critiqued not only white supremacy but also the smugness and certainty of the entire Western humanist apparatus" (9, emphasis in original). Drawing on Hortense Spillers's distinction between body and flesh and a renewed sense of the archive as a location for interpreting alternate accounts of social life that find their conceptual coordinates in historically lived difference, Reid-Pharr names the responsive object of his posthumanist practice "archives of flesh" (10–11). Rather than taking the ejection of blackness from the human as the final word on the matter, these archives of flesh bring to the fore "many moments of illogic, indeed of wildness and bestiality, that one finds in humanist discourse" (10), inviting its undermining through archival interpretative practices attuned to alternate forms of the human already existent in the past.[96]

If this book's archives of black trans childhood are, to a considerable extent, overwhelmed by the sheer force of medicine as a domineering form of humanism, yielding only the slightest glimpses of the situated perspective of black trans childhood, this is, as Reid-Pharr importantly reminds, less a reason to abandon the archive than an invitation to invent better interpretive practices that break from dominant epistemes and ontologies by recognizing that domination has to be historically produced but is never a done deal. It is also, however, a reminder that this book provides only one account of black trans childhood's historicity. We need more of these histories, and we do need different archives that produce alternate forms of knowledge richer in the grain of black trans and trans of color embodied objectivities than what this book can provide by focusing on the history of medicine.[97]

I turned to S.T.A.R. to frame my thinking about the collective project of trans of color studies not only because it provides subjugated historical knowledge from before the contemporary liberal LGBT movement but also because Rivera's life as a street kid reminds us that there are countless untold stories latent in the past that could be what Snorton terms "fugitive moments in the hollow of fungibility's embrace."[98] And even when they contrast with or outright contradict the account that I provide in this book, that contributes toward displacing the whiteness and rationality of transsexuality, suggesting black trans and trans of color futures that do not reiterate the exhausted closure of humanism. It matters, but precisely in ways that we can scarcely yet imagine in their profundity, that as some of the trans children I write about in the last chapter of this book were visiting Harry Benjamin's private practice on the Upper West Side of Manhattan in 1970, across town and some thirty-odd blocks south Rivera was picketing Bellevue Hospital, where she had been held by medical authorities as a child.

With these methodological and historiographical coordinates in mind, this book's conclusion argues against the etiological framing of trans children, whether by medicine, the helping professions, or the media. As I began to suggest in the preface, *Histories of the Transgender Child* asks us to turn against and away from figurative thinking about trans children in general. Trans children must no longer bring us to some new knowledge of trans life or sex and gender, making them a means to some other abstract end. Rather, through the twentieth-century history of the chapters that follow I propose an ethical relation that calls upon adults to stop questioning the being of trans children and affirm instead that there *are* trans children, that trans childhood is a happy and desired form—not a new form of life and experience but one richly, beautifully historical and multiple.

CHAPTER 1

The Racial Plasticity of Gender
and the Child

IN THE LATE NINETEENTH- AND EARLY TWENTIETH-CENTURY life sciences, sex underwent two key transformations: sex became synonymous with a concept of biological plasticity that made it an alterable morphology, and, through experiments by largely eugenic scientists, it was racialized as a phenotype. The framing of sex through racial plasticity occurred in a broader scientific milieu in Europe and the United States that defined living organisms, both human and nonhuman, as naturally "bisexual," a mix of masculine and feminine forms. First operationalized through experiments in changing the sex and phenotype of animals, this racial plasticity was adapted for altering the human body by the emergent field of endocrinology between the two world wars. Yet if plasticity named the inherent indeterminacy of sex as a biological form, scientists also began to wonder if that meant it might *not* be inclined to take on binary form, at least in certain cases. On the one hand, defining sex in the terms of racial plasticity granted unprecedented technical access to altering living morphology. On the other hand, the material reach afforded by plasticity held open the door to biological *resistance* to the imposition of rigid forms, such as mutually exclusive masculinity and femininity. Since plasticity is a *quality*—a capacity to generate and receive imprints of form—and not a visibly discrete "part" of the body, endocrinology called upon the figure of the developing child to serve as a stabilizing metaphor. As a metaphor for an invisible but material plasticity, the child organized sex and growth along parallel phylogenetic and ontogenetic scales. Yet this metaphor also preserved and kept alive the tension between indeterminacy and form at the core of sex. As a result, the sex binary moved closer to conceptual collapse the more it became scientifically alterable.

By returning to the era that precedes the emergence of the medical category "transsexuality," what Henry Rubin calls the "pre-history of experimental endocrinology," we encounter "sex" as a wide-open field of biological form with highly racialized significance in the heyday of eugenic science.[1] Early twentieth-century endocrinology contextualized how the child's body became a central living laboratory for trans medicine over the rest of the twentieth century, while at the same time actual children were rendered passive and invisible within the closure of its discourse. This chapter, then, is not about trans children directly but rather works to open up the key concept of plasticity that shaped the trans twentieth century. This chapter is not quite, for that matter, about many actual children at all, but more so about the strangeness of "the child" as a figurative form of life. One of the historical problems endemic to Western childhood is that an abstract concept of "the child" has profoundly overlaid—sometimes, overdetermined— the lives of actual children. The tension between abstraction and material life is, precisely, incorporated into the child as a strangely *living figure*, or what Claudia Castañeda aptly calls a "figuration."[2] One of the key historical effects of this figuration is that it allows for the child to serve as a metaphorical representation of other concepts, often ones that are too inhuman to stand on their own—including plasticity.

By calling attention to how scientific cultivation of the racial plasticity of sex relies on a metaphor, I do not mean to suggest that it is for that reason unreal or some kind of ruse. On the contrary, as we will see, it is precisely the partial misfit between plasticity and the child greased by the mechanics of metaphor that was so productive for medical science over the ensuing century. Metaphor is, after all, a well-established explanatory technique in the sciences. The rhetoric of science has been investigated through the metaphors that govern its composition, while the techniques of scientific research and theoretical inquiry have been read in terms of the metaphorical relationships between models and the phenomena under investigation.[3] The history and philosophy of science have also paid close attention to the ways in which metaphor, among many literary, poetic, and aesthetic commitments, explains the emergence of European science from a specific Romantic tradition in the eighteenth and nineteenth centuries.[4] Still, in those accounts metaphor tells us much more about language and the practice of science than about the objects, animals, and silenced bodies subjugated through scientific practice. The point is to reassess not only the position of the scientific observer but also the object of observation and scientific discourse. As Gillian Beer observes in *Darwin's Plots*, a focus on metaphor is not an argument that scientific discourse is a set of literal fictions. In the case of Darwin, Beer argues that it was precisely his awareness, conscious or otherwise, of his use of metaphor in his writing that allowed him to generate a theory of evolution through natural selection that, read closely, continues to exceed totalization.[5]

Donna Haraway also investigates the central function of metaphor in biology in *Crystals, Fabrics, and Fields*, her first book.[6] The premise is perhaps deceptively simple: science is not a transcendently objective description of the real world, nor should it be. Drawing on Thomas Kuhn's *The Structure of Scientific Revolutions* and Mary Hesse's *Models and Analogies in Science*, Haraway undertakes an analysis of metaphor that is the launch point for a postpositivist study of science.[7] For Haraway, a "metaphor is generally related to a sense object—such as a machine, crystal, or organism. A metaphor is *an image that gives concrete coherence to even highly abstract thought*" (9 n., emphasis added). In other words, metaphors in science operate much in the same way as metaphors in literature, but with rather distinct effects given the putative purchase of science on real-world objects—or, in the case of biology, on living organisms. Metaphor is also a crucial way for humanists to access the *practice* of science, rather than only the critique of its epistemological basis, as metaphor illuminates the active role of language and form in the production of scientific knowledge *and* their entanglement with the material world being described or observed— they are mutually informing. Biological metaphor, Haraway explains, "gives boundaries to worlds and helps scientists using real language to push against those bounds" (10). In so doing, it ensures that language is neither outside those worlds nor an imposition on or misrepresentation of them. Although metaphor imports ostensibly nonscientific or nonobjective meanings that shape the intelligibility of scientific data (10) and for that reason is of concern to critiques of biology, this originary contamination is not itself a problem to be overcome. In offering an account of production in the history or the life sciences, the analysis of shifting metaphors opens up its discourses, data, and historical effects to a kind of dynamic analysis that includes critique, contestation, and the potential for creative mutation and difference.

The point Haraway raises is that a better metaphor can make an epistemological and political difference. In the production of situated knowledges, struggle over operative metaphors is a method for producing responsible, relational perspectives that emphasize the entanglement of the so-called object of a scientific discourse with the scientific observer. An exclusively cultural analysis, which would regard metaphor as contamination or a by-product of ideology, avoids responsibility to objects and beings, such as children, who have been made into poorly fitted metaphors. Metaphor remains a vital avenue for the production of nonteleological, nonreductionist branches of biology and science as much as it has been the historical vehicle of its dominant, objectivizing forms. Rather than opposing metaphors entirely, the task is to imagine different ones that would reshape the practice of science and the production of biological knowledge from the situated perspective of the long-presumed passive object.

If biological metaphors are images or ideas that guide the life sciences without corresponding to an actual object, we could understand almost any abstraction of human or nonhuman life through this framework. Sex and gender, certainly, could be considered rather broad metaphors for human form. More precisely, as *phenotypes* that pretend to derive themselves straightforwardly from an imagined genotype, they are metaphors that go *too* far in relation to biological life, overdetermining it with poorly fitted meaning. The endocrine system, as an anatomical abstraction, would also qualify well as metaphorical. When it was first conceived in the late nineteenth and very early twentieth centuries, the endocrine system was proposed as a way of differentiating certain bodily functions from the popular nervous models of the era. The supposition that "chemical messengers" secreted by organs traveled the blood system, integrating and coordinating disparate parts of the body, was founded on an abstract image of the circulatory system and accessory glands.[8]

This chapter turns to two related but far less obvious metaphors, ones that have *no* correspondence to the visual anatomy of sex. They are instead implicit or latent metaphors for life as it becomes human: animality and child development. Since the plasticity of living organisms cannot be isolated as a discrete physiological object, endocrinologists relied on metaphors from the inhuman constituents of the human to animate its coherence as an endocrine *system* that could be partially manipulated.[9] Given that medical science has been able to leverage that metaphorically animal or childish plasticity to induce real changes in the phenotypic form of the human body, it matters quite little whether plasticity "really exists" somewhere in the flesh. Or, to put it differently, the impossibility of disarticulating actual, material plasticity from the discourse of plasticity is not a hard limit on thinking critically. Plasticity has already had real historical effects through the work of metaphor.

The child and the animal are metaphors as formal ideas and material actors, as Haraway suggests. To say that sex and gender are "metaphors" for the human comprehends the historically specific material, biological effects of those images on, in, and *as* the animal and child body in the lab: the chemical, technical, and affective forms of masculinity and femininity that have invested and sculpted the flesh down to the tiniest of scales. Yet biological life and the objects of research are also *involved* in the metaphors medical science deploys to engage with them. The "organic" names precisely that paradoxical entanglement of indeterminacy and form that a metaphor gets just right enough to do something real in the body, without ever controlling or exhausting what it can do. Animals and children were much more than abstract referents that rhetorically directed scientific and medical accounts of endocrine system (although that is, in part, what they were) in the early twentieth century. Animals predominantly but also infants and children, as we will see in the next two chapters, were the experimental objects in the laboratories and clinics of endocrinologists during the first half of the twentieth century. Theirs was the flesh through which the endocrine system was abstracted as raw material and given new form as plastic sex. For this reason, the child and animal metaphors cannot be the vehicle of an exclusively discursive critique of the ideological basis of science and medicine but instead insist on the organic centrality of animality and childishness to sex, gender, and the forms that they keep alive.

Life's Bisexuality in the Nineteenth Century

The emergence of a concept of biological plasticity in endocrinology and elsewhere is embedded in much larger nineteenth-century debates between mechanist and vitalist views on life. A range of emergent European and American disciplines and fields collecting under the umbrella of biology sought to investigate a set of common questions about the relations between form and genesis, inheritance and impressibility, and the individual and the species.[10] While the mechanists retained a faith in atomism, chemistry or, later, physics to describe the basic unit of processes that made organic matter, the vitalists explored a range of explanatory concepts for the special addition or force that made the inorganic alive. Over this time period the metaphor of the organism was proposed to resolve the entrenched opposition of both camps.[11] Meanwhile, the study of sex in anatomy, physiology, embryology, and endocrinology refined the focus to center around life's apparent natural bisexuality, the conceptual predicate to plasticity. "Sex," a concept broad enough to signify in this era both sexual differentiation in organisms and sexual reproduction, was made accessible to science to the degree that it was intrinsically amenable to alterations in form, a capacity verified by and rooted in its originally bisexual disposition.

The earliest figures in European endocrinology came to this consensus by way of animal experiments. Arnold Adolph Berthold's study, in 1848 and 1849, of chickens in Germany significantly advanced the hypothesis that a unique system of internal secretions governed much of the biological life of the animal. In technique, Berthold was repeating a set of experiments on the gonads of fowl that had been undertaken countless times before, perhaps most famously in the eighteenth century by the English physician John Hunter.[12] Berthold first "caponized" a group of cocks by surgically removing their testes, observing that they subsequently underwent a radical "feminization" in morphology and behavior, not only looking like hens but also acting like them. He also transplanted some of the removed testes back into the birds from which they were taken, but in their stomachs. Berthold's goal was to disprove an older somatic model of sex by demonstrating that the gonads were not part of the nervous system. By severing any potential nervous connection at the moment of excision and placing the gonads in an entirely separate part of the body, Berthold sought to determine whether they were able to continue functioning by some means other than nerves. When these birds "exhibited the normal behavior of uncastrated fowls" after the testes were placed in the stomach, he argued, "it follows that no specific spermatic nerves exist." Instead, Berthold explained, "it follows that the results in question are determined by the productive function of the testes [*productive Verhältniss der Hoden*], i.e., by their action on the blood stream, and then by corresponding reaction of the blood upon the entire organism."[13] The concept of a system of chemical communication between various "ductless glands" in the body by means of the circulatory system laid the basis for a specifically endocrine body. And for Berthold, sex, directed by the gonads, was the primary means of access to that body.

Berthold's choice of animal subjects was not made exclusively to avoid the much more complex possibility of human experiments. Rather, endocrinology drew on centuries of informal knowledge in animal husbandry; farmers had long cultivated sex, breed, and phenotype to maximize certain characteristics over others. The notion that "sex changes" were possible by rationally manipulating the chemical output and communication of the endocrine system was well established by the end of the nineteenth century, if still based on a great deal of speculation (namely, the hormone molecule was unknown). The theory of life's natural bisexuality and its amenability to cultivation simply jumped, by analogy, to the human species. In *The Variation of Plants and Animals under Domestication*, for instance, Charles Darwin explains matter-of-factly that "in every female all the secondary male characters, and in every male all the secondary female characters, apparently exist in a latent state, ready to be evolved under certain conditions," citing the earlier studies in birds. Before moving on, he adds, "We see something of an analogous nature in the human species."[14]

The key transformation indexed by Darwin's reference to research in birds and its applicability to human form is that the persistent *latency* of bisexual characteristics, which could "revert" under "certain conditions," carried a *primitivist* meaning. Such latency of sexual form in humans was almost entirely metaphorical—it had never been directly observed, nor had researchers yet removed the testes or ovaries of humans in analogous experiments. If the latency to which Darwin referred had no physiological correlate in the human, then it could be imagined as a stored primitive capacity that was actually observed in "lower" animals. Hence, only under those metaphorical "certain conditions" would a sex change like the ones achieved by Berthold take place in humans. This primitivist sense of a latent bisexual animality on an evolutionary scale (phylogenesis) is important because it would soon be recoded and extended through a parallel timescale: the individual development of the child (ontogenesis). Sex would become the form that could bind evolutionary time and individual life span through a materialist concept of plasticity.

By the time of Darwin's remarks, the natural bisexuality of life seemed poised to herald a new era for medicine and scientific research: the simultaneous transformation of the individual body and the species through the hormonal manipulation of sex.[15] It is worth emphasizing again that "sex," in this era, meant both sexual differentiation of the organism (its growth from one cell to maturity) and sexual reproduction. Ernest Starling, who coined the term "hormone" in 1905 and worked to introduce the new field of endocrinology to medical science in the first several decades of the twentieth century, stressed that the function of the endocrine system was precisely to integrate differentiation and reproduction. Sex, which was governed by hormones, simultaneously regulated the metabolism and the phenotypic form of the body (height, weight, bone structure, genitals, secondary sex characteristics), while ensuring the transmission of these traits to the next generation, employing the same organs for both tasks.[16] If in its regular somatic commerce sex was originally and naturally bisexual, this suggested that sex granted access to the real manipulation of form and the transmission of that form's heredity to future generations. As the twentieth century wore on, then, this bisexuality identified in lower animals was recoded into a general concept of biological plasticity that would direct endocrinologists toward the child.

The identification and naming of the hormone took place at the start of the twentieth century. In the course of research on the role of the pancreas in digestion, William Bayliss and Ernest Starling aimed, much as Berthold had, to disprove a reigning nervous theory of the organ. That view held that some form of nervous reflex governed each stage of the digestion of food, analogous to the secretion of saliva triggered by the presence of food into the mouth. Bayliss and Starling looked at the relation of the pancreas to the small intestine in dogs by surgically removing part of the latter during digestion, scraping off its surface, and distilling the chemicals there present. They hypothesized that some chemical agent produced in the mucous membrane, activated by the entry of stomach acid into the small intestine, was responsible for the secretions of the pancreas during digestion. When they injected the distilled solution into a dog, they found that it induced the pancreas to secrete in the absence of stomach acid. Bayliss and Starling named this speculative chemical "secretin" in 1902.[17] Although they were unable to speak either to its molecular composition or to its actual mechanism of action on the pancreas, in their findings they speculate on the possibility that "there are similar mechanisms in relation to other secretions" throughout the animal body.[18]

Starling, who, in the 1905 Croonian Lectures to the Royal College of Physicians of London provided an important sketch of the new field of endocrine medicine to his peers, extrapolated "secretin" into the broader category of the "hormone." While the nervous system had dominated the medical conception of the body for some time, Starling ambitiously proposed that the hormonal body was of a more fundamental evolutionary organization. Many organisms lacked a nervous system, after all, whereas chemical communication was ubiquitous down to the unicellular level of life.[19] Even in complex forms like humans, he suggested that the role of "chemical reflexes," rather than nervous reflexes, had been greatly underappreciated, in spite of the continuing ignorance of the actual operations of hormones (16–17). Starling described hormones as "the chemical messengers which, speeding from cell to cell along the blood stream, may coordinate the activities and growth of different parts of the body" (16). The hormonal economy of the body is distinguished for him by two modes: the increase and decrease of specific organ activities and the growth of tissues or organs. "One cannot, however," he cautioned, "draw a sharp line between reactions involving increased activity or dissimilation [of an organ] and those which involved increased assimilation or growth, since under physiological circumstances the latter is always the immediate sequence or accompaniment of the former" (25). The endocrine system rather incorporates a vital, if strangely mixed, degree of growth and transformation of the biological body into its quotidian operations.

While the original research into the pancreas had no obvious connection to sex, in the Croonian lectures Starling stressed its comparative importance. "The largest group of correlations between the activity of one organ and the growth of others," he said confidently, "is formed by those widespread influences exercised by the generative organs" (26). As Darwin had earlier claimed without the model of the hormone, so too did Starling posit sex as the most intense site of the endocrine body's intrinsic transformability. His final Croonian Lecture focused on the largely speculative but alluring and growing consensus that there exists a homology between sex and growth as hormonally regulated aspects of human form. Beginning with the long-standing experiments on the removal of the testes in birds, Starling then reviewed contemporary work that had established the ovaries as hormone-secreting organs. Research into the mammary glands and pregnancy seemed to him to promise in 1905 the most densely entangled amalgam of sexual differentiation and somatic growth, combining fetal, placental, gonadal, and possibly neurological dimensions of the endocrine system (27–33). "As is well known," Starling pointed out, in a nod to the theory of natural bisexuality, "at birth these [mammary] glands are . . . equal in extent in both sexes" (28).

While the suggestion of a homology between bisexuality and plasticity was largely latent in Starling's 1905 lectures because the actual mechanisms of hormonal synthesis and communication remained almost entirely speculative and based in analogies, near the end of his career, in 1923, he reflected in much stronger terms on the potential of the endocrine body to experimental medicine: "It seems almost a fairly tale that such widespread results, affecting every aspect of a man's life, should be conditioned by the presence or absence in the body of infinitesimal quantities of a substance which by its formula does not seem to stand out from the thousands of other substances with which organic chemistry has made us familiar."[20] With the passage of time, his confidence in the primacy of sex in the endocrine system had only increased. Speculating that "the reproductive organs are possibly even more marvellous" than any other hormone-secreting glands, Starling sums up nicely the consensus of the life sciences of the 1920s: "The whole differentiation of sex, and the formation of secondary sexual characteristics, are determined by the circulation in the blood produced either in the germ cells themselves or, as seems more probable, in the interstitial cells.... Thus, it is possible by operating *at an early age* to transfer male into female and *vice versa*."[21] Berthold's experimental sex change in chickens had been concretized into a fully fledged model of an endocrine body whose sex and growth were governed by the circulation of specific hormones. What's more, as chemicals, if sex hormones could be synthesized, that economy could be directly manipulated by science and medicine, altering the sexual differentiation and reproduction of the species. To understand how, in several decades, a vague and largely metaphorical picture of "chemical messengers" could lead to confidence in the scientific changeability of sex in animals and possibly humans, we need to examine more closely the recoding of bisexuality as plasticity. Starling's qualification of "at an early age" is key: the still vague developmental language growing in endocrinology would be made explicit by the introduction of the child as a metaphor.

From Bisexuality to Plasticity

At this early twentieth-century juncture, the metaphor of primitive animality used to explain the plasticity of sex was transformed into a much more potent metaphor of child development. Drawing from the closely related field of embryology, early twentieth-century endocrinologists wagered that the receptivity to transformation of sexed life was much higher in its juvenile stages—indeed, the embryo was probably the most plastic of all life, with that quantum of plasticity diminishing gradually during fetal life, infancy, and childhood until it was nearly gone in adulthood and old age. In doubling animality's primitivism from a phylogenetic temporality to a second, ontogenetic temporality, developmental plasticity offered a clear, material target for medical science: intervene into the growing organism before it has finished sexual differentiation and its eventual form could be cultivated rationally.

As microscopic technology grew in refinement and cell theory began to take shape in the nineteenth century, a pointed interest had arisen in "protoplasm," the direct conceptual predecessor to plasticity. The Czech anatomist J. E. Purkyne had coined the term in 1839 through microscopic examination of an animal embryo.[22] In 1846, the German physiologist Hugo von Mohl, who also proposed the theory of cell division, described the "tough, slimy, granular semi-fluid" in plant cells as protoplasm, arguing it was the original material out of which the nucleus of new cells is formed.[23] While protoplasm's material referent was, in a literal sense, that observable liquid, speculation simultaneously arose as to its *invisible* action as the possible abstract force of life, a potential correspondence between cell division and organismic growth. This interest in the protoplasmic qualities of the cell and, by analogy, of living creatures composed of many cells, fed into a broader theory of the plastic materiality of biology by the turn of the twentieth century. Given how conceptually abstract and unrepresentable protoplasm was as a force (although cell division could be observed, the actual mechanism by which it took place could not), the theory of biological plasticity would find itself in need of a more compelling metaphor were it to become alterable in the lab.

While researchers in the mechanist camp of the life sciences still hoped to identify a specific chemical or physiological basis of protoplasm and to picture how it drove cell division and the growth of life forms, they were continually frustrated by its recalcitrance. The field of embryology therefore began to adopt techniques of experimental anatomy and physiology rather than merely describing biological structures, diffusing the interest in protoplasm and plasticity throughout the rest of the life sciences. In an important experiment in 1891, Hans Driesch artificially shook apart two-cell sea urchin embryos. In the dominant mechanist paradigm of the era, he expected that the two now-separated cells would grow into deformed half-organisms, for each would have been otherwise destined to grow into a specific, predetermined part of the adult sea urchin. When the two separated cells instead went on to form whole embryos, albeit about half their normal size, Driesch was forced to reconceive of the embryo as an equipotential system where each part has the material capacity to grow into a whole. In other words, a distinct field of plasticity seemed to pervade the embryo, allowing it to radically adapt to changes from its environment and to maintain a certain form, although this plasticity could not, strictly speaking, be observed under the microscope.[24] Driesch could see only its effects.

In 1907, Ross Granville Harrison, an embryologist at Johns Hopkins University, published a paper on his success in the first culturing of live tissue without an attached body. Adapting what was known as the "hanging drop" method, Harrison removed neural tissue from a frog and was able to culture it in a liquid solution so that it grew in three dimensions. His summary of the implications of this experiment dwells on how the cultured nerve fiber "develops by the outflowing of protoplasm from the central cells"—in other words, an intrinsic plasticity is the vital engine of live tissue, coaxed by the hanging drop apparatus to grow into an incipient form out of its embryonic indeterminacy and without the body of the frog organizing it.[25] The absence of a body in tissue culture suggested that plasticity was a fundamental quality of life at various scales, rather than a property or part of specific biological structures, like the organism or the body.

The Harrison technique went on to play a central role in a massive amount of scientific and medical research over the twentieth century: on cancer, organ regeneration, and transplants, for instance. The plasticity of living tissue, now successfully cultivated in the lab, promised to grant a new mode of access to the biological body for the life sciences. Yet as an invisible, latent force of both growth and receptivity to form, this emergent sense of plasticity still lacked coherence. Protoplasm or, as it was increasingly rendered, plasticity, needed a metaphor because, in its visual absence to researchers except in its effects it was unable to break the deadlock between mechanist and vitalists. Either the plastic quality of life was a series of chemical reactions that had yet to be observed due to inadequate scientific instruments or else plasticity was just another name for a metaphysical, vital force of life that was beyond rational influence of alteration. Neither of those options had provided much opportunity to work with and cultivate plasticity in the lab. And work by embryologists like Driesch or Granville could definitely prove neither. In this context, the child could serve as a much better metaphor for plasticity, combining cell theory with the concept of life's natural bisexuality through the narrative drama of development. As the child study movement grew on both sides of the Atlantic alongside the development biologists of the *Entwickslungmechanik* school, the traffic between fields was favorable to the production of the child as a particular kind of metaphor.[26]

Within the child study movement, G. Stanley Hall looms large not only because he established the category of "adolescence" but because of his dedicated interest in the life sciences.[27] His 1904 foundational work *Adolescence* is grounded in a psychobiological and rigidly evolutionist materialism. Borrowing heavily from physiology, embryology, and endocrinology, Hall made of adolescence a critical period of plasticity, where the natural openness of children's growing bodies and minds *demanded* to be cultivated for the teleological ends of his narrow and racist vision of the human species. Hall grounded the psychological and spiritual development of children and young people in a direct analogy to biological development, so that the psychic and somatic unfolded as part of the same material process. *Adolescence* also reflects the consolidation of a strict teleology of child development. Growth was coded as unidirectional *and* parallel at the individual and species levels, binding childhood to a highly charged evolutionary concept of race as inheritable phenotype. The discourse of development registered as a problem of timing, in the multiple senses of pacing, stages, and thresholds after which plasticity waned and could no longer be manipulated. In Hall's ardently recapitulationist view, children and adolescents were "neo-atavistic," much like ancient human ancestors in form and structure but ready to grow to "higher" ends in a rapid period with the right environmental input.[28] Childhood and adolescence were henceforth incarnations of a temporary plasticity subject to natural and artificial variation that could produce correspondingly normal or abnormal growth. Yet even as he offered this plasticity as an object to be governed by scientific technique, Hall had to concede a certain agency to its unpredictability. "Some linger long in the childish stage and advance late or slowly," as Hall put it, "while others push on with a sudden outburst of impulsion to early maturity" (xiii). Without the intervention of science, medicine, and education, that plastic indeterminacy could not be counted upon to achieve the specific (and fundamentally racist) form of the human that Hall advocated. Biology alone was not enough; it had to be cultivated. At the same time, it might resist or thwart cultivation.

Hall defined adolescence precisely as "the age of modification and plasticity" (128), and his characteristic overconfidence in the material basis of plasticity indexed its widespread acceptance at the turn of the century:

> For biology the plasmata in general and the protoplasms in
> particular, under many names and aspects, occupy a position of

ever-increasing interest and preeminence. Unlike ether, the still more
hypothetical background of all physical existence, protoplasm is a
tangible reality accessible to many and ever more subtle methods
of study, and . . . its all-dominant impulse is to progressive self-
expression. It is the creator of the ascending series of types and
species of plants and animal, which become its habits of self-
formulation. . . . It unites successive generations into an unbroken
continuum, so that they bud, the later from the earlier, each
ontological line organizing a soma of gradually lessening vitality
doomed to death, while it remains immortal in the phylum. (411)

This account of the protoplasmic élan of life from the cell upward
to the species verges on an imaginative vitalism. More important is that
Hall identified the plasticity of life as its vector of material growth, one that
is temporarily impressible during childhood.[29] Hall saw the science of
child study as leading directly to the practice of cultivating children and
adolescents into normative adults, for nature alone was insufficient to the
project of evolution. "Even if it be prematurely," he explained in the case
of schooling the growing child, "he must be subjected to special disciplines
and be apprenticed to the higher qualities of adulthood, for he is not only
a product of nature, but a candidate for a highly developed humanity" (xii).
Such "apprenticeship" could be straightforwardly educational, but even that
was based for Hall in a biological metaphor for the apprenticeship of natural plasticity, the directed cultivation of an ideal, mature form or phenotype
for the human—for Hall, not surprisingly a white, binary, male body.[30]

Timing asserted itself as the most important problem here because plasticity was neither permanent nor constant.[31] "Never again" after the ages of
eight to twelve, Hall felt, "will there be such susceptibility to drill and dis-
cipline, such plasticity to habituation, or such ready adjustment to new
conditions" (xii). Disease was recoded in this developmental sense as a
pathology of precocity, arrest, or belatedness, all indigenous to childhood:
"Some disorders of arrest and defect as well as of excessive unfoldment in
some function, part, or organ may now, after long study and controversy,
be said to be established as peculiar to this period" (xiv). Moreover, and
quite importantly, nature alone could not ensure the normal development
of children, for corrupt or abnormal growth was stored and transmitted to
the next generation by sexual reproduction. "The momentum of heredity
often seems insufficient to enable the child to achieve this great revolution

and come to complete maturity," Hall opines, and "there is not only arrest, but perversion, at every stage, and hoodlumism, juvenile crime, and secret vice" (xiv). The slip from "arrest" in developmental progress to "perversion" and "secret vice" is hardly incidental, for sexual differentiation was of uniquely intense concern to Hall, who borrowed from endocrinology the view that sex housed the primary plasticity of life during development and its method of transmission to future generations through reproduction.[32] For that reason, sex was at once the most robustly powerful and fragile dimension of the growing child's body. In matters of sexual development, Hall pronounced, "life reaches its maximal intensity" (412).[33]

Hall's concept of development places plasticity in a staged model, according to which different moments of differentiation express plasticity to different degrees, while the overall trend is toward the withering of plasticity by adulthood and old age. Describing the sexual differentiation of body parts during puberty, Hall reasoned, "Such changes are far more numerous and more rapid in the infant, and still more so in the growth of the embryo; but in these respects *they are analogous in their nature, although later growths are less predetermined, rapid, or transforming*" (127, emphasis added). The protoplasmic quality of the embryo was as an ever-diminishing return as it accomplished the growth of the human, with important spikes in infancy, childhood, and, finally, adolescence, before firming up into an adult morphology. "So puberty is not unlike a new birth," Hall could say, "when the lines of development take new directions" (127). With a nod to the neo-Lamarckian camp in biology, he adds: "There is much reason to believe that the influence of the environment in producing acquired traits transmissible by heredity is greatest now" (127). Hall's work on child development provided a stable way to imagine the alteration of racial plasticity in human bodies in endocrinology, which would take up his work in an abstract, metaphorical form, to move closer to the point of being able to alter human sex.

The Racial Cultivation of the Developing Endocrine Body

By the early twentieth century, human development had been rendered as a biological declension narrative of plasticity into form. The intrinsic tension between indeterminacy and form had not actually been resolved but was given new life in the body of the child, with the temporal frame of development ostensibly providing organization and justification for the incredibly narrow phenotypes that scientists like Hall judged to be the proper end of the human. As endocrinology came into its own during the first several decades of the twentieth century, the child as metaphor for plasticity enabled the field to move from animal experimentation toward imagining the hormonal alteration of the human body, a prospect that eugenicist endocrinologists greeted with enthusiasm.

In Europe, Vienna became the anchor of a socialist and eugenic community of endocrine research. During the first several decades of the twentieth century, experimental organotherapy, glandular transplants, and early attempts at hormone administration attempted to modify the plasticity of animals and humans during their juvenile stages, as well as encourage the passing on of more refined, normative phenotypes to future generations. For Eugen Steinach, who would achieve world renown for his endocrine therapies, sex was therefore nothing less than "an integrating component of the life concept."[34] Steinach's fame came in large part from his incredibly popular "rejuvenation" surgery, offered to aging men to revitalize and reawaken their physical and psychological youth by reactivating the dormant plasticity of the gonads. In reality, the surgical procedure amounted to a vasectomy, but testimonies of dramatic revitalization from legions of men around the world led to great demand for endocrine rejuvenation in the 1920s and 1930s, and Steinach's personal clients included the likes of Freud, who was also an avid consumer of Steinach's published work on bisexuality.[35]

Prior to his acclaim, Steinach began his career by re-creating the animal castration experiments of his predecessors, including Hunter and Berthold. Preferring to work on small rodents, through gonadal transplantation he reaffirmed in a series of papers in 1912 and 1913 that "the implantation of the gonad of the opposite sex" in guinea pigs "transformed the original sex of the animal" (66). A hormonally induced sex change reinforced the thesis of life's fundamental bisexuality, which he quickly analogized to humans: "Absolute masculinity or absolute femininity in any individual represents an imaginary ideal. A one hundred percent man is as non-existent as a one hundred percent woman" (7). Retracing the line of thought that had emerged from the child study movement, Steinach narrated endocrine development as a teleological arc from natural bisexuality to a stable sexed form. "Long before puberty, at the dawn of their individual existence, male and female human beings show no sharp differentiation of form, apart from their organs of generation." Rather, "differentiation appears later, and is at first gradual"

(45). Steinach often referred to the gonads as "the puberty gland," and in his references to "the cubhood of young boys and the difficult 'teens' of girls" he was fully enmeshed in a discourse of puberty as "crisis" that shared much with Hall (46). The physiological and psychological tumult of growth and adolescence, for Steinach, was "a case of external manifestation of extensive workings under the surface, a secret and fateful activity of internally functioning glands" (46). In his endocrine model, the hormonal body was developmental in organization, and his experiments on animals were interpreted through the metaphor of the child.

Steinach's interest in the racial plasticity of puberty was expanded in his work with his colleague, the biologist Paul Kammerer, with whom he co-authored a paper titled "Climate and Puberty" in 1920.[36] Kammerer was a strong partisan of the neo-Lamarckian theory of the inheritance of acquired characteristics. Together with Steinach, he hoped to draw on the newly developmental model of the endocrine body to demonstrate *how* morphological characteristics were both acquired *and* inherited. Unsurprisingly, they argued that sex, comprising both differentiation and reproduction, played host to that process. They also proposed that the endocrine system, which also played such an important role in metabolism, effectively mediated between the living organism and its environment. In two parts, the essay draws an analogy from their experiments on rat growth to human development through a superficial reading of colonial anthropology. Their experiments had demonstrated that rats reared in warmer temperatures developed quicker than those in temperate environments. Equally important, the warm-temperature rats apparently grew more prominent secondary sexual characteristics. These sexed forms also appeared to be heritable. When after several generations of warm climate the rats were moved to a cooler environment, their offspring continued to grow into the morphology of their warm-weather ancestors. The second half of the essay makes the leap to human populations described in anthropology to argue that warm climate resulted in the hypersexualization attributed to non-European peoples by encouraging the overdevelopment, first, of the puberty glands and, consequently, of the secondary sex characteristics. Similarly, the authors asserted, the neurasthenic exhaustion of European settler colonists from the endocrine overactivity induced by warm climates explains their frequently neurotic sexual pathologies.[37]

This theory of the inheritance of acquired characteristics through the sexed form of the endocrine system had two important effects. First, it reaffirmed a racist evolutionary hierarchy of human societies through the hormonal body, drawing a homology between a hypersexualized body of color and species-level primitivism. The sexed form of the internal and external body was coded as an explicitly racial form. Second, and quite importantly, the binding of sex and race relied on the concept of plasticity. If environmental information such as heat could influence the sexed form of the growing body and be transmitted to offspring, a feat replicated in rats in the lab, then the possibility of effecting analogous changes in humans was opened. Steinach and Kammerer mobilized the endocrine system's now established developmental plasticity to bind sex to race. In so doing, it was no coincidence that puberty was the object of their analysis, for the child metaphor animating their version of the endocrine body made the plastic period of growth prior to adulthood the sensitive moment of environmental input that led to the acquisition and transmission of new sexed characteristics.

This binding of sex to race gave plasticity a eugenic significance. Both Steinach and Kammerer were involved in a community of socialist eugenicists in interwar Vienna, attempting to apply their research to uplift the "stock" of the working class through manipulation of the inheritance of acquired characteristics at the population level.[38] In the United States, endocrinology also took on a eugenic logic during this period, albeit without the same politics. And in its earliest forms eugenic science in America aimed itself at children. In turn-of-the-century California, for instance, the botanist Luther Burbank argued that children were like not rats but plants. Independent of the circulation of Gregor Mendel's work and the rise of genetics, Burbank undertook countless plant hybridization experiments at his Santa Rosa farm. Not only did his hybrid plants have a major impact on the practice of U.S. agriculture, but also his emphasis on the cultivation of biological form in plants lent itself to a great deal of eugenic writing and advocacy. His curious 1907 book, *The Training of the Human Plant,* is dedicated to "the sixteen million public school children of America." Combining his expertise in the crossing of plant species with the principle of natural selection and a neo-Lamarckian understanding of environmental impressibility, Burbank argues for "the adaptation of the principles of plant culture and improvement in a more or less modified form to the human being."[39] Burbank felt that the United States was aptly suited to creating what he called "the race of the future" (12) because of the widespread "mingling" (33) encouraged by immigration.

While sex as reproduction alone would provide for some hybridization, it was in the planned cultivation of children's developing bodies that
Burbank saw the greatest potential and most urgent matter for eugenicists.
"All animal life is sensitive to environment," he wrote, "but of all living
things the child is the most sensitive. . . . Every possible influence will leave
its impress upon the child, and the traits which it inherited will be overcome to a certain extent" (14–15). In other words: "A child absorbs environment" (14–15). Were that absorption to be scientifically directed toward
the perfection of human phenotype, the racial stock of America could be
enhanced through each generation of children to come. At the heart of this
earliest American eugenics was the assumption that in the body of the child,
as Burbank put it, "no where else is there material so plastic" (26). While
Burbank could not advance much further than romantic naturalism, suggesting good sunshine, clean air, and good food as the basis for cultivating
children like plants, endocrinologists could turn to the newly modeled
hormonal body for a more precise program of human enhancement.

One such important figure for endocrinology in the early twentieth
century was the biologist Oscar Riddle, remembered most for the discovery of the hormone prolactin and its function in the pituitary gland. Riddle
joined the Cold Spring Harbor eugenic research station in Long Island,
New York, in 1913 as a research associate. Although he did not get along
very well politically or intellectually with Charles Davenport, the station's
director and the de facto figurehead of American eugenics, the two co-
existed for many years.[40] Prior to joining the premier American eugenics
research lab, Riddle had spent time in recently annexed Puerto Rico with
the U.S. commissioner of fisheries, cataloging and examining the island's
fish in the service of colonial science. He had also spent time teaching in
Berlin in 1910 after completing graduate school, where he became well
versed in the broader European life sciences.[41]

At Cold Spring Harbor, Riddle's research was broader in scope than the
pituitary gland. His interest in the racial plasticity of sex led him to countless experiments in the alteration of animal phenotype through endocrine
experimentation. For years he bred ringdoves, experimenting with the
planned refinement of different forms and morphologies.[42] Riddle's long-
term study of pigeons, likewise, translated the promise of plasticity into
a critique of the rising field of genetics, with its chromosomally determinist account of life. "The field of modifiability"—his phrase for plasticity—
"is not only the more alluring aspect of development—it promises results

of more practical importance," he explained. "Though we may not hope to take from or give to the chromosomes of mankind, the temporary transformability—not mere modifiability—of probably all alternative genes of every human being and of every organism is a scientific possibility which awaits only the work of the investigator."[43] In connecting sexual differentiation and reproduction to the metabolic activities of the rest of the body's ductless glands, Riddle's research intensified the still largely enigmatic relationship between sex and growth first identified by Bayliss and Sterling's work on the hormone.

In rats and pigeons, Riddle also examined the specific effects of nascent synthetic hormone therapy on growth and sex through the gonads, the pituitary, and the adrenal glands. In an experimental "sex-reversal" in the pigeon, the findings of which he published in 1924, he explained that "the sex of numerous pigeons has been reversed in the earliest (gamete) or egg stage" by the application of partially synthesized hormone compounds. Among his conclusions was that this could mean that the "'hermaphrodite' birds might actually be a sex-reversal that had yet to complete."[44] Although he never conducted research in humans directly, he referred to the child as metaphor for plasticity to lend a developmental organization to sex in the pigeon studies. The sheer plasticity of the pigeon embryo was understood to constitute the "right" moment of sensitivity to induce a "sex reversal" by the application of hormones. Riddle's technical approach was underwritten by the embryo's naturally bisexual character, primed for the influence of hormones to develop into a distinctly sexed form. By applying hormones, Riddle understood himself to be artificially inducing sexual development in the direction of his design.

Riddle's confidence that sex change in animals was both a common occurrence in nature and achievable in the lab by technical means had major implications for trans and intersex medicine during the early twentieth century, as the next two chapters explore in detail. The concept of a mutually exclusive, biologically grounded two-sex binary popular today was simply not an established concept in the early twentieth century. In this era, "sex" was commonly and scientifically understood to mean an original bisexuality that, although quite capable of differentiating into male or female, nevertheless retained the latent possibility of reversal—a revision of Darwin's concept of "reversion." At the same time, the growing medical interest in intersex bodies and sexual inverts suggested that the human species, too, harbored a dramatic range of sexed morphologies, rather than hewing strictly to a binary. For endocrinologists, the application of the child metaphor to work with animals established the viability of "sex-reversal" as a possible future endocrine therapy in humans, where it would seem quite natural to begin with children. The tensions in the child metaphor between indeterminacy and form remained latent, hiding just underneath the veneer of a developmental timescale that purported to convert sex into phenotype. A purely mixed bisexuality would never obey a doctor and differentiate into male or female, so the notion of progressive sequence was added to bring a temporal order to sex. Yet the material actions of plasticity in laboratories simultaneously undermined that developmental schema, leading to confusion that was well summarized by the biologist Allen Ezra in the 1920s: "One may well ask: Is any human being completely sexed?"[45] In the face of that increasingly complex question, Ezra reflects the growing consensus of the interwar era, claiming that that "sex is the expression of *a combination of male or female* characteristics within an individual,"[46] so that "a completely sexed individual is the result of a variety of forces acting in sequence on a progressively changing substratum."[47] The tension in this account between the notion of "a completely sexed individual" and the "progressively changing substratum" of sex preserved a significant conceptual paradox at the heart of endocrinology's interest in plasticity.

While the era of normative bisexuality seems to have been largely forgotten or overlooked in the history of gender, sexuality, and trans medicine, so too have its eugenic foundations. Although children occupied a rather visible place within the project of the American eugenics movement in the early twentieth century, notably in "better baby contests" and public health and education campaigns, Riddle's or Steinach's reliance on an abstract metaphor of the child to developmentally organize research speaks to a less visible historical role played by the child. Children do figure in the historiography of American eugenics, but their importance is framed mostly in the sense of being born or not being born. While the more visible and violent forms of race hygiene and eugenic medicine were contested in the aftermath of the Second World War, recent scholarship has dismantled that declension narrative, arguing that eugenic ideas and practices in fact have found their most pervasive reach in the postwar era. There is no meaningful, nonideological difference between so-called positive and negative eugenics, and the historical binding of race to reproduction remains largely unchallenged, which is to say unmarked and unspoken, in medical science to this day.[48] The modern endocrine body incarnates one important instance of the persistence of eugenic logics after the war, as later chapters in this book explore in greater detail. The child metaphor was in large part what allowed the cultivation of sexual plasticity through development to proceed without reference to its eugenic heritage and without much acknowledgement of children at all. The figurative purchase of the child in endocrinology brought plasticity under the jurisdiction of experimental medicine, and the potential for more complex "sex reversals," including in humans, grew over the next fifty years in ways that Riddle or Steinach could scarcely have imagined.

Figurative Life

Toward the end of *Strange Dislocations*, Carolyn Steedman makes an enigmatic claim about the relation of literary figures of the child to the life sciences in the nineteenth century, explaining that she has "attempted a partial description of some of the knowledge . . . by which strange acts of personification took place, that is, *the giving of abstract information about children and children's bodies, shape and form in actual children*, not by bringing statues to life through the force of prosopopeia, but by *using living bodies as expressions*."[49] To clarify, she adds: "Meaning and knowledge, remembering and affect, actually *come into existence in human bodies*. I have chosen a literary figure or trope, that of personification, to describe that kind of active making of something out of ideas," an "act of embodiment."[50] The figurative existence of the child is always premised on abstraction, but, as Steedman notes, it is an abstraction whose form is paradoxically expressed in the real, living bodies of children. Something about children's bodies incarnates and takes living form in large part as the personification distilled from an abstract concept. The child, paradoxical as it may sound, is a living figure. Or, in her incisive words, one of the defining characteristics of the history of modern Western childhood is that "children became the problem they represented."[51] This is so in one sense because "the child" does not exist without relation to actual, living children. As this chapter has examined, it is also so because the child has been made a metaphor, in Haraway's sense, for the plasticity of sex. The child has been made a living figure in biology because children can metaphorically accommodate the ultimately paradoxical relationship between form and plasticity that, somehow, grows into the human and can be altered by medical science. This is a *historical* situation, not an ontological one: children are not intrinsically prone to figurative life, nor is that form the only one to which they are perpetually consigned. In the same way, the twentieth-century association of children with the racial plasticity of sex was not inevitable, nor must it necessarily endure into the future.

Steedman's choice of personification over metaphor to describe this historical process, however, implies a unidirectional account of the materialization of children's bodies *by* abstract knowledge. Perhaps matters are less straightforward than that. We might say that the growing child was a compelling metaphor in the late nineteenth and early twentieth centuries not merely because plasticity was, strictly speaking, an invisible quality of biological life or that protoplasm was too abstract an idea to guide the life sciences. More important, the child metaphor granted real access to altering the human body for science and medicine. By turning to the developmental model refined by the child study movement, endocrinology was able to redescribe the life of the cell and the unfinished organism's glands as pervaded by a plastic field sensitive to hormonal information, whether natural or synthetic, even if that field could not be seen under the microscope or in the clinic. At the same time, however, this child figure made to slide from the cell to infant, to adolescent, to adult, and back, was only a partial success. As Haraway reminds, metaphors work only insofar as they are imperfect descriptions, linking two disparate concepts together. For that reason they remain unstable and open to contestation, including from the situated perspective of the disavowed object, in this case the child. The metaphor of the child was meant to manage the paradox between indeterminacy and form that sex's racial plasticity ignited, but it actually served to keep that tension alive, including in actual children's bodies as their sex was medicalized in the early twentieth century. Plasticity, as a concept that has no literal or physiological referent, would turn out to be more unruly than Starling, Hall, Steinach, Kammerer, or Riddle might have wished. The child is an alluring living figure of racial plasticity because children grow so quickly and dramatically before the eyes of adults, but the distinction between "the child" as a figure and "children" as actual biological bodies produces an ineffable gap in knowledge about race and sex, rather than extinguishing it. Some of the many historical consequences of this choice of metaphor are taken up in the next chapters.

I have spent so long on the details of turn-of-the-century endocrinology because the clinical histories that follow in subsequent chapters rely directly on the key concepts that were invented and experimentally established in this era. The rest of this book shifts focus from the child as a metaphor in medical scientific discourse to actual children's bodies in specific clinical settings, examining how plasticity ramified in the medicalization of intersex and trans children over the twentieth century. As the endocrinologists in this chapter began to imagine a transfer of the concept of plasticity from the animal to the human body via the child, physicians in the United States started to make that jump clinically through the early twentieth-century treatment of intersex children, who seemed to literally represent the thesis of natural bisexuality, while finding themselves in the course of that work confronted with some of the first trans people to seek medical support for altering their sex. As the trans early twentieth century took shape, the involvement of biological life in the metaphors used to describe it began to frustrate clinicians and children alike. Scientists and doctors maintained no pretense of being in control of sex and growth, as much as they clung to dogmatically binary and racialized definitions of sex. They could hope only to influence, nudge, and contour still largely metaphorical processes that began in natural bisexuality and, according to them, were meant to end in binary form. For the eugenicists, meanwhile, this indeterminacy of sex occasioned a litany of racist anxieties over individual pathology and population-level degeneration.

In opening up plasticity to its historical context—something so often missing from its celebration in recent years by feminist science studies, neuroscientific work, and neo materialisms[52]—Haraway's suggestion that the referent of a metaphor has its own organic agencies is useful. The eugenic heritage of endocrinology informs the medicalization of sex, gender, and trans life in the twentieth century, but it hardly exhausts plasticity's meanings for forms. If intersex and trans children, as we will see in the next several chapters, have been forced to grow in the dislocation between the figurative and the material existence of race, sex, and plasticity, they may have accrued or encountered strange and unexpected plastic agencies along the way. If, as Steedman speculates, "figurative existence is a form of historical existence," we cannot assume that the overriding power of the child metaphor was able to completely disenfranchise children—even if, most of the time, it nearly did.[53]

CHAPTER 2

Before Transsexuality

The Transgender Child from the 1900s to the 1930s

H OW CAN WE NAME A *TRANS* early twentieth century given the myopia of the medical archive in the era before transsexuality? For all the zealous attention focused on the plasticity of sex in the life sciences, particularly between the two World Wars, the practice of medicine was by comparison quite conservative on the question of changing sex in the absence of physiological "abnormality." While endocrinologists carried out the idealistic and eugenic sex experiments on nonhuman animals explored in the preceding chapter, surgeons, physicians, and psychiatrists confronted with human bodies remained reluctant to adopt the ethos of their scientific colleagues. At least, that was the prevailing situation in the United States. The dominant context for changing the sex of the human body in American medicine prior to the 1950s was a chaotic matrix of intersex diagnoses, gathered under the catchall term "hermaphroditism," whose morphology was as elusive as it was visible in medical discourse. Synthetic hormone therapies were not practically available until the mid- to late 1930s, and even then it took a great many years of research just to establish a basic sense of how the administration of estrogens, testosterone, and cortical steroids could affect the body's plasticity. For most of the first four decades of the twentieth century, urological and plastic surgeons, rather than clinical endocrinologists, directed the medicalization of sex and plasticity. And they remained largely dismissive of otherwise "normal" people who wished to change their sex.

In Europe, particularly Germany, the sexological paradigm championed by Magnus Hirschfeld's Institut fur Sexualwissenschaft provided medical transition for trans people as early as the 1920s.[1] Hirschfeld's sexological community fostered a productive dialogue between the German sense of "intersexuality" and a new category, "transvestism," which referred not only to the desire to cross-dress but also to the desire to live as a sex different from the one assigned at birth.[2] American medicine, by contrast,

showed little practical interest in the concept. As a consequence, the slip-
pery diagnostic matrix that attempted to manage the relations that linked
homosexuality, sexual inversion, hermaphroditism, and transvestism, all
of which shared core connotations, is a very complex place to read recognizably trans life, unless we emphasize that discourses of transness in this
era were not confined by the limited, binary vision of the postwar model
of transsexuality and so were free to take on multiple forms. Sex change,
transformation, and transition were ostensibly split in the United States
between experiments in the life sciences on animals on the one hand and
the mostly surgical approach to hermaphroditism in medicine on the other.
The lives of people we might read as transvestite or transgender were meant
by medical design to be excluded from those two projects, putting up an
archived obstacle to locating early twentieth-century trans life. This gatekeeping is the source of the challenge for historical work on trans life in the
early twentieth century, and this chapter works to address both the affordances of an era without the narrow terms of the postwar medical model
and the limits of an archive in which doctors very clearly did not wish for
trans people to be identified with the concept of changing sex.

    Despite the brusqueness of American medicine, the archive still holds
the traces of many people we can read as trans. In 1917 and 1918, Alan Hart
became one of the first trans men anywhere to transition with medical
support. Upon graduating from medical school at the University of Oregon, in 1917, Hart had consulted a psychiatrist "and with him made a complete study of my case, my individual history and that of my family." After
a physical examination, the diagnosis was, in Hart's words, "Complete,
congenital and incurable homosexuality together with a marked modification of the physical organization from the feminine type." Life having
"become so unbearable that I felt myself confronted by only two alternative courses—either to kill myself or refuse to live longer in my misfit role
of a woman," Hart decided on the second. After an exploratory laparotomy
surgery "for the purpose of establishing definitely and indisputably my
proper role," Hart achieved through an "operation" and "transformation"
that included a hysterectomy "the result that I left the hospital as a man."
Despite facing slander, discrimination, and prejudice from colleagues, Hart
went on to a distinguished medical career in Oregon, Montana, and California as a radiologist and tuberculosis researcher. Despite an earlier claim by
the historian Jonathan Ned Katz that Hart was a lesbian, scholars now agree
that Hart's profession of being a man and his having pursued a medical sex

change ought to be taken seriously and that the term "homosexuality" in these documents cannot be taken literally through its contemporary definition. The fact that trans life could fall under the sign of "homosexuality" is actually an important clue for how to read the early twentieth-century medical archive, for the wider category of sexual inversion regularly mixed gay and trans connotations.[3]

Hart, of course, had access to medicine by virtue of education and vocation. The possibility of reading trans *children* in the early twentieth century is more complex. Some of the first trans people to collaborate with doctors in the 1940s and 1950s in the emergent field of transsexual medicine recalled their childhoods lived during the 1920s and 1930s. And among them were a few experiences with medicine, like that of "Val." One of the first trans women to try, albeit unsuccessfully, to obtain access to surgery in the United States in the 1940s, Val had the blue-chip endorsements of the endocrinologist Harry Benjamin, the sexologist Alfred Kinsey, and Karl Bowman of the Langley Porter Psychiatric Clinic in San Francisco. In 1948, while dozens of doctors at the University of Wisconsin–Madison's General Hospital quarreled over whether to grant permission for surgery, Val, who was then in her early twenties, recounted her childhood to a psychiatrist. At age two she had become unwilling to wear boy's clothes, and her parents relented, letting her dress full time as a girl. When she started school, around 1930, her parents, who were on the local school board and who were close to the county judge, arranged for her to officially attend school as a girl. "Special arrangements for toilet, etc. were made," and even though classmates knew Val "was actually a boy," they treated her "with respect and apparently did not tease or shun" her.[4] When she was ten, Val even joined the 4H Club "and took cooking and flower gardening."[5] A local doctor, probably drawing on the developmental theory of human bisexuality, advised the family that the condition was one she "would normally grow out of at puberty." When that did not happen and the local high school was more hostile, Val dropped out and had "spent the subsequent time at home doing a woman's work."[6] Later reading "a good deal" about her "condition," including "several books and articles on operative procedures which feminize men"[7] by sexologists like Havelock Ellis and Hirschfeld,[8] Val decided to pursue surgery and hormone therapy. Repeatedly, however, hospital boards including the one in Wisconsin forbade any procedure, so she later tried, with the help of Kinsey and Benjamin, to find options in Europe.[9]

Hart and Val are rare evident examples of the interaction between trans people and medicine in the first half of the twentieth century. But their childhoods can be established only retrospectively. Most trans childhoods, like much of trans life in the era before the term "transsexuality," remain *implicit*. We are left to wonder just how many more trans people had no reason at all to be archived.[10] This is not to say that self-identified trans adults from the midcentury necessarily understood themselves in those terms during their childhood, either. Val seems to have understood herself from a young age to be a girl, convincing her parents to let her live and attend school as such. Whether she, her family, her doctor, or her school entertained a concept of her belonging to a distinct "sex" category seems unlikely. Unlike in Europe, "transvestism" was a rarified concept in the United States until around the 1940s, and it is hard to imagine that many children had access to sexological texts that, rarely translated into English, had a minuscule readership among professional adults. Indeed, even Val did not encounter them until she was twenty years old. Other than the vaguely general pronouncements of a local doctor, her trans childhood had no substantive relation to medicine, nor did it evidently need one.

In spite of these epistemological and archival challenges, this chapter takes Val's childhood as a launch point for investigating trans life and trans children in the medical archive of the first half of the twentieth century. There are compelling, if partial, records from this era that suggest inter-action among trans adults, children, and doctors. The fragmented quality of this archive is *not* a flaw or symptom of damage to the historical record but a valuable interruption of how the trans twentieth century has been too often narrated by beginning in the 1950s with transsexuality. Return-ing to the decades that precede that moment opens a complex field of medicine and its interaction with trans people, one in which intersex chil-dren occupy the stage with trans children. The abstract value of the child's growing body as a guiding metaphor in the life sciences and the process through which its plasticity was brought under the jurisdiction of medi-cine hold our attention. Intersex children were forced during these decades into a decisive role as the experimental subjects in whose bodies the abstract theories of endocrinology were translated into real medical technique for altering human sex. The very medical feasibility of Val's request for surgery in 1948 was predicated on decades of medical sex reassignments performed on infants, children, and teenagers diagnosed as "hermaphrodites." This chapter and the next explore the various impacts of the medicalization of intersex children on our understanding of trans history. Intersex children are just as much a part of the history of transgender children as they are an integral part of the broader twentieth-century history of sex and gender. Another important reason to consider intersex and trans people together is that they visited the same doctors. At the Johns Hopkins Hospital, in Baltimore, the paramount American institution for medical research on sex, children's growing bodies were made to manifest what had remained speculative in endocrine theorizing about the plasticity of sex and its racialized meaning as human phenotype. Experimenting on intersex children's unfinished bodies provided the founding protocols of sex assignment *and* reassignment for all human bodies, including for those who would be called transvestites and transsexuals with regularity only later. Some early twentieth-century trans people attempted to claim a space for themselves in that medical discourse, drawing on the relative porosity of categories like intersex and "inversion" to argue that their bodies represented a mix of masculinity and femininity that could be altered by doctors too. While the impulse, looking back from the present day, may be to separate trans and intersex life, this was precisely the undecided tension at hand between doctors and patients in the early twentieth century.

This chapter shows that as sex became more alterable through experiments on intersex bodies, it became less obvious why trans people's requests to change their sex would be disqualified from the same procedures, because in the absence of a medical discourse like transvestism, the sheer similarity between trans and intersex embodiment empowered some trans people to simply argue that they *were* intersex. In the face of this situation, doctors could only scramble to mobilize an ill-fitting narrative of psychological homosexuality to deflect trans people from the clinic. And within this complex field of diagnosis and experimental treatment are key archival traces of trans children from the early twentieth century. The trans child *before* transsexuality, however, does not tie up all of these leakage points between categories. In fact, the trans child casts significant doubt on the utility of a "before transsexuality" paradigm altogether. This chapter shows how the disorganized field of sexual inversion, hermaphroditism, homosexuality, and transvestism in which children were caught *undoes* the presumption that modern medicine played a causal role in defining the parameters of trans life. Rather than serving as a "prehistory" of what came "before" transsexuality, then, this chapter moves toward framing *multiple* trans childhoods, with multiple definitions of transness (including

nonmedical forms of knowledge and identity), each with competing definitions that *exceed* the binary terms to which transness in general and trans
childhood have been confined in the postwar medical model.

The Transatlantic Circulation of Endocrinology, Sexology, and Eugenics

One of the reasons that it is difficult to look in the early twentieth-century
medical archive for legibly trans life is that the most visible Western sexological category through which it circulated—transvestism—appeared only
on the margins of American medicine. One practical obstacle was that major
works of German sexology like Hirschfeld's lengthy study, *Die Transvestit-
enin*, were not translated into English.[11] The British sexologist Ellis, who
coined the term "eonism" to describe the desire to dress and live as a sex
different from the one assigned at birth, did write in English, but his terminology never really caught on.[12] Sexology was also regarded quite differently on the two sides of the Atlantic. While in Europe many physicians,
endocrinologists, and surgeons who practiced medicine found it intuitive
to stay apprised of the work undertaken at Hirschfeld's Institut, in the United
States sexology remained mostly the province of psychiatrists and social scientists, who were rarely well versed in the German literature. In an era when
Freud's reception was both slow among and highly contested by Americans, Hirschfeld and Ellis were likewise regarded with skepticism.[13] When
Val read sexological work on transvestism in the late 1940s, she was actually at the avant-garde of the American reading public, professional or lay.

Nevertheless, clinical experiments at Johns Hopkins on intersex and
trans bodies did not happen in isolation. And, despite a general resistance
to German sexology, there is one endocrinologist who in his biography
and career worked to bridge the European and American paradigms: Harry
Benjamin. Perhaps best known as a founding figure in the 1950s and 1960s
of transsexual medicine, which he pursued from a private practice on the
Upper West Side of Manhattan, Benjamin early in his career as a physician
specializing in endocrinology blended German and American approaches.
Benjamin anchored his view of the endocrine system in the German concept of "intersexuality."[14] He felt strongly that sex, although it was entangled with the psyche, should be understood as a foundationally biological
form. For instance, he maintained throughout his career in the United States,
and quite against the prevailing mood, that "Freud was not a Freudian" but

rather that "he would be shocked if he saw what went on today; he was much more of a biologist."[15]

Graduating from German medical school in 1912, Benjamin traveled to the United States a year later, lured by the promise of a treatment for tuberculosis. When that did not pan out, he decided to return home, but the outbreak of World War I prevented his boat from passing a Royal Navy blockade. Forced into temporary exile, he settled in New York City and opened an endocrine and geriatrics practice.[16] After the war ended, Benjamin immersed himself in the cutting edge of European research on sex and hormones. During the 1920s and 1930s he made almost annual summer trips to Vienna, where he spent months working in Eugen Steinach's endocrine lab.[17] He also befriended Paul Kammerer, the eugenicist biologist who collaborated with Steinach on hormonal rejuvenation and the theory of the inheritance of acquired characteristics.[18] Benjamin led the effort to circulate the pair's work in the United States, bringing both on lecture tours in the 1920s.[19] He was also a major proponent of Steinach's "rejuvenation procedure" in the United States, promoting the cause of endocrine therapeutics as offering eugenic improvement of virility in old age.[20]

While keeping up with the latest in experimental endocrinology, Benjamin also embedded himself in the German sexological circles in which transvestism was being studied and medicalized. Benjamin had first met Hirschfeld in 1906 or 1907, through a mutual friend, and had been taken by him to visit gay and transvestite bars in Berlin. During the 1920s he visited Berlin frequently during his summer trips to Europe, spending a great deal of time at the Institut and attending Hirschfeld's lectures.[21] In 1930 he also helped arrange for Hirschfeld to visit the United States.[22] In the late 1920s Benjamin met someone he considered his first transvestite patient. Otto Spengler was a German immigrant living in New York City who, at the opening of the twentieth century, had been briefly involved with Hirschfeld's circle of transvestite researchers. In 1906 Spengler had given a lecture on "sexual intermediaries" to the German Scientific Society of New York City, perhaps the first public lecture on a trans subject in the United States.[23] Spengler was also one of the transvestite cases profiled by the sexologist Bernard Talmey in a lecture given to the New York Society of Medical Jurisprudence in 1913, published the following year as an article in the *New York Medical Journal* and also in his 1919 medical manual, *Love: A Treatise on the Science of Sex-Attraction*, which contained five case studies of Talmey's transvestite patients.[24]

Talmey did not do much other than observe, describe, and try to theorize the potential meaning of transvestism. He did not discourage his patients from dressing and living as women or men, but neither did he offer much concrete medical support. When Spengler became Benjamin's patient in the late 1920s, they began to collaborate on experiments with hormonal transition and feminization. Benjamin prescribed the earliest version of an estrogenic compound, as well as x-ray treatments to sterilize the testicles and, it was hoped, deactivate their endocrine activities. Spengler explained the treatment in a letter as aimed "not so much [at] rejuvenation, but femininization, as belong to the class of Transvestites."[25] When the recipient of that letter forwarded it to Benjamin, annotating, "Is this a man, a woman, or a lunatic?" Benjamin replied somewhat tongue-in-cheek: "Believe it or not, this person is a man, a woman and somewhat of a lunatic, so you guessed 100% right. To be serious: he is a married man, father of several children but is a transvestit [sic], that is, his passion is to go in women's clothes."[26] Despite the humorous tone, Benjamin's characterization of Spengler as at once a man, a woman, and "somewhat of a lunatic" points to how much the first two categories were not mutually exclusive when the third was present. In the 1930s Benjamin also worked to arrange funding for research into the isolation of "male" hormones, advancing the path toward the synthesis of testosterone for clinical experimentation.[27]

As he built a career as a practical bridge between German sexology and American endocrine medicine, Benjamin was also actively involved with eugenics research and institutions. More precisely, the endeavors overlapped. In the mid-1930s Paul Popenoe, the secretary of the Human Betterment Foundation, began corresponding with Benjamin to inquire about the physiological effects of the "Steinach procedure" and the hormonal theory of sexual and racial rejuvenation.[28] Benjamin also struck up a relationship with the decorated biologist Oscar Riddle. Based out of the Cold Spring Harbor eugenics laboratory on Long Island, New York, Riddle is remembered best for his work on the pituitary gland. The eugenic context of his research has been less appreciated, despite his long-term residence at the premier American eugenics research institution. Riddle undertook decades of "sex change" studies on pigeons and other birds at Cold Spring Harbor, speculating on how the endocrine system's plasticity could be scientifically manipulated to predictably alter the racial phenotype of a species.[29]

Benjamin had met Riddle in Berlin in 1926 while both were presenting at a conference. A few years later he wrote to Riddle after reading an article of his in the *Journal of the American Medical Association*. Benjamin expressed interest in translating Riddle's relatively abstract sex change experiments on birds into medical therapy for humans. "You know of my interest in Steinach's researches and—being a practicing physician—in their practical application to men," he explained. "You speak in your article at some length of the importance of these experiments that proved the reversibility of sex." Benjamin goes on to make a rather petty point—that Riddle unfairly did not cite Steinach's animal experiments in his article.[30] Riddle was gracious in accepting the criticism but pointed out the advance of his work over Steinach's. "But now note carefully that from my standpoint, and that of the biologist generally," as he put it, that "*sex reversal* is demonstrated only by a forced developmental reversal of testis into ovary, or reverse. Of course Steinach's beautiful studies do not even touch this point. His results showed the reversal of secondary sexual characteristics."[31] Riddle claimed to be able to induce sex change in the actual gonads of animals, rather that the "secondary" morphology of sex influenced only later by hormone circulation. Whether there was a viable way to translate this method into a process for changing human sex, however, was unclear. Benjamin invited Riddle, in 1931, to join his newly formed Medical Society for Sexual Sciences, which he explained would consist of a "Research Committee," a "Committee for Medicine and Therapy (dealing in the fields of urology, endocrinology, psychoanalysts, etc.)," and a "Sociological Committee (dealing with such problems as birth control, eugenics, sex education, etc.)."[32] The invitation was refused, as Riddle felt "I am not myself a medical man," reflecting the American norm of maintaining a gap between the life sciences and the practice of medicine.[33] While the two never collaborated more closely, they still found themselves in dialogue, often at the same conferences.[34]

Benjamin's career is an important backdrop to the early twentieth century because it took shape at an atypical convergence of intellectual and research traditions: German sexology, experimental sex change research in animals, early endocrine therapies in humans, the eugenics movement, and work with the transvestite community. By traveling to Europe nearly every year between the two World Wars, Benjamin imported a great deal of speculative thinking about the plasticity of sex and the viability of changing sex in humans to the United States. He also helped to import the European racialization of plasticity as the eugenic alterability of sex as phenotype from colleagues like Steinach and Kammerer. This latter point seemed to get the most traction with American eugenicists, who during the 1920s and 1930s were very interested in the potential medical applications of research on sex in the biological sciences.[35] Ultimately, Benjamin's work during these decades was not widely diffused. Other than Spengler, and unlike his colleague Talmey, he did not see other transvestite patients, nor did he succeed in widely popularizing Hirschfeld's, much less Steinach's, work. These decades would prove germane only later, at the end of the 1940s, when Kinsey introduced Benjamin to a young trans girl in San Francisco who, with the support of her mother, was looking for access to sex reassignment surgery.[36]

The reason for turning to Benjamin first in this chapter is to underline a deferred continuity from the era before transsexuality to the postwar era. The early twentieth-century theory of the plasticity of sex, its eugenic racialization as alterable phenotype, and the German category "transvestism" were all preserved and carried forward into the category "transsexuality" by Benjamin, who, extremely long lived, continued to practice medicine until 1979. The emergence of transsexuality in the midcentury was not the result of a major paradigm shift or a technical advance in medicine but actually took up multiple, competing early twentieth-century concepts, dressing them in new terminology without being able to extinguish their internal tensions. Benjamin will return in the chapters of this book that look at the 1950s through the 1970s. While his attempts to merge animal experiments and human medicine found limited success in this era, experimental research on children at the Johns Hopkins Hospital *did* translate the abstract plasticity of sex from experiments in endocrinology into clinical medical technique—yet, strangely enough, at first *without* hormones.

Sex Reassignment without Hormones

The earliest cases of hermaphroditism seen at the Brady Urological Institute of the Johns Hopkins Hospital established the basic protocol, followed for the next four decades, for producing a binary sex out of the intersex body. Hugh Hampton Young, the surgeon in charge of the Institute, always began with a head-to-toe physical exam, recording in great detail the appearance of the entire body and vital organs, with emphasis on the appearance of the genitals. Through external and internal palpitation he attempted to ascertain the existence and position of any gonads, glands, and organs governing sex, including a phallus/clitoris, testes and/or ovaries, a prostate, uterus and fallopian tubes, and/or vagina. The physical exam was usually followed by a cystoscopy, during which an instrument was introduced inside the front of the bladder to illuminate it and search for a vaginal cavity.[37] Frequently an x-ray would follow in an attempt to picture the rest of the inside of the abdomen. These initial procedures to map the external and internal sexual anatomy of the body were typically followed by an exploratory laparotomy. The rationale for this surgery was that it represented more or less cutting open the abdomen to look inside for a truth to sex. Young began his tenure at the Institute in a gonadocentric paradigm according to which the presence of a testis or ovary was interpreted as the arbiter of a "true" sex, regardless of the rest of the body or the patient's sense of self. This scopic regime of surgical technique produced a truth by looking inside the body, and biopsied microanalysis of gonadal tissue was given great weight in Young's advice for sex reassignment.

The Institute opened its doors in 1915. As Hopkins rapidly expanded in the early twentieth century, it was an integral part of the hospital's modernizing program for clinical research, experimental practice, and the training of medical professionals.[38] Young helmed the Institute in an attempt to standardize the field of urology in the United States. It was responsible for popularizing new techniques for picturing the inside of the body, such as the cystoscope, and for surgically altering internal and external anatomy under increasingly controlled and sanitary conditions.[39] It also reflected the prevailing ethos of Hopkins as a medical institution that, as much as it was run on an ostensibly "charitable" mission to serve the poor, expected in return total access to those bodies, particularly those of the local African American population in East Baltimore. Research at Hopkins was as often coercive and nontherapeutic as it was curative, and from the facility's opening rumors spread through the black community in Baltimore that warned of the danger of "night doctors" and other medical men who would rob graves, kidnap people off the street, and treat black patients as disposable experimental objects rather than as persons.[40]

The Institute's eight floors were divided equally between wards for patients and a set of laboratories—"clinical, pathological, chemical, bacteriological, physical and experimental surgical."[41] A machine shop on-site provided the ability to design and build new diagnostic and surgical instruments as needed for experimental procedures.[42] A basement wing housed labs for experiments on animals.[43] As a urological surgeon, Young directed the Institute to conduct clinical research, train medical students, and undertake experimental medicine on a massive range of conditions involving the urological anatomy.[44] His work with the kidneys, prostate, adrenals, gonads, bladder, and genitals became the most well known. The Institute's capacious understanding of internal medicine also meant that it saw many women, not just men, as patients. Children were also frequent patients, especially for conditions involving sex, despite the existence of the pediatric Harriet Lane Home at Hopkins. In fact, the Institute was the primary place that intersex children were admitted from the 1910s to the 1930s because during these decades the Harriet Lane Home had neither an endocrine nor a psychiatric ward. In the 1920s only two children at Harriet Lane were diagnosed with hermaphroditism—and both ended up being sent to the Brady Institute for consultation with Young—while in the 1930s there were a mere four. The advent of synthetic hormones and the hiring of Lawson Wilkins to head pediatric endocrine research in the mid-1930s eventually shifted admissions. In the 1940s the number of hermaphroditism admissions at Harriet Lane jumped fivefold. And in the 1950s the number admitted soared to 150.[45] The difference has to do with the dominant medical techniques for altering sex in these two moments. Young employed a surgical, urological model, while Wilkins preferred hormone therapies, to be followed by surgery as a supplement. There was also sporadic involvement with Leo Kanner, the canonized child psychiatrist who reshaped much of his field in the United States from his position in the Harriet Lane Home. This chapter focuses on the era without widely available, synthetic hormones, from roughly 1915 through 1940, while the next chapter examines Wilkins's hormonal work in detail.

Young was not well versed in endocrinology, relying on colleagues for advice.[46] Yet from its opening the Brady Institute began to see so-called hermaphrodites among its patients, making the endocrine system an important part of its clinical work.[47] From 1915 to the 1950s the Brady Institute recorded 139 admissions for hermaphroditism.[48] Some admissions overlapped with the Harriet Lane Home, so the total number of intersex patients at Hopkins is somewhat unclear, although it numbered in the hundreds. The vast majority were children. Young was not especially interested in providing a theoretical explanation of hermaphroditism. His focus was the medical production of binary sex. And while hermaphroditism and sex were only two areas that the Institute's work covered, intersex bodies seemed to hold a particular fascination for him and his colleagues. This extended to making some patients submit to motion picture filming of their bodies, a rarity usually reserved for operations. "We have now numerous motion pictures in color of those patients who come in female dress, are discovered to be males, and undergo operations to transform their status so that they finally leave in masculine attire," Young wrote in 1940, with typical condescension. "Some of these 'strip-teases' are most amusing."[49]

Prior to the 1930s, at a time when synthetic hormones did not exist, Young practiced a certain flexibility with sex reassignment after laparotomy, unable to influence the plasticity of intersex children's bodies to a great extent. Particularly when patients were very young children, he often followed a sort of "wait-and-see" policy, letting them grow into puberty.[50] At that time Young would try to follow the lead of the patient's body, so to speak, suggesting plastic operations that conformed to whatever sex seemed to him to have become "dominant." This was hardly a concession to the autonomy of the patient. Young's was a highly developmental reading of childhood plasticity, and he intensely aestheticized the morphology of the body to match idealizations of masculinity and femininity. He developed a series of surgeries to straighten out and lengthen hypospadiac penises, as well as to amputate the vagina, in patients assigned as male, while standardizing clitoral amputation and vaginoplastic procedures for patients assigned as female.[51] As the historian Alison Redick argues, Young also felt perfectly justified in contradicting the "dominant" sex of children if their romantic and sexual desires might turn out to be homosexual. Sex reassignment was in many cases an attempt to medically produce and enforce heterosexuality.[52]

One of the Institute's very first patients in 1915 was a child named Robert Stonestreet, who was diagnosed with hermaphroditism. Because his life was made a spectacle in the press years later, Stonestreet's name is a matter of public record. For that same reason, however, twenty-first-century federal privacy regulations governing health records also prevent disclosure of the contents of his original medical file. I can draw only on information already published to narrate his time spent at Hopkins, despite the existence of unredacted information in his medical records that might undermine Young's and his colleagues' published account.[53] Still, even with that limitation, Stonestreet's life illustrates the way that the Brady Institute's founding protocols for sex reassignment translated the laboratory isolation of sex's plasticity in animal life into practical medical technique. Where researchers like Riddle had found methods of altering the endocrine system in juvenile animals, effecting changes in their racial phenotype, Young began to assemble a set of techniques that could attempt the same in children's plastic bodies.

In his memoir Young describes a "case that did not end happily" to introduce Stonestreet. As Young remembers it: "A 'boy' was brought to us years ago for operation on account of a genital defect. Dr. William Quinby... discovered that the patient was a girl, and advised the father to allow him to carry out operations to make his child normal."[54] Quinby, a surgeon at the Institute, eventually published an article on the case in the *Bulletin of the Johns Hopkins Hospital*.[55] Like Young, Quinby was most interested in the possibility that overactivity of the adrenal glands from fetal life on had resulted in the masculinization of Stonestreet's body, leading to his assignment as male at birth despite his having "female" gonads. Stonestreet had been raised without question as a boy for ten years and unambiguously understood himself to be a boy. Indeed, when the Stonestreets brought their child to the Institute, the reason was "hypospadias [a condition in which the tip of the penis is located on its underside] and undescended testicles," not hesitation over his sex (50).

Young and Quinby undertook an external and internal physical exam, followed by radiographs, a urine test to establish kidney function, a syphilis test, a blood pressure check, and a blood count (51). Suspecting that the adrenal glands were involved, they also administered pharmacodynamic tests, injecting Stonestreet with different doses of adrenaline and measuring the reaction in his blood pressure (51). Finding nothing out of the ordinary, aside from the appearance of the genitals, they moved on to an exploratory laparotomy. Finding "an infantile uterus with tubes and ovaries of normal appearance," Young and Quinby were faced with a contradiction (52). According to the gonadocentric paradigm, the presence of ovaries would trigger a diagnosis of "female pseudohermaphroditism" and sex reassignment as a girl. "The sex of an individual must always be determined by the nature of the gonads, regardless of the presence of abnormalities either of other parts of the genital system or the secondary sexual manifestations of the body as a whole," Quinby explained in his *Bulletin* article (52). "Consequently," he argued, "this patient is of the female sex; and this is in spite of so many secondary sexual characteristics of the opposite, male sex" (52). Yet the masculine forms of evidence were numerous, including "voice, the hair on the face," "the general bodily habitus," and "the mental processes" (52). In every way, biologically and psychologically,

Stonestreet appeared, felt, and expressed himself as a boy. His life seemed to openly defy the gonadocentric paradigm.

Despite Quinby's confident assertion of the meaning of Stonestreet's ovaries, it is evident even in his published account that the gonadocentric paradigm had to be ignored in clinical practice, for too many intersex children exceeded its narrow definition of "true" binary sex. Quinby therefore had to look elsewhere and turned to endocrinology. The rest of his article attempts to translate that field's thesis on the plasticity of sex into urological practice:

> There has been of late years a rapidly increasing amount of evidence, both experimental and clinical, tending to show that the proper development of those attributes which constitute the *sexe-ensemble* is dependent on normal activity of the endocrine system. Though it is to be doubted that internal secretory processes play any rôle in the primary determination of the sex of the gonad itself, it is certain that such processes are responsible for the normal progress of events from a very early age. The present teaching is well stated by Barker when he says: "We are simultaneously, in a sense, the beneficiaries and the victims of the chemical correlations of our endocrine organs." (52–53, emphasis in original)

This is one of the earliest attempts to translate abstract endocrine research on the plasticity of sex in animals into a practical framework for human medicine. Quinby's bibliographic citations in this paragraph are to works by German and French endocrinologists. His reference to hormonal "processes" that "are responsible *for the normal progress of events from a very early age*" indexes his adoption from them of the abstract metaphor of child development. A child's growth, defined as the developmental trajectory that unfolds from the fetal stages through puberty, was understood to be the material axis through which sex incrementally achieved a recognizable bodily form—in other words, became a phenotype—out of an originally plastic potential for either sex. The ideal itinerary of the child was from plasticity (mixed sex) to a single-sexed form, and the economy of internal secretions functioned to regulate that process in controlled stages. If most children were binary "beneficiaries" of these various "chemical correlations" during development, then, according to Quinby, Stonestreet was one of "the victims" for whom growth had gone astray somehow. The plasticity of his sex had become receptive to a form that strayed from the normative developmental path; it had formed into a body that was masculine despite having "female" gonads.

If the ovaries alone were not the guarantors of femininity, Quinby suspected it was Stonestreet's adrenal glands that had intervened at a developmentally sensitive moment to form masculinity out of his body's plastic potential for either sex. "It will be recalled that the adrenal cortex is developed from the Wollfian ridge—that is, from the same rudimentary tissue as the sex-gland" (53), he noted, turning to embryology. "Clinical and pathological evidence demonstrates the remarkable effect that lesions of the adrenal cortex exert on various factors constituting sex," as well as the regulation of "growth, nutrition, and especially the reproductive organs" (53). The adrenal-gonad relation was evidence of the way that sex and general development were intimately bound together, mixed in the timeline of a child's growth from plasticity into form. The functioning of the adrenals therefore could have produced developmental effects in Stonestreet's plasticity, altering his sex from female to male. Since he was now approaching puberty, the developmental imperative to intervene had only grown stronger: the window for medically altering his plasticity was closing.

Quinby's attempted translation of endocrine experiments into urological practice did not have the chance to move beyond theory, however. According to Young, when Quinby advised Stonestreet's father "that the patient was a girl," the response was "that he had six girls and that this 'boy,' although only ten, was a valuable worker on the farm. He refused to have another girl added to his family and departed."[56] Young may have invented that explanation to render the refusal of diagnosis irrational, or perhaps it really did happen that way. The Stonestreets might have also recognized their child's self-identity as a boy as real, choosing to reject the medical model. Either way, they left Baltimore, although not before nude photographs were made of Robert's body for Young's and Quinby's research. In one of the photos, the ten-year-old's expression is painfully agitated as he tries to cover his chest with his hands, as if to resist being made an object and spectacle by the doctor and the camera's gaze. In a second photo the doctors have forced him to put his hands at his side, exposing his entire body. Quinby published the photos in his *Bulletin* article, without comment.[57]

Twenty-one years later, Stonestreet returned to the Brady Institute. Now in his thirties, he had lived his whole life as a man and was engaged to marry a woman. Their priest, however, had refused to perform the ceremony because Stonestreet's father had told him about the childhood hermaphroditism diagnosis. Stonestreet now demanded that Young provide medical proof that he was a man, not a woman. "After a careful study I had to tell 'him,'" Young claims, "that no mistake had been made. The two left in tears."[58] Three days later Young was summoned to the Institute. He found Robert there, on his deathbed. An autopsy found that he had committed suicide by taking a lethal dose of mercury. Young took advantage of his death to verify his theory of adrenal hyperplasia during the autopsy. A few years later he published photographs of Stonestreet's autopsied adrenal glands in his memoir.[59]

Ending in suicide, Stonestreet's experience testifies to the violent and often traumatic effects of medicalizing intersex children as living laboratories of plasticity. Even in circumstances where no medical sex reassignment took place, the obsessive production of binary sex frequently went against the personal feelings, lived experience, or family wishes of those subject to research in exchange for medical care. The protocol for determining and reassigning sex fundamentally relied on the plasticity of children's bodies for its biological footing, even as it simultaneously disqualified their autonomy and self-knowledge as lacking scientificity. It is not surprising, then, that patients and families were frequently critical of Young's advice or refused to comply with his recommendations.[60] Other times the costs of medical treatments were prohibitive, leading families to leave before surgery could be performed or unable to pay when bills arrived.[61] Intersex children were also seen for years on end without closure, often because plastic surgery operations fell short of Young's aesthetic and functional ideals, leading to painful complications like incontinence and the development of fistulae. Young also insisted that children return to the Institute annually for a physical exam in order to contribute to his research program. If that was not possible he would sometimes correspond with their family physician for updates.[62]

When Young's diagnosis went contrary to a child's self-identity or how the child had been raised, the labor of forcibly resocializing the child and parents was often tortured. The Social Work Department at Hopkins might get involved, as well local children's aid societies or religious charities, trying to strictly govern how families announced the "new" sex of their child and paying visits to their home to ensure compliance with the doctor's orders. These organizations also kept records on the bullying, ostracism, and trauma faced by some of these children at school.[63] Social workers and charity workers spoke condescendingly of any resistance to the medical model from children, their family members, or the community—especially when it came from black residents of Baltimore. In many instances black families and their communities in Baltimore were evidently quite accepting of intersex children, to the point of being skeptical of the need to accept a medical decision and binary sex. In response, physicians and social workers tried to disqualify their beliefs as unscientific or irrational.[64] And in the detached language of case files there was little room for children to speak in their own voice. Every so often a chilling, indirect vignette appears, as in the case of a child who had been reassigned to a sex that contradicted their[65] sense of self and who was referred to an ophthalmologist. The ophthalmologist found nothing wrong with their eyes and was puzzled. The recorded complaint from the Brady Institute staff was that this child's "eyes tear" constantly.[66] Apparently the doctors could not even imagine that constant crying might have been a traumatic effect of their aggressive medical protocol.

As Young saw more and more cases of intersex children whose adrenal glands, in particular, had caused them to "change sex" from female to male, his decision on whether to pursue sex reassignment began to crystallize not around gonads but around age. Young began to attempt to reverse the masculinization of adrenal hyperplasia in *younger* children. The surgical procedure he developed involved an invasive entrance through the back to expose the adrenal glands. Using a clamp tool he had designed, Young was able to hold open the back cavity and access both glands during long surgeries. In patients with hyperplasia the adrenals grew massively large, often to more than a dozen times their typical size. At first Young excised a portion of each adrenal, trying to return each of them to a normal size. Later he found it safer for the patient to instead remove one adrenal entirely and leave the other.[67] The procedure yielded tepid "success." Although the removal of one of the overactive glands would result in a major decrease in the amount of adrenal androgens in the bloodstream that led to masculinization, Young had to admit that this did not seem to necessarily stop, let alone reverse, childhood growth into masculinity. What's more, the surgery was risky, involving a difficult recovery that killed some children.[68] Having performed a number of adrenalectomies in the 1920s and 1930s without being able to definitively "change" the sex of his intersex patients from male to female, Young was able only to effectively alter the appearance of the genitals. The intersex plasticity of the children at the Institute flatly refused to yield any more of its autonomy.

In the mid-1930s a toddler who had been assigned female at birth was brought to Baltimore from Pennsylvania for a second opinion on their genitalia. Young felt that at this age the infant's body was too small for a proper cystoscopy. He recommended waiting for the child to grow a few more years before continuing. "Until we know definitely the condition of the ovaries," he specified, "I think no treatment is indicated. Should later examination show fairly normal ovaries present, operation to remove the enlarged clitoris and bring down the vagina to its proper position would be indicated.... My recommendation is to do nothing at present, and to encourage the parents to understand the situation is not serious and that it can be corrected at a proper time."[69] Two years later the family returned, and Young felt he was observing "a very unusually developed child. The phallus," in particular, "is larger than before." Still, he felt this child was too small for a safe laparotomy and asked the parents to return again in another year. James Howard, who consulted with Young, suspected that "this patient is one of adrenal hyperplasia and not a male." At the end of the 1930s, the laparotomy and plastic surgeries were finally carried out. Young amputated the clitoris/phallus and performed a vaginoplasty. He felt the operation was a "perfect" success, following exactly the model for sex reassignment as female outlined in his recently published textbook, *Genital Abnormalities, Hermaphroditism, and Related Adrenal Diseases*.[70] Two years later the family returned so that Young could make a definitive diagnosis of adrenal hyperplasia. This involved his bilateral exploratory surgery procedure. When he found two very large adrenals as predicted, he removed one. The recovery from surgery was extremely difficult. The child was constantly sick, and the wounds became infected.[71]

Why did Young decide to put this child through the severe process of bilateral adrenal surgery, when in other cases he simply left the adrenals alone? While it was true that the presence of ovaries and a uterus found during laparotomy were a factor, this had not been enough in many other cases, including Stonestreet's. Young could have removed the ovaries and the uterus and performed a plastic surgery to lengthen and straighten the phallus into a penis. Instead, he decided to amputate it and undertake a vaginoplasty. What made the difference? This child was very young, under ten at the time of the adrenalectomy. This meant that the masculinization caused by the adrenals had not yet solidified during puberty. There remained a developmental window of opportunity to intervene in their plasticity and attempt to direct their phenotype toward a feminine form.

At least, that was Young's theory. Translating the alterability of plasticity from the abstract realm of endocrinology into an actual child's body proved quite difficult. The adrenalectomy alone, he knew, would not be enough to make the child's body normatively feminine. Even with plastic surgeries on the genitals, by the time puberty arrived the body would undergo an intense masculinization. A few months after the surgery, then, Young had this child return for a follow-up and to consider a prescription for stilbestrol, a new synthetic estrogen. A six-week trial of daily doses, Young hoped, would "encourage breast development, enlargement of the internal genitalia and may decrease masculinity. It is also intended to depress the activity of the adrenal cortex." The patient's family doctor in New Jersey, where the family now lived, administered the hormones.[72]

Stilbestrol was an extremely new hormone. It had not yet even received FDA approval, and it took some doing to get access to it from a lab in New Jersey. After six weeks had elapsed, Young and the family doctor decided to continue with the therapy. A few months later the doctor reported that there had been some visibly feminine development, but not much. Young recommended keeping the child on the hormone for the rest of their childhood. Even though this would induce an early puberty, he felt it was better to preempt the inevitable masculine puberty caused by adrenal hyperplasia. The effects of this speculative therapy on the child's plasticity were, however, unpredictable. Severe back acne, as well as rapid growth of breasts, led to harsh criticism from their mother, who wrote to Young to complain. He then decided to stop the stilbestrol and try another newly synthesized hormone, lutecylol, which he thought might "suppress the production of adrenal androgens by inhibiting the pituitary hormone." When it did nothing at all, he abandoned the idea. Toward the end of the 1940s, as urine analyses were developed, it became possible to verify the precise degree of overactivity of the adrenals. By now, all of Young's attempts at sex reassignment had been resisted by this child's actual growth. He wrote to the patient's mother and suggested the family see Lawson Wilkins, the new head of pediatric endocrinology at the Harriet Lane Home. As the next chapter explores, this shift in clinics represented a broader movement toward a hormonal paradigm that sharply redefined Young's role in altering children's sex. Although Young had adapted an endocrine perspective and had translated it into a basic model for surgically altering children's sex according to the relative plasticity of age, his approach was met with a great deal of resistance in the body to binary sex.[73]

Young's protocol banked on a naturally available plasticity in the growing body that would induce phenotypic changes during childhood growth. Yet sex was not given by plasticity—it had to be grown. If it was plastic, then there were no guarantees that the originally mixed character of an embryo or infant would inevitably reach a binary form. This instability was precisely what drew researchers to experiments on intersex bodies in the first place, for in displacing the gonadocentric paradigm they cast serious doubt on whether humans were really sexually dimorphic, even as medicine promised to capitalize on their plasticity to produce a binary. To resolve this instability, the plasticity of sex was coded in this clinical research as an abstracted form of whiteness, a latent capacity to be reformed and transformed into something new. That most of Young's intersex patients were white indexes how the "abnormal" body of a child diagnosed with hermaphroditism could be made valuable through its plasticity, the promise of alteration and normalization through medical intervention. That the few black intersex children and families who spent time at the Institute were regarded by its staff as more "difficult," combative, irrational, and ultimately disposable points to the racialization of plasticity in this era. Young saw an abstract sense of alterability in white children, while he projected a fungibility onto black children that has a genealogy in American medicine stretching back to slavery.[74] As was the case more broadly at Hopkins, doctors like Young regarded black children as suitable experimental subjects because of presumed access and disposability, whereas white children who were subject to similar procedures were framed as exhibiting the potential for a normative cure or at least improved normality.

The movement in these decades from research on sex in animals to practicing on humans was also highly charged with racial significance. In a 1935 letter to Young about a black child diagnosed with hermaphroditism, Edwards A. Park, the head of the Harriet Lane Home, enclosed two scientific articles about sex and evolution, which were meant to help Young with a paper he was writing. Park explained that "one contains a complete review of the subject in different forms of life, [while] the other discusses the basis of hermaphrodism in animals. From the picture [of the patient] I judge that *the condition which you found in the little colored girl has been duplicated in mammals.*"[75] Park analogizes intersex embodiment in this black child to a form of primitive animality, imagining an evolutionary regression through a supposed visual equivalence between the black intersex body and the sexed bodies of nonhuman mammals. He also sees in this black human body an equivalent to a laboratory experiment on animal sex. Where the plasticity of white children's intersex bodies, in spite of being abnormal, was nevertheless valuable for its biological potentiality that medicine could cultivate, black children's sexed plasticity was framed as atavistic. This differential between the abstract whiteness of plasticity and the visual regimes of race and antiblackness that inflected the clinical treatment of actual children is a central feature of the modern medicalization of sex, one whose change over time this book follows across the rest of its chapters.

As Hopkins became the principal American hospital for experiments on intersex children, by the 1930s it had to deal with the fact that word was spreading that Young could change a person's sex. Soon, the first recognizably trans patients came to the Institute.

Sexual Inversion and the First Trans Patients at Hopkins

From the 1910s to the 1940s, a messy set of ambiguous diagnoses that included "sexual perversion," "sexual inversion," and "homosexuality" was applied to a wide range of patients at the Brady Institute for reasons that included sexual impotence in heterosexual men, lesbian and gay feelings, accusations of homosexuality, masturbation, and concerns about individuals we can read as trans. The Harriet Lane Home, by contrast, did not use any of these categories, so there is no particularly visible evidence that children who came through its doors might have wished, like Val, to live as a sex different from the one assigned at birth. Looking globally at the hundreds of cases of children diagnosed with hermaphroditism at Hopkins during the first half of the twentieth century, it seems unlikely that any of them invite a strong trans reading. This is not to say that there is no relation between the categories intersex and trans. On the contrary, for many trans people the idea of overlap was central to their requests for transition and surgery. Until well into the 1950s and 1960s, many publicly trans figures in the United States and Europe used the language of intersex or endocrine "abnormality" to legitimize their transitions in the public eye as a question of medicine "repairing" mistakes made by nature.[76] Despite that, physicians at Hopkins demonstrated a strong gatekeeping impulse to keep anyone lacking visibly abnormal physiology out of the orbit of intersex medicine and especially sex reassignment.

Doctors employed the medical category of homosexuality, not hermaphroditism or transvestism, to frame trans life in a way that could justify rejecting requests for support. This was possible because of the tangled meaning of "sexual inversion," the nineteenth-century sexological progenitor of both homosexuality and transvestism.[77] That being said, the prevailing use of homosexuality at Hopkins is best described as confused. In his 1937 textbook, *Genital Abnormalities*, Young pondered how some of his patients seemed to mix homosexuality and intersex conditions. "Individuals, apparently not otherwise abnormal, occasionally assume the attire, mannerisms and habits of the opposite sex," he admitted. "Some of these cases also become homosexual. The etiology is often obscure and may possibly be due to glandular and endocrine abnormalities as complex as those encountered in hermaphroditism."[78] Young's description of these "individuals" sounds quite a bit like Hirschfeld's definition of transvestism, which blended sexual inversion and a vaguely intersex notion of some unknown "glandular" component.[79] At the Institute, however, Young called upon not sexology but psychiatry to adapt a vaguely Freudian model of inversion for trans people diagnosed as homosexual. Despite this psychological turn, Young's small gesture toward the endocrine system held open the door to an overlap between intersex and trans sex reassignment surgery, a detail that did not go unnoticed by trans people seeking medical support.

The earliest diagnosis of sexual inversion at the Institute was recorded in 1916, for an army officer complaining of "sexual impotence."[80] In the 1920s there were a few scattered diagnoses, but Young's interpretation of them was highly improvised. Endocrine medicine was in an experimental moment defined by organotherapies that used living tissues from nonhuman animals or "normal" human bodies to try to influence the body's plasticity. In that context, although he was by no means an expert, Young came closest to integrating the insights he was generating around the intersex body into the possibility of altering the homosexual and trans body. One of these cases involved a child. In 1922 an important figure in a national rabbinical organization arrived in Baltimore with his teenage son in tow. Delivering him to the Institute, the father reported that his son's problem with masturbation had forced their trip to Hopkins, but Young's recorded diagnosis was "Perversion, homosexual type." Apparently their stay was brief. The father quickly left town on business, and after being evaluated the teenager was sent home to Virginia without any treatment.[81]

Not long afterward Young received a letter from a hospital superintendent in Virginia who was very close to the family. Apparently the superintendent had also been the one who referred them to Young. "Possibly

I should have sent you the boy's history before he came to see you," he explains in this letter, for "upon his return to the city . . . [the father] told me the only report you made was that the boy could get married, from which I judge you meant that he was free of Syphilis or Gonorrhoea." The superintendent was convinced "that you do not know the exact state of affairs. It is quite probable that the boy did not tell you the whole truth and that you were mislead [sic] in the real object of my sending him to you. The boy's history is as follows." According to the superintendent, about a month after the family sent their teenage child to a religious school in Ohio, the parents received a telegram informing them that he had been expelled. "The Doctor [father] telephoned the head of the college and asked the reason for the telegram. The answer came 'a very serious charge and he would not be permitted to return.'"[82]

Since the father was stuck on business in the Southwest at the time, the superintendent traveled to Ohio in his place to investigate, finding "a most distressing state of affairs." "To save himself from the reformatory (being under twenty one) I learned that he had to leave the city at once, by request of the mother of a boy whom he had assaulted." The superintendent did not shy away from spelling out the content of that "assault." Apparently the teenager had "told the mother [of his schoolmate] that he was homo-sexual. He told the president of the college that it was a disease with him and that his father knew it, which was, of course, untrue." What's more, he went on, "Since returning to the city, I have been told that this frightful practice had been going on before he left [Virginia]" and "these facts lead me to believe that mentally he is a pathological type, possibility inheriting some glandular deficiency." Yet the superintendent also added that "the boy is not the type that you would think homo-sexual, as he is fond of out-door sports, likes to be in the company of nice boys and girls and is won-derfully kind to his invalid mother. He possesses a very lovable personality withal."[83]

While I find this episode interesting on its own terms as part of the his-tory of queer sexuality, I am not arguing for reading this child as trans. Rather, the important detail is Young's reaction to the letter. After thank-ing the superintendent for "putt[ing] an entirely different light on the case" and agreeing that "the problem [is] much more serious and difficult" than originally thought, he conceded, "I hardly know what to suggest. If his homo-sexual desires should continue *it might be well to try transplanta-tion of the testes from some normal individual* who might die as a result of an accident. In a recent case we obtained testes from a man who was hung in our penitentiary, and the transformation of the individual was remarkable."[84] Young was exaggerating the "remarkable" effects of testicular transplant. Nevertheless, he was following the lead of other medical researchers in the 1920s, using incarcerated bodies for organotherapy experiments. Young hoped that replacement of supposedly "abnormal" testicles with "normal" ones—although it is not clear why Young considered a criminal sentenced to death "normal"—would result in a more virile, masculine endocrine system. Young did not end up pursuing this idea with the teenager from Virginia, but the fact that he could imagine hormonal organotherapy for cases of sexual inversion illustrates how the experimental environment of the 1920s harbored a short-lived mixing of intersex and inversion models. While the teenager from Virginia reads as gay, not trans, the categorical overlap between homosexuality and trans life in the early twentieth century makes this case an important reference for Young's later trans patients, who took note of such possibilities.

Organotherapy quickly fell out of fashion. Once synthetic hormones became available, on the rare occasion that Young did prescribe hormones to patients diagnosed with sexual inversion it was only to encourage a gender-normative, heterosexual effect. When testosterone therapy failed to do so, as it inevitably did, Young referred patients to Thomas Rennie, a resident psychiatrist at the Hopkins Phipps Clinic, who had similarly little success.[85] As improvised attempts to hormonally treat inversion failed, Rennie's psychiatric model became the dominant lens through which the Brady Institute framed inversion. By the mid-1930s the psychological perspective seems to have totally won out over endocrine experiments. For instance, when Young and his colleague John Howard saw a gay man in his early twenties from Washington, D.C., in 1936, Howard expressed a confident consensus. "My impression is that so far as endocrine abnormalities of secretion are concerned they probably do not exist," he wrote in his case notes, "and that the disorder is entirely a psychological one. Therefore, it does not seem to me that there would be any benefit from the possible use of androsterone or other endocrine products."[86] This swing in the pendulum over ten years from an organic, endocrine hypothesis to a psychological one, however, brought little efficacy to the clinician's toolkit.

The psychiatric approach was weakest in the face of trans patients who, fluent in the idioms of intersex and endocrine plasticity, sought out Young hoping to undergo sex reassignment, rather than be "cured." In 1938

"Bernard," a textile worker in his late twenties, journeyed from Alabama to Baltimore complaining vaguely of a "congenital malformation." Performing a physical exam on Bernard, who was assigned female at birth but identified as a man, Young recorded an "enlarged phallus" and that he "had sexual relations with one young woman and [his] definite gratification and sexual desires have always been towards the female sex." What's more, "Patient has always been jealous of her [sic] brothers because they are boys.... She feels the phallus is bound down [i.e., hypospadiac, an intersex condition]. She believes she urinates through the phallus.... She has felt definite mass or testicle in right groin. Patient's voice changed at an early age. She shaves once a week and definitely wants to be a man."[87]

Bernard, in other words, was hardly the typical case of "homosexuality," claiming what looked much more like intersex embodiment. When Young consulted his colleague in endocrinology Samuel Vest for a second opinion, however, Vest put a great deal of pressure on Bernard's intersex narrative. "I think the patient is deluding herself concerning the growth of hair," he argued. "Clitoris is of normal size and appearance, as are both labia" he added, questioning Young's evaluation. "No palpable masses in inguinal area. Urethral and vaginal orifices normal." While Bernard had presented himself using a legibly intersex narrative, implying that he might have been mistakenly assigned as female at birth and apparently convincing Young, Vest felt this was some kind of front. "I believe this case is entirely mental, & homosexual," he concluded. "She has a very typical mannish haircut, wears a stiff, man's shirt, with tie, etc."[88]

Vest was probably not aware of the details of how Bernard found his way to Baltimore. Young had received a letter from him "concerning what is to me, a most vital subject. I have been reading recently of sex-changing operations such as the Mark Weston[89] case in England and others. I wrote to Dr. David H. Keller, editor of Sexology Magazine and his reply that you were the foremost authority on this subject reached me today." Bernard explained that "I have always liked boyish things such as games, books and clothes. I wear my hair cut short, and tailored clothes all the time. I feel much more at ease in men's clothes than in women's."[90] Putting his main question to Young, he mixed the endocrine language of hermaphroditism, inversion, and the plasticity of sex, rather than a psychological theory of homosexuality:

As I understand it, a person may have secondary sexual organs
which control his mental and emotional life; while the primary

organs are of the opposite sex. What I want to know is can these secondary organs really be developed in such a way that a person who has been known as a female becomes a male? I know that sex books say that no one is really 100% of either sex. If this can be done, I would like to know about what the cost would be and the time required. I have read that most of these operations are yet in the experimental stage, but I am perfectly willing to become a part of the experiment.[91]

To conclude, he clarified: "I hope that this letter does not seem too foolish to you and that you will not regard it as a mere whim. I think that you can understand I need help badly and if it can be attained in this country that you can give it." Young replied by asking him to come to Hopkins for an appointment.[92]

The letter cuts a fascinating line through the web of hermaphroditism, sexual inversion, homosexuality, and transvestism. Presenting himself as intersex, Bernard comes across as well read on the theory of natural bisexuality and expertly deploys it to legitimize sex reassignment. Although it seems that he had no actual endocrine or physiological evidence of being intersex, beyond a phenomenological feeling, he made a strong connection between news reports of "sex-changing operations" happening across the Atlantic and Young's surgical experiments on intersex children at Hopkins. *Sexology Magazine*, like many other popular sources of scientific information on sex in the 1930s, would have been a productive relay point between the trans reading public and institutional medicine, reaching as remote a location as small-town Alabama. Hoping for medical support "in this country," Bernard may have reasoned that using the language of an intersex condition would be the best way to get Young's attention. Hence, his claim to have undergone an organic voice change, to need to shave regularly, and to feel a potential testicle in his abdomen may have been part of a strategy. Or he may have really believed himself to be intersex and felt each of those things about his body to be true. There is no way to be sure. Regardless, the effect is clear: he succeeded in getting Young's attention.

After two physical exams, Young decided to refer Bernard to Rennie. In his report, evidently overwhelmed, Rennie took the opportunity for a long attempt at theorizing, in the absence of a concept of transsexuality or even transvestism, what Bernard's claims about his sex might mean. Using the only frameworks he could muster, Rennie assembled a roughshod

mélange of Freudian psychology and endocrine theories of plasticity, all
the while trying to drive a hard wedge between them and to recuperate
Bernard into the archetype of homosexuality. The resulting document is
a fascinating look into the confounded state American medicine had created for itself. Given the stubborn resistance of psychiatrists and physicians to accepting a patient's embodied self-knowledge as meaningful,
Rennie could only attempt to aggressively theorize his way through Bernard's life.[93]

Rennie began by characterizing Bernard in terms that read as legibly
trans, rather than lesbian, and by adding an important detail to his biography. Bernard "has come to Johns Hopkins because she [sic] feels that
she is really a man in spite of her female body build," Rennie explained,
"and because she wishes to have an operation to give her male organs. She
says she must have this done because she has been in love with a young
lady in her home town for the past five years and now wishes to marry her."
In recounting his biography, Rennie noted that Bernard "was of Dutch and
also of native Indian extraction," although he attributed no particular meaning to either. He went on to confirm a long-standing wish to be a boy, one
that stretched back to early childhood. "When she was told as a child that
she could turn into a boy by kissing her elbow," for example, "she remembers doing it hundreds of times." Rennie noted also that he "liked to wear
her younger brother's overalls and trousers as a child as her parents never
objected." Bernard's father was a physician, and he "states with evident plea-
sure that she looks exactly like her father, that she has pictures taken of
herself wearing his clothes and that people are always fooled by these pictures into thinking it is her father." Like his father, Bernard "once hoped
she would be able to study medicine," but it "was not possible." Rennie
corroborated that he "always had the feeling as a little child that she must
have male sex parts somewhere inside and says she often gets the sensation
to this day that she must have a male organ concealed somewhere inside."
In one of the rare moments that he quoted Bernard directly, Rennie wrote:
"'For years,' the patient states, 'I have thought I was the only person in the
world like that and I have only lately heard that there are people with the
same feelings.'"[94]

As for Bernard's explanation of trans embodiment, Rennie reported
that he "feels that she must be a peculiar biological mixture and suggests
that since twins run in her family she might have been intended originally
to have been a pair of mixed twins, but that somehow both sexes have been

combined in her." This was not an entirely idiosyncratic theory. "This feeling is reinforced by some popular scientific readings she indulged in," Rennie explained. He was probably referring to the biologist Frank R. Lillie's paradigm-shattering 1916 study on "free-martin" calves, a condition in which a specific fetal endocrine situation in a cow pregnant with opposite-sex twins causes the female in the pair to masculinize under the circulatory influence of androgens from the male twin.[95] The study had been incredibly consequential in reshaping endocrine theories of the plasticity of sex, for it suggested, much as this patient did about himself, that biological organisms could be female in some ways and yet be masculinized enough to change their sex. Lillie's work was widely read outside professional medicine, and it is easy to imagine Bernard accessing it in Alabama through something like *Sexology Magazine*.[96]

Rennie, of course, did not subscribe in the least to this theory. Yet neither did he make any prescription for trying to "cure" this case of "homosexuality." "Because of the fact that the patient wanted to return home at once and because she was not interested at all in any psychotherapy, but merely in the matter of surgical intervention," he explained that "not much could be undertaken.... It was merely suggested to the patient that in view of her own history there might have been strong psychological influences which led her to wish to be a man." Bernard left for Alabama, never to return to the Brady Institute.[97]

Rennie, however, continued rambling for several more pages in his report to Young, scrambling for an expert opinion. "There are many conflicting theories for the origins of a condition like this," he noted, although he again failed to name what, precisely, that condition was if not textbook homosexuality. "One stresses the constitutional ingrained aspect of the problem; another, the psychogenic origins based on various types of life experience." Reflecting on how "the tendency has been present from earliest life" for Bernard, he wagered that "we are perhaps more justified in speaking of a constitutional type." Rennie was, as a psychiatrist, quite skeptical of endocrine bases for inversion. "As with hormonal status, where we find both male and female sex hormones in every individual, there are those who claim that every person has a homo- and heterosexual component in the make-up," he observed, "and that the difference depends upon the balance of the two components." Unconvinced, Rennie believed that the presence of estrogen and testosterone in varying degrees might correspond instead to the difference between "an active homosexual type" and "a passive, more

feminine type." He added, moreover, that "the homosexual is often immature and infantile looking." Here, inversion was translated into a developmental condition:

> The psychoanalysts sketch the development of mature sexuality as
> follows: the infantile phase is one of curiosity and manipulation,
> essentially hedonistic and self-gratification. There is then a latent
> phase beginning around five or six, extending to the age of 10, 11 or
> 12 (puberty), when the average child shows little or no interest in
> girls. With a pre-pubertal phase, he is strongly homosexual and that
> is the period when young girls get 'crushes' on each other and boys
> gang together having no interest in girls. With adolescence, there
> comes a burst of heterosexual interest and a slow maturing of the
> adult pattern. Homosexuality, therefore, in some case is *the failure
> to develop beyond a certain phase*. . . . Thus it will be seen that in
> early adolescence homosexuality is not so serious and is certainly a
> fairly common casual experience in boys' schools, etc.[98]

Rennie's reliance on a Freudian model that takes the male child as universal reads as sloppy considering that Bernard was raised as a girl. But
the passage executes the key maneuver of making inversion "the failure to
develop beyond a certain phase." Much like the reigning theory of hermaphroditism, it is the plasticity of sexual development that underwrites
both the normal outcome of childhood (heterosexuality) and its abnormal, arrested version (homosexuality). This line of thinking clarifies why
the Harriet Lane Home did not diagnose children with sexual perversion,
inversion, or homosexuality and why Hopkins kept intersex children as
separate as possible from homosexual or trans cases of inversion. If children were *naturally* inverted to some degree during childhood, then there
was little reason to assign them diagnoses like homosexuality that were
understood to be meaningful only insofar as they indicated arrest. Inversion, in other words, was significant only in adults. In children it was not
(yet) pathological. One of the consequences of this developmental model
is that trans children who might have passed through Hopkins would not
have been very visible within the epistemology of inversion.

This expansive review of the medical literature spanning hermaphroditism, inversion, and homosexuality notwithstanding, Rennie ended his
report as deprived of an object as when he began. "In our patient," he

emphasized, "the tendency is fixed and probably unmodifiable." Bernard's
rich account of his self and his biological body dissolved in the hands of
a psychiatrist who could not fit him into the American medical model that
separated intersex life from inverted life. Yet by spending so much time
redirecting an obvious request for sex reassignment and transition into the
psychoanalytic framework of arrested homosexual development, Rennie
produced an effective justification for refusing Bernard's request to change
his sex. Indeed, the deployment of homosexuality in this case and the
practiced ignorance of the staff of Hopkins over the concept of transvestism were powerful forms of gatekeeping. I read this case as evidence of
how American medical science produced for itself an advantageous state
of ignorance. A trans man from small-town Alabama, who had some college education and was employed as a textile worker, produced a far more
sophisticated theory of trans life and the feasibility of transition than anyone at Hopkins wanted to imagine. Bernard's self-taught expertise was,
precisely, the reason for which he was disqualified from the medical support he requested.[99]

During the same period that Bernard visited the Institute, "Karen," a
trans woman in her midthirties, made the trip to Baltimore from Michigan. Young coded her through the category of homosexuality too, noting
that "patient comes for advice and possible correction of his [sic] tendency
to seek satisfaction sexually with members of his own sex, which has been
present for as long as he can remember." Wary of any diagnostic overlap
with hermaphroditism, he added that "to the best of his knowledge he has
no physical deformity sexually but has noticed female fat distribution and
small hands." When Dr. Drew, a Hopkins psychiatrist, was brought in for
a consultation, he likewise paid the most attention to her sexual history,
recording it in great detail. But Drew also recorded that her "real desire is
to have his [sic] external organs altered to match his personality and permit
normal relationships with a loved one." Rather than being a homosexual
man, Karen "classifies himself as a male physically with female passive personality." In Michigan she had owned a small business and later taught music
"but is not doing anything now" in the middle of the Great Depression.[100]

For reasons that are not recorded, Karen left after these initial exams
but returned to the Institute two years later, when John Howard examined
her. In his report Howard notes that she "is quite concerned about the
social and moral stigma of his chief complaint. However, he feels that the
tendency developed 'naturally' in him about 20 years ago and, except for

the worry attached, he has no desire to change his status. He thinks psychiatrists could do him no good. *He came here hoping that Dr. Young could perform an operation on him.*"[101] Howard agreed with her that psychiatric treatment would be irrelevant. "Whether or not alterations of circulating sex hormones are present in homosexual individuals," he continued, "is, so far as I am aware, still an unknown point. We could do determination [*sic*] of male and female sex hormones, if Dr. Young feels this is indicated. It would be a far cry, but, perhaps, worth trying to see how testosterone might influence this patient."[102] Howard's suggestion that they explore hormonal treatment found no audience. As was the case with Bernard, Young ignored the possibility. Karen left Baltimore after her second exam. Considering that her request for surgery was rejected, we can imagine why she did not return.

The Archive of Early Twentieth-Century Trans Childhood

While some trans adults who were well versed in medicine, like Bernard and Karen, personally sought out Young, embodying the overlap between intersex and trans embodiment, physicians and psychiatrists consistently refused to take their requests seriously, pushing them into a model of homosexuality that obviously did not fit. Where does this leave the question that opens this chapter? What case can be made for a distinctly trans early twentieth century, before the category of transsexuality, if we rely on a medical archived limited by the partial perspectives of its categories and our retrospective investments in them? Bernard and Karen, like Alan Hart, had to travel under the medical sign of "homosexuality" but stood apart from its growing psychological framing, grounding their self-account of sex in a plastic narrative that borrowed extensively from the medicalization of intersex children. Each of them had the means to inform themselves about medical models and technique and to seek out leading clinicians in the United States.

    What about trans children from this era? Given that inversion, like intersex conditions, was defined in increasingly developmental terms, it was easy for Young and his colleagues, including Rennie, to imagine that trans life was meaningful only in adults. Children's bodies held a different sort of value to them as indeterminate, unfinished, and plastic, and the line between normative and abnormal growth needed to remain blurry to float their experimental agendas. It seems likely that most children who

understood themselves in terms that we might read as trans did not interact nearly as much as adults with medicine. As in the case of Val, evidence
for trans childhood in the early twentieth century remains mostly implicit
or retrospective.[103]

Although the records of the Brady Institute *do* include the diagnostic
category "transvestism," its use was both belated and brief. John Money
likely brought it with him to Hopkins, where in the early 1950s he took
over research on intersex children. The earliest records date from around
1953 and 1954, but only a mere eight patients were ever given this diagnosis. Overlapping with Christine Jorgensen's media storm and the moment
in which Harry Benjamin published his first articles on "transsexualism,"
these trans men and women were able to get much closer to obtaining
hormones and surgery in the United States than anyone before them. Half
of them continued on in the Hopkins Gender Clinic that Money would go
on to cofound in 1965, but by then the term "transsexuality" and its various
cognates had come into widespread usage, supplanting "transvestism."[104]
A few of them also described their childhoods. By far the oldest was a
retired trans woman from Ohio who was interviewed by John Money in
1954 and who recounted her early childhood in the 1890s. "'When but a few
years old,'" she explained, in order to establish the longevity of her knowledge that she was a woman, "I wanted a doll and doll buggy very much,
and enjoyed it,'" although she had not found the social possibility to live
full time as a woman until her retirement.[105]

In 1959 a trans man in his midthirties contacted the Brady Institute
from his home in New York, wondering "if it would be possible for me
to enter your hospital for a complete medical examination. I have read several times of the work done at this hospital to help persons who appear
to be male or female but feel like a member of the opposite sex." When
he arrived in Baltimore and visited the Institute, the urologist W. W. Scott
recorded the initial confusion of the staff, because this man "had been
accepted for admission to Brady because of a breast abscess and in the
belief there was a problem of hermaphroditism. Actually the patient was
recognized by the admitting doctor as a transvestite." It turned out that the
"breast abscess" was probably a strategic complaint. When the psychologist John Hampson interviewed the man, he noted that he "had hoped
a penis might be fashioned through some miracle of plastic surgery" but
most of all "considered that her [*sic*] emotional burden would be eased if
her large pendulous breasts could be removed. In fantasy, she had come to

Hopkins hoping the breast abscess might provide an acceptable surgical rationale for breast amputation."[106]

Hampson's interview also recorded a partial account of this trans man's childhood in rural New York. In the late 1930s he "left school because of the excruciating sense of embarrassment at being obliged to wear girl's clothes." Scott's case notes add a more complete picture. At age thirteen he dropped out of school but also began working in his family's lumber business "and has dressed as a man since then," without interruption. "Patient's father," the report continues, "was disappointed that she was female, and was always 'proud' that he had a daughter who could 'work so hard.' Patient has dated girls, and several have begun to hint at marriage; at that point, he explains his condition of biological female, but 'feelings' of a man."[107] It seems that this trans man had lived his teenage years in the 1930s and 1940s as a boy, with at least the tacit support of his family, working in a male-dominated profession, and without much difficulty, in a rural town. He did not seek out medicine until much later, in the 1950s, when transsexuality had become a highly visible subject to the American public.

A trans woman in her thirties, referred by a doctor in New York in 1959, told Hopkins plastic surgeon Milton Edgerton of an experience with medicalization during her childhood in the early 1940s. Although she had felt herself to be a girl since a very young age, her family was not very tolerant. "There was some argument on the part of the father and mother," Edgerton surmised. Having dropped out of school at the ninth-grade level, as soon as she turned eighteen she decided to leave home and began living full time as a woman, building a well-paying career as a professional dancer in the Midwest and Northeast. Not long before leaving home, at age seventeen, she had been to see a local doctor in her Missouri town. This doctor apparently "found 'a large portion of circulating female hormone'" and "it was his idea that an exploratory operation should be performed in order to determine whether or not ovarian tissue was present." Presented with this medical opinion, "a good bit of correspondence was carried out with the parents at the time but the operation was not carried out because the patient's father felt the doctor did not know what he was talking about."[108]

These two patients recalled living openly as a trans boy and a trans girl in rural spaces from their teenage years on, in the 1930s and 1940s. In this they share a similarity with Val, whose childhood opened this chapter. They found livable ways to grow up as trans children without needing a sexological category like transvestism or requiring any particular medical discourse to set the terms of their lives. Interestingly, however, both also interacted with intersex discourse to a degree that strongly undermines the gatekeeping logic that doctors at Hopkins tried to impose during those decades. The trans man from New York who had lived publicly as a boy since age thirteen took on the language of the intersex body to seek out top surgery and possibly bottom surgery, while the trans girl in Missouri was framed *by* a doctor through intersex language at seventeen. What these brief pieces of evidence point to is how the trans child and the intersex child traveled together in the early twentieth century. Despite the ostensibly discursive separation of "hermaphroditism" from "sexual inversion," "homosexuality," and "transvestism," in reality there was an informal understanding on the part of trans children, adults, and some doctors that there was reason to see trans life in at least partially intersex terms.

As the thesis of the plasticity of sex migrated from endocrine experiments in animals to medical technique at hospitals and clinics, it knit the fate of intersex and trans children together in a way that became a major point of tension between medical gatekeepers and laypersons. On the one hand, the measurable plasticity of intersex bodies provided proof that it was possible for someone's sense of self to differ entirely from their body's morphology. In a moment where there was no dominant medical explanation for trans life in the United States, "hermaphroditism" offered a compelling source of information on inversion and transvestism to medical professionals and lay people alike. To be clear, then, I am not arguing that trans people in this era were actually intersex or even perceived themselves to be truly intersex. The development of a protocol for altering the plastic sex of intersex infants and children, rather, served as proof to interested trans people that they, too, might change their sex. The growing collision of these concerns from the 1910s to the 1940s led to the situation in which Young and his colleagues tried to keep trans and intersex patients separate in the face of their demands for medical support.

Given this overlapping and ambiguous terrain, what are the stakes of claiming a specifically trans early twentieth century for children? Does the fact that it was intersex children whose bodies were largely medicalized, while trans bodies were intentionally misrecognized as homosexual, not weaken the case? My argument is slightly different and follows the historiographical lead of Emma Heaney's rereading of trans feminine life in the early twentieth century in *The New Woman*.[109] This chapter serves not just to provide sorely needed detail for our understanding of the first four decades of the trans twentieth century but also to undermine any over-reliance on the midcentury parameters of transsexuality to direct histori-ography. The issue is not that the 1950s are not important but that the decade has accrued too much causal force in trans historiography. In *Testo Junkie*, for instance, Paul B. Preciado frames his concept of the "pharmaco-pornographic" mode of biopolitics through an impressive litany of trans-sexuality collected at the end of World War II: "John Money coined the term 'gender'" and "famously affirms that it is possible (using surgical, endocri-nological, and cultural techniques) to 'change the gender of any baby up to 18 months'"; "Harold Gillies was performing the first phalloplastic surger-ies in the UK, including work on Michael Dillon, the first female-to-male-transsexual to have taken testosterone"; "US soldier George W. Jorgensen was transformed into Christine, the first transsexual person discussed widely in the popular press"; and "Harry Benjamin systematized the clinical use of hormone molecules in the treatment of 'sex change' and defined 'trans-sexualism,' a term first introduced in 1954, as a curable condition."[110]

Preciado is right that the Cold War military, scientific, political, and capitalist milieu of state and medical biopolitics resulted in a new diffusion of techniques for making sexuality and the sexed body productive, and to that extent transsexuality was an artifact of that midcentury moment. And this book will turn to that era, too. Yet beginning with World War II and its aftermath overlooks that sex reassignment was practiced long before the concept of gender existed, that phalloplasties were performed by sur-geons like Young before Gillies, that Jorgensen was not the first celebrity trans figure, and that Benjamin's work with trans people actually had begun three decades earlier, in the 1920s. Perhaps more important, framing the twentieth century through the time frame of transsexuality can reinforce an implicit technodeterminism, perhaps most infamously demonstrated in Bernice Hausman's dehumanizing argument in *Changing Sex* that medi-cal discourse somehow *literally* produced trans subjectivity.[111] Although Hausman's work has been roundly critiqued, the underlying problem of drawing on the authority and rationality of the medical archive to narrate the past is not so easily overcome. Writing the history of transsexuality is inherently risky for the ways that it can serve to reinforce that category's colonizing form, rather than undermine it.[112]

A different way to understand both the fragmentary, ephemeral qual-ity of these trans childhoods lived at a great distance from medicine and their overlap with intersex discourses is to insist that trans childhood, or children's transness, has no ontological reliance on medicine at all for definition. The trans child *before* transsexuality, then, offers no grand narrative to supplant a history of transsexuality that begins in the 1950s. Nor should it. Rather, this chapter's archival detail, its long parsing of an entangled field of inversion, hermaphroditism, homosexuality, and transvestism, means to undo the stubborn presumption that modern medicine played a causal role in defining the parameters of trans life. It did not. Trans life evidently preexisted any early twentieth-century medical discourse that could claim to know it. Trans children and adults in this era lived at a fairly wide distance from doctors, but this distance was not a product of a lack of knowledge or language to describe themselves, considering that the archive records a boy living out his teenage years in a lumber mill in New York, a girl in Missouri moving out on her own at eighteen, and a girl attending elementary school in rural Wisconsin. None of these children began living a trans life after encountering medicine. On the contrary, medicine was significantly challenged by its encounters with them. Rather than looking for a "specific" trans childhood in the early twentieth century, then, it is better to say that there were *multiple* trans childhoods in play in this era, that the definition of transness characterizing children takes a range of differing and competing forms, without any discursive resolution. While this may feel like shaky ground to stand on historiographically or even a dilution of the meaning of transness, those feelings are actually retrospective ideological effects of the medical model of transsexuality, which has worked so hard to confine trans life to a singular, binary-driven definition. Our inability to grasp exactly what the trans childhood of a teenage boy in New York, a teenage girl in Missouri, or a young girl in rural Wisconsin might be distilled into is not an epistemological problem if we recognize that there is an opacity to transness in its multiple and, especially, non-medical forms. It becomes a problem only when trans historiography concedes to a limiting medical model that was not even in play in this era.

When trans children did interact with doctors prior to the 1950s, their embodied plasticity was hardly domesticated by the medical model. Instead, the informal mixing of intersex and inversion models in their lived experience threatened to disrupt the very architecture of the sex binary. If all children were naturally intersex or inverted to a certain degree, as doctors and psychiatrists at Hopkins had begun to speculate, then the rationality of binary sex itself was put in question. Perhaps trans childhood and trans life were important but not pathological or even exceptional forms of

humanity. This looming epistemological crisis of sex was acute enough
as the midcentury approached that it would motivate two of the psychologists who conducted interviews with trans people at Hopkins in the 1950s,
John Money and John Hampson, to craft a new category of embodiment
and psychology called "gender" that, they hoped, might finally achieve
a level of control over plasticity, cementing the sex binary once and for
all. The inevitable failure and widespread impact of that project, to which
I turn next, is largely responsible for the ways in which we have failed to
see the richness of trans life and trans childhood in the early twentieth
century.

CHAPTER 3

Sex in Crisis

Intersex Children in the 1950s and the Invention of Gender

B Y 1950, SEX WAS IN CRISIS. After a half-century of research on its plasticity in the life sciences and clinical sex reassignment of intersex children, both biology and medicine had worked themselves into the position of being perilously close to lacking a rationale for the sex binary altogether. When trans people began to seek out doctors like Hugh Hampton Young in the 1930s, hoping to change their sex, the intersex narratives they presented to enhance their medical requests may have been rebuffed, but they were hardly received as groundless. Sex had become an unwieldy biological category, now composed of genotype, gonads, hormones, genitals, internal organs, secondary anatomical features, and psychology, with none of them exerting what amounted to a deterministic influence. If human sex *naturally* started out life in infancy and childhood as indeterminate, harboring the potential for both masculine and feminine growth, then it was quite plausible that the plasticity medical science had come to operationalize in the service of producing and reassigning sex under a binary model might endorse the opposite conclusion. It increasingly seemed plausible that human life might *not* be binary, that intersex and trans embodiment were but two facets of life's natural variation. While scientists and physicians fell short of actually promoting that viewpoint, they were certainly anxious that it was becoming an irrefutable interpretation of their work.

It was under the backdrop of this looming epistemological crisis that John Money, a doctoral student in psychology at Harvard University, visited the Judge Baker Guidance Center at the university children's hospital in the late 1940s. During the visit, which Money's graduate seminar had undertaken in order to meet with some of the intersex children on the ward, he and his peers encountered a teenager who, raised a boy from birth, had grown increasingly feminine during childhood and now, during puberty, passed as a girl. Many years later, Money suspected in retrospect that this child likely experienced a form of androgen insensitivity syndrome, which left their body unable to make use of the androgen the endocrine system produced. As a result, from the fetal stage through childhood and puberty their body's plasticity would have grown into an increasingly feminine form, dramatically transforming sex.[1]

At the end of the 1940s such a diagnostic framework did not exist, however. Money was instead struck by the child's living contradiction of reigning endocrinology and psychology. In the gonadocentric paradigm of the moment, doctors conventionally assigned a body with testes as male, but nothing else about this child's body seemed masculine. Since the parents had been advised by doctors at birth to raise their child as a boy, there was a second, psychological complication that caught Money's attention. "Independently of this hormonally feminized body," he felt from observation that "her mind has masculinized."[2] The intersex body of this child incorporated a growing paradox of sex, caught between hormones and psychology: by gonadal definition "male," this child nevertheless appeared morphologically and hormonally a "girl" and yet also felt psychologically more of a "boy."[3] The doctors at the Baker Center were unable to settle on a medical sex assignment. Money left the hospital intending to write a term paper that would challenge the Freudian theory of sexual differentiation through the intersex body. This unnamed child was one catalyst for the subsequent invention of a new category of sexed life that we now call "gender."

Although gender has come to be associated with cultural malleability and feminist political projects, as far as its conditions of emergence are concerned it is better described as a medical device mobilized to face the potential conceptual collapse of binary sex. As Jennifer Germon explains, feminists in the 1970s who popularized the term "gender" outside medicine turned to the work of sexologists, psychologists, and psychiatrists, especially Money and his colleague, Robert Stoller, to leverage the category against patriarchal definitions of sex as biologically determined. Yet at the same time, as she points out, "it has become something of a received wisdom that gender was the invention of feminism."[4] In reality, however, even the analytic separation of sex and gender was actually a product of Stoller's work in the 1960s.[5] For Money and Stoller, of course, the distinction between sex and gender was never meant to undermine sex or advance feminist projects. On the contrary, the concept of gender was meant to *save* the sex binary from imminent collapse by offering a new developmental justification for coercive and normalizing medical intervention into intersex children's bodies. Gender would make nonbinary morphology into under-development, allowing medicine to claim that sex assignment was merely its normal completion. Yet from the 1970s on, feminist and, later, queer and trans projects seem to have increasingly lost sight of the conservative historical context of gender's invention. Work at the crossroads of trans and intersex studies by Sharon E. Preves, David A. Rubin, Jemima Repo, and Paul B. Preciado has only recently begun to revisit the significance of gender's historicity and to revise its misattribution to politically progressive projects.[6]

While the impact of gender on human embodiment, psychology, and subjectivity is monumental, it also has a particularly important place in the history of transgender children, which is why it figures so prominently in this book. Although the overlap of intersex and trans life had proven productive in the early twentieth century, the increasingly aggressive gate-keeping of clinicians had by the 1950s more or less extinguished that avenue of access to medicine. What changed at the same time is that Money's protocol for assigning a gender to intersex children laid the immediate foundation of the protocols of American transsexual medicine, which was just emerging and finally beginning to catch up to its European counterparts. The consolidation of hormonal, psychological, and surgical standards for transition and changes to the sex of intersex children were transposed to the new medical category of transsexuality, even as it abandoned the older sense that trans embodiment might have some sort of intersex basis. Even though trans children do not explicitly surface in this chapter, then, the invention of gender was a signal event that set the context in which the trans children in the rest of this book engaged with medicine. Given the contemporary stakes for trans children in defining what counts as "gender," moreover, a return to the category's emergence is an important part of contextualizing present-day pediatric endocrinology and its critics; both sides tend to rely on an implicit reading of Money's work.

Although the conservative import of gender has been forgotten in certain ways since the 1970s, Money's historiographical role in its invention has at the same time been given far too much weight.[7] Picking up where the previous chapter ended, at the Johns Hopkins Hospital in the 1940s, I claim that we should locate the emergence of gender in work with intersex children with adrenal conditions *before* Money arrived at Hopkins. This chapter underlines the connection of the 1950s to the early twentieth-century work of Hugh Hampton Young at the Brady Institute and focuses on the endocrine clinic run by Lawson Wilkins at the Harriet Lane Home for children. More important than the earliness of gender's emergence, however, is my argument that the clinical medicalization of intersex children in the 1940s and 1950s shows *how* the concept of gender was able to stabilize the crisis in the concept of binary sex: by promulgating a developmental framework that made gender identity the endpoint of a teleology of growth out of plasticity. At the same time, this clinical history shows that the actual plastic bodies of intersex children constantly undermined the fiction of that temporal order. In other words, the discursive uptake of intersex plasticity into the concept of gender as a racialized discourse of malleability became haunted in clinical practice by the embodied plasticity of children. Although I insist heuristically in this chapter, then, on the gap between the discourse of plasticity and the actual embodied plasticity of the children seen at Hopkins, my argument is that the indissociability of discourse *about* plasticity from the body's material plasticity is, precisely, the problem that gender's emergence marks. While gender may have redefined the terrain of sexed embodiment, signaling the close of an early twentieth-century era in which trans and intersex life were entangled, it still rested on a tenuous and volatile clinical relationship to plasticity in the bodies of children that undermined its apparent resolution of the crisis of binary sex. The refusal of children's embodied plasticity to fully cooperate with the theory of gender has been seriously underestimated. And the racialized meanings of plasticity from the early twentieth century were smuggled into the postwar era by attempts to resolve that issue through defining gender in severely developmental terms. In this chapter's reading of the invention of gender, Money is hardly a singular historical force, while the concept of gender is simultaneously a signal event but one that fails to live up to its own discursive claims. The broader point of this chapter within this book is to show how Money and the concept of gender serve as more of a functional relay point between early twentieth-century intersex medicine and postwar transsexual medicine.

Racializing the Plasticity of Gender

Iain Morland has argued that the medicalization of intersex bodies and Money's uptake of clinical research into a theory of gender was a form of medical humanism that equated "humanity" with a racialized plasticity, an abstract whiteness that signals the capacity for the scientific transformation of the body and mind in the broader service of the human species. Looking at the postwar shift in the sciences away from scientific racism associated with biological reductionism and evolutionary hierarchies, Morland found definitions of the plasticity of humanity in important venues such as the UNESCO statements on race, as well as the model of psychological development emblematized in Alfred Adler's work, each of which informed gender laterally.[8] As he put it, "The congruence between Money's claim about gender and contemporary scientific debate about race gave his work a self-evidence that was crucial to its broader uptake."[9] Gender was able to present itself without an acknowledgment of the racial normativity of plasticity precisely because the postwar episteme of cultural or population science, rather than removing biology from race as it claimed, actually made it more intangible and latent than it had been before.

The equation of humanity with plasticity helps to explain why the violent and nonconsensual surgical alteration of infant and children's bodies in the 1950s was still, after so many decades, considered not harmful or traumatic but *humane*. The whiteness of intersex children's bodies, at both the abstract level of their hormonal plasticity and the concrete level of demography (the vast majority of intersex children seen at Hopkins were white), signified to doctors their *need* to be instrumentalized in the service of a broader medical "improvement" of the human form. Morland cautions, therefore, that "I am unconvinced that we can straightforwardly demarcate inhumane from humane treatment, even though it would be reassuring to do so. I argue that the history of humanism cannot decide the meaning of a humane response to atypical genitalia. In other words, we cannot discover the right way to treat individuals with intersex anomalies by determining what it means to be human."[10] So long as the universalized "human" equals plasticity racialized as whiteness, critiques of the inhumanity of medical normalization remain trapped inside the postwar turn to cultural forms of race.

Yet the abstract whiteness of medicalized plasticity has deeper roots if we trace its clinical operationalization from the previous chapter into the 1940s, before Money arrived at Hopkins. The "humane" meaning attached to nontherapeutic and painful surgeries was based in a metonymic slide from life-threatening circumstances that sometimes accompanied intersex conditions to benign variations in morphology. This slide, as metonymic, was ontologically groundless, but it took advantage of a powerful material foothold because the plasticity of intersex children's actual bodies, as we

will see, made the two fields inseparable. In the gap between physiological conditions that greatly affected quality of life and arbitrarily binary
models of sexual differentiation grew the abstract whiteness that Morland
named "humanist." Clinicians continued to try to cultivate intersex children's plasticity, as they had since the early twentieth century, into forms
that equated sex with human phenotype, the proper end form of normal
development. In this way the older, eugenic connotation of plasticity that
originated in the life sciences was not extinguished by the events of World
War II and as scientific bodies such as UNESCO purported to do, but were
actually translated into new forms at the level of medical technique.

The plasticity that Money worked with in the early 1950s had been isolated and operationalized over the preceding decade by Lawson Wilkins,
the head of pediatric endocrinology at Hopkins. Wilkins's clinical work in
the 1940s and early 1950s shows how two concepts that we might presume
are separable from gender's malleability—technicity and race—were in fact
grown out of the same organic milieu, the bodies of intersex children. In
that context the apparent paradigm shift of gender, its aggressive reconsolidation of the sex binary, was shadowed by the threat of its own undoing
in children's bodies in the clinic. Wilkins spent years developing a potent
new hormonal therapy for children with intersex conditions caused by the
overactivity of the adrenal glands, a condition that had frustrated doctors
at Hopkins since Young's adrenalectomies in the 1920s. When a new synthetic hormone came on the market that could directly address the hyperplasia of the adrenal glands and their sexed effects, it seemed to reframe the
field of clinical endocrinology, effecting what looked like the first primarily
hormonal (rather than surgical) "sex change." This event proved decisive for
Money's model of gender, which interpreted Wilkins's data on the assumption that children's bodies were radically plastic before gender imprinted
at a certain developmental moment.

While Money presumed intersex children's biological plasticity in his
theory of gender, the actual clinical history of pediatric endocrinology at
Hopkins undermines his foundation. The treatment of what was by the
1940s called "Congenital Adrenal Hyperplasia" (CAH) confronts us with
unruly, indifferent, and volatile forms of embodied plasticity that express
the capacity to cause death as much as to alter sex. Wilkins did not simply
impose a binary form on intersex bodies through a new hormonal protocol of sex reassignment. He was embroiled in a constant negotiation with
plasticity, an inescapable need to solicit biological consent *from* the sexed

body of patients for new hormone therapies to produce predictable and reliable effects. The emergence of gender, which began not with Money but with adrenal hyperplasia in the 1940s, leads us to a different sense of the malleability or political potential of gender as plastic, for Money had to solicit that same consent from the body before imposing a gender assignment. The problems generated by this reliance on plasticity would carry forward into transsexual medicine, too, significantly shaping the terrain for trans children in the postwar era.[11]

Pediatric Endocrinology at the Harriet Lane Home

Although it was only one of many intersex conditions medicalized at the Harriet Lane Home, CAH captured Wilkins's attention because of the sheer number of admissions in whom it was present, as well as its persistent resistance to the treatment approach Young had developed over the preceding twenty years.[12] One variation of CAH also included a dangerous salt-losing symptom that led to immediate metabolic health crisis and, if left untreated, almost certain death.[13] Most other intersex conditions, especially nonnormative or nonbinary genital appearance, had no life-threatening implications at all.[14]

One of the reasons that Young had never found a way to directly remedy the hyperactivity of the adrenals is that the physiology of CAH remained poorly understood until it was retheorized in light of more precise hormonal analyses in the 1940s. Wilkins now knew that CAH was a metabolic disorder in which the adrenal glands were congenitally unable to produce the steroid hormone cortisol or could only produce it in small amounts. In the absence of adequate quantities of cortisol circulating in the blood, the pituitary gland's compensatory response would be to secrete massive amounts of an adrenocorticotropic hormone that, in turn, causes the adrenal glands to secrete very large amounts of androgens.[15] The regular circulation of so many androgens causes profound transformations in growth and a "virilization" or "masculinization" of the body, including the genitals and the so-called secondary sex characteristics. In children who would otherwise be assigned as male at birth, CAH causes a form of precocious puberty, including the premature fusion of the bones, stunting eventual height. More common at the Harriet Lane Home were cases of CAH in children who would otherwise be assigned as female at birth. In these children, masculinization of the genitals sometimes occurred in utero, so that the baby was assigned at birth as a boy until doubts arose during childhood. Other times this visible masculinization occurred rapidly during the first months or years of life. Children assigned as female at birth and raised as girls would begin, seemingly without warning, to dramatically masculinize. Only in cases accompanied by a life-threatening inability to retain salt would immediate hospitalization be almost guaranteed to bring a child into a clinic. Otherwise, many children with CAH lived as boys and never saw a doctor unless complications arose or changes in their sexed body caused enough concern in parents or other adults that they sought out medical attention.[16]

When Wilkins was hired to head the Harriet Lane Home's new Endocrine Clinic, in 1935, admissions of intersex children began to shift from the Brady Institute to the clinic because of Wilkins's research program centering on hormones. However, it took many years of improvisation and trial and error just to establish how hormones could affect children's plasticity. While intersex embodiment was far from the only area in which he worked, Wilkins devoted a great deal of time to this area of research. Many of the infants and children he worked with were local, referred from elsewhere in the hospital or from Baltimore, but by then Hopkins had built such a reputation that families seeking a medical sex assignment would come from around the country. In 1942 a family made the trip from California with their child, "Alex," who was less than ten years old. Assigned as a girl at birth, Alex had begun to rapidly masculinize and outpace their peers developmentally around age five. A local doctor consulted by the parents suggested that they already had "the bone age" of a nine-year-old. That doctor wrote to Hugh Hampton Young for advice, and Young referred the family to a urologist in their hometown. After finding that Alex had no vagina, the urologist made a diagnosis of "female pseudohermaphroditism due to adrenal hyperplasia" but, unlike what Young would have done, added that he "strongly advised against adrenalectomy or plastic operation."[17]

Upon arriving at the Harriet Lane Home, Wilkins ordered a daily urine analysis and an adrenal function test to establish a data flow on Alex's endocrine system. In his case notes he questioned the older surgical framework for CAH, reasoning that it "seems more logical to try to stimulate female development by the use of large doses of estrogens. In this way the male characteristics can be suppressed." Although he added that it "is questionable whether such treatment will suppress the activity of the adrenals" and that long-term estrogen therapy "would probably lead to atrophy [of the ovaries] and sterility," he argued that "the principle objective should be the development of the secondary sex characteristics and the suppression of the male." With these rigidly binary aesthetic criteria in mind, he added that "surgical removal of the clitoris and possibly later plastic operations on the vagina seem desirable." Wilkins sent Alex for an exam by a gynecologist, who felt that an exploratory laparotomy was still needed to see if "the intra-abdominal structure felt" during palpitation "proves to be an ovary," in which case "nothing should be done." If, however, "it should prove to be a testicle . . . it should be removed," after which "patient could go through life quite normally as a female, except, of course, for her sterility." After the laparotomy was scheduled and found normal ovaries, the surgeon amputated Alex's phallus and Wilkins prescribed a daily estrogen regimen.[18]

Wilkins also asked a child psychiatrist to interview Alex, providing a more intimate, if still highly mediated, account of Alex's experience at Hopkins. The psychiatrist used a "mental standardization" test, thereby archiving something of their perspective, although it is highly obscured by adult fears around innocence. Apparently Alex's mother was very anxious about whether they knew they were intersex, so Dr. Tietze, the psychiatrist, asked only vague questions, like "Why did you come [to Hopkins]?" to which Alex replied, "Because I am so tall. Rather be a little smaller. Have trouble finding shoes that fit me. Children of my age are smaller. . . . Would rather look young." Tietze also interviewed Alex's mother, gendering her concerns over medicalization as a hysterical symptom of "constant emotional strain." She mentioned to him that she had read as many books on hermaphroditism as she could "and is up to date." Her biggest worry "is how to break the news to the child, whom she believes is not aware of her condition," followed by "whether or not [child's name] will not finally turn out to be a boy" instead of a girl.[19]

After Alex had recovered from the laparotomy and phallic amputation, Wilkins sent the family back to California with a 5-milligram daily dose of stilbestrol, noting that it was "very high and probably smaller doses" would be found effective over time. Their family doctor was to oversee the hormone therapy, and Wilkins remarked that stilbestrol had the value of "ease of administration" for "treatment at home." Not long after returning home, the mother sent Wilkins a letter after Alex had to be hospitalized for a sinus infection and bronchitis, followed by the measles. During these illnesses the estrogen had produced a severe side effect of abdominal pain and nausea. The family doctor halved the daily dosage to reduce the discomfort. As for changes in sex, the mother reported that "her voice is a little higher and her appearance is more feminine."[20]

Alex's medicalization indexes the shift in approach from Young's older, surgical paradigm to a hormonal one. Wilkins led with hormones, despite the unpredictability of their effects, and turned to surgeries only as a supplement to medical sex assignment. Yet both Young and Wilkins knew well that estrogen therapy would not do very much other than cause slight changes in appearance for children with CAH. Chemically it did nothing to address the underlying adrenal condition. The specific hormone to address in treating CAH was the absence of cortisol. During World War II, Lewis Sarett, a chemist working for the pharmaceutical company Merck and Company, was successful in partially synthesizing cortisol in a lab, something desired by the military for the potential biological enhancement of soldiers. After the war ended Merck decided to make the synthetic version of cortisol, which they termed "cortisone," available for medical research, having also significantly improved its chemical quality and reliability over the intervening several years. The initial trial application of the synthetic hormone was in rheumatoid arthritis, which seemed to be miraculously cured with regular cortisone administration. Wilkins speculated that it would probably be highly useful in treating CAH, too. A team of doctors working with intersex children at the Massachusetts General Hospital in Boston pursued the same avenue, and both those doctors and Wilkins announced their findings in December 1949 that cortisone could treat CAH.[21]

The clinical difference made by cortisone was astonishing. Many of the Harriet Lane Home's existing patients, who, like Alex, had undergone surgeries and received mostly ineffective estrogen prescriptions, were now prescribed cortisone, inducing what amounted in many cases to binary sex reassignment. Cortisone's effectiveness even changed Wilkins's decision about medical sex reassignment itself. For instance, a child raised as a girl in Appalachian coal country arrived at the Endocrine Clinic in 1947, just before cortisone became available. Wilkins was certain "that this is a case of female pseudo-hermaphroditism due to congenital hyperplasia of the adrenals" and ordered urine analysis that confirmed the correlate androgen levels. In his case notes, Wilkins pointed out that "the correction of the adrenal condition by the removal of 1½ adrenals has frequently been tried by Dr. Hugh Young and others without any benefit." With a lack of other options, given the relatively uselessness of estrogen therapy, Wilkins was "face[d] with the question of whether one should attempt by means of surgical and hormonal treatment to feminize or masculinize this patient." Unconvinced by the soundness of either option, he deferred to the child psychiatrist Leo Kanner, who "indicate[s] that she would probably be happier as a boy and living a male life." Wilkins echoed the "wait and see" policy that Young had often employed since the 1910s, writing "that the wisest, most successful and easiest course to follow is that of following the direction of the predominant sex hormone which is being produced," legitimizing this child's masculinity. The parents apparently agreed, and "the case was referred to social service to help . . . make plans for this major adjustment in their lives."[22]

For reasons that are unrecorded, when the family returned to West Virginia their child did not socially transition to being a boy but continued to live as a girl. In 1953 the family retuned to Baltimore because puberty was causing so much masculinization that the child was finding it socially difficult to continue living as a girl.[23] Wilkins now offered his new cortisone therapy. For three weeks the child submitted to daily urine tests to establish a baseline for their androgen levels. Wilkins then prescribed 50 milligrams a day of cortisone. After observing the initially slow fall in androgen levels, he increased the dosage twice over the following three months. About six weeks into the therapy a clitoral amputation and vaginoplasty were also undertaken to feminize the genitals. After the child spent three months on the ward receiving cortisone, Wilkins reported "some beginning development of breast tissue," as the adrenal glands shrunk and masculinization morphologically converted into femininization. Sent home with an individualized cortisone regimen based on exhaustive study of the daily urine samples, this child continued to return to the Harriet Lane Home about once a year, while Wilkins corresponded with their family doctor to stay apprised of the course of their femininization. By the mid-1950s, when the child was in their midteens, their CAH had been dramatically mitigated by cortisone therapy, and Wilkins was satisfied that their body was going through a feminine puberty. Years of medicalization, social ostracism at the hands of other children, and the alternation between medical assignment as a boy and a girl had also taken a toll, however. When Money interviewed this child and followed up with them in the mid-1950s, he noted a serious depression that showed no signs of abating.[24]

Many other patients that Wilkins had seen since infancy and who had been originally medicalized under Young's surgical paradigm returned to the Harriet Lane Home in the 1950s to receive cortisone because of its potential to effect a medical sex reassignment as a girl. A newborn from New York who in 1935 had undergone plastic surgeries by Young to feminize the genitals, for instance, returned in 1950 to see Wilkins for the first time. During the 1940s this child had been given "intermittent" prescriptions for stilbestrol, but they had failed to inhibit masculine growth. The cortisone treatments, however, effected a rapid reversal into femininity. By 1956, as the patient was completing college and applying to medical school, Wilkins noted in his follow-up notes that they were easily socially recognized as a woman.[25] Wilkins and his team analyzed changes in breast development, the vagina, the clitoris, menstruation, basal temperature, hair, acne, and voice in order to track the transformation of the body's plasticity during cortisone therapy.[26] In children older than infants, whose genitalia were not regarded as very plastic, normalizing surgery was often recommended to achieve the rigid aesthetic standards governing the morphological appearance of the "female" body. The reduction of the size of the clitoris or phallus was the most common, even though there was no medical necessity at all for the procedure.[27] While not a "cure" for CAH insofar as therapy would probably be required for the rest of childhood and puberty, cortisone had the profoundly visible effect of normalizing the sex of the intersex child into a binary form.

CAH was not a singularly "sexed" condition but carried with it certain long-term cardiac and cancer risks from exceptionally high androgen circulation, which cortisone therapy minimized as it changed the body's sex. Still, cortisone therapy to reverse the masculinization of children that doctors felt "should" have been assigned female at birth cannot be disentangled from the purely surgical interventions with the genitals that had no medical justification beyond aesthetic norms. Such surgeries produced their own justification only retroactively by locating the normality of the sex binary out of altered genital appearance. Raising children with CAH as boys when they might have been assigned as girls or letting girls grow into a partially masculine body, whether with body hair, a "large" clitoris, or the latent specter of same-sex desire, were all considered self-evident pathologies, akin to cancer or cardiac arrest risk. As intersex studies scholars have argued so well, this normalizing slippage justified the coercive and nontherapeutic alteration of intersex children's bodies at the same time as it let doctors also claim normalization as proof that sex *should* be rendered binary *even when it did not always grow that way on its own*.[28] This is how the abstract whiteness of intersex children's plasticity was already well established before the 1950s moment that Morland examines. In the slippage between medical conditions that could affect the livability of intersex children's lives, including cancer and cardiac complications, and the entirely benign question of their sexed morphology, especially their genitals, Wilkins framed binary sex as the proper phenotypic outcome of cortisone treatment by including genital surgeries in his protocol—something that, strictly speaking, did *not* affect the course of adrenal hyperplasia. Hormonal plasticity gave cortisone its traction, reversing hyperplasia, but it was also given a second meaning through the inclusion of genital surgeries, as if both were equally relevant to the long-term health of an intersex child.

This slide from the adrenals to the genitals in sex reassignment, however, was less a perfect accomplishment of cortisone therapy than a speculative gambit. The entanglement of the part of Wilkins's protocol concerning "sex change" and the part concerning the general metabolism of the adrenals also raised the specter of biological resistance to medicine from the intersex child's embodied plasticity. While genital surgeries were meant to shore up the normative boundaries between masculine and feminine, the treatment of CAH in the specific case of its salt-losing variation illustrates the very weak basis for these medical interventions because of the partial refusal, if not radical indifference, of embodied plasticity in some cases. This autonomy of the plastic body profoundly undermines Money's subsequent interpretation of Wilkins's work into a theory of gender acquisition and reassignment.

Salt-Losing CAH and Embodied Plasticity's Autonomy

When children with a salt-losing version of CAH were admitted to the Harriet Lane Home, the stakes were high, for without immediate treatment they would inevitably die of dehydration or heart attack. While Wilkins noted in detail atypical genitalia as part of the diagnostic assessment of these children, the lion's share of his attention was drawn to stabilizing the electrolyte balance of the body while simultaneously suppressing the adrenals and, *only* if both of those could be harmonized, subsequently focusing on an aesthetic sex reassignment. The immediate priority was to resolve the salt crisis through massive doses of sodium. Once imminent death was no longer a concern, Wilkins would add cortisone to the daily regime, usually starting with a high dose. During their stay at the Harriet Lane

Home, children would have their urine analyzed exactly every twenty-four hours, on two data points: the excretion of 17-Ketosteroids (which measured the androgens being produced by the adrenal glands) and the various electrolyte levels that indicated to what degree salt was being retained.[29] The practical difficulty of analyzing urine from newborn babies on precise daily cycles was in and of itself a massive undertaking for the clinic's staff.[30] Growth rate and bone development were also tracked over a longer term. With this continuous flow of data established, the main task became to work to find the minimum effective dose of cortisone that would suppress the adrenals while also figuring out how salt intake could be reduced in the same proportion as its retention increased (since too much salt was also dangerous). Crucially, Wilkins found that, although he could not explain how or why, cortisone *improved* salt retention in some incalculable way. Although cortisone could not alone cure the electrolyte problem, its effects could not be separated from it, either.[31]

Integrating the interpretation of these two sets of daily readings while simultaneously guiding them toward the electrolyte and androgenic statistical norms for a child's age was exceedingly difficult work because the exact relation between cortisone and salt retention was unknowable. Wilkins found that sex and general metabolism were deeply entangled in a way that the binary discourse of sexed plasticity could not contain. In the face of this practical epistemological and material limit, he created an elaborate metabolic chart system to try to bring the two indeterminate data sets under his jurisdiction. Charting daily, monthly, and long-term changes (some infants remained hospitalized for years), he would constantly adjust the dosage of cortisone, salt, and, for some patients, a second corticosterone hormone given to enhance salt retention.[32] Relying on his ability to partially graph the moving relation between the input of hormones and salt and the output of data, Wilkins attempted to calibrate the therapeutic regimen to harmonize the child's electrolytes, growth, and sex.

Anything less than *resonance* between the moving parts of this clinical apparatus would put the child's life at risk again. Unfortunately for Wilkins, the conversion of daily urine analysis into separate data fields of electrolytes and androgens was a poor predictor of how adjusting hormonal and salt dosage would move the numbers the following day. The constant threat of dehydration, infection, vomiting, loss of appetite, rapid weight loss *or* massive weight gain, growth, and irritability rarely subsided or could start up again without warning. Trying to harmonize the resonance between general endocrine metabolism and the specific dimension of sex in a child admitted at seven weeks old, for instance, Wilkins significantly changed the treatment regime *nineteen times in eighteen months* before achieving sufficient stability to warrant discharge from the Harriet Lane Home.[33]

Colleagues and students who worked with Wilkins noted the fastidiousness and long hours required for his strenuous commitment to the technology of patient charts. "Normalization" of the child's CAH body, far from imposing a binary on a nonbinary intersex body, consisted of a chaotic, nonlinear engagement with the organic entanglement of sex and salt materialized in living metabolism. Claude Migeon, at the time a visiting research fellow, recalled the process thusly many years later:

> In the evening of each working day, the ketos [17-KS] results
> were posted on each patient file. The files were pinned on bulletin
> boards in the secretaries' office. After the secretaries had left,
> Dr. Wilkins was joined by Lytt Gardner, John Crigler and me.
> Often, there would be one or two interns as well as one of the
> numerous visitors [to the clinic]. Long discussions would take
> place about modifying the treatment of each patient. . . . *It seems
> that* out of these daily meetings came the elaboration of the proper
> treatment for CAH patients.[34]

Migeon's reminiscence that "it seems that" this rumination on data and its relation to dosage led to "the proper treatment" evokes the central problem at hand in this clinical history. The method developed by Wilkins's team never came close to a hormonal *control* of somatic and sexual growth, where control would mean the imposition of a binary form as an orthopedic device, or the suppression of nonbinary form. Wilkins and his team never found a stable relation between salt and cortisone that could function predictively. The clinical reality amounted much less coherently (and much less confidently, as Migeon's choice of phrase reveals) to a kind of *chasing after the plasticity* of the child's growing body through its doubled metabolic forms. Cortisone was a chemically potent but highly indeterminate tool that acted simultaneously on the electrolyte and the sexual dimensions of the metabolism, but without a clear relation between the two. In salt-losing cases of CAH, Wilkins relied profoundly on the biological consent of the child's plastic body to transform salt and sex, a consent that he could hardly count upon.

We often frame the medicalization of intersex children, as Preves puts it, as based in an "impetus to *control* intersexual 'deviance' [that] stems from cultural tendencies towards gender binarism, homophobia, and fear of difference."[35] Yet the clinical history of the Harriet Lane Home leads to a different argument. Wilkins's labored attempts to reconcile electrolyte metabolism and its sexual version through the technologies of hormones, salt, and patient charts describe a scenario where "control" is at most a perpetually deferred horizon, not an outcome. Cortisone therapy is more consonant with Repo's argument that "the hermaphroditic subject was a subject of biopolitical *potentiality*: a subject who, through the surgical alteration of genitals, could be psychologically managed into a different-sex desiring subject and hence become a subject useful for the reproduction of social order."[36] Cortisone therapy was meant to address the young child's plasticity in a normalizing sense, to remedy the adrenals at the same time that it feminized the body, recalibrating development along a binary trajectory. However, in its salt-losing version, incredibly virulent embodied plasticity constantly interfered with the isolation of "sex" as a distinct "part" of the body, frustrating the metonymic slide from life-threatening medical conditions to arbitrary binary models of human phenotype and genitals. This inability to isolate sex was a dramatic incarnation of the epistemological crisis of sex that plasticity had generated over the first half of the twentieth century, and it manifested specifically on the endocrine ward as a radical metabolic openness to the environment. As Wilkins so often found, diet and stress in the clinical setting often overrode the action of cortisone in the midst of treatment, throwing resonance off without advance warning.[37]

There are two entangled modes of embodied plasticity at hand that Wilkins struggled to put into discourse. First, there is the sexual plasticity of the adrenal glands, whose masculinizing effects could be suppressed and transformed by cortisone, changing the outward morphology of the sexed body from masculine to feminine. Second, there is the much more volatile plasticity of general metabolism, partially regulated by salt. While those two forms of plasticity were not coincident in the child's body, their invisible relation as "parts" of the endocrine system was given a metonymic relation in patient charts. The entanglement of these two modes frustrated Wilkins's attempt to govern either, preempting the question of genital surgery altogether and revealing it as an arbitrary add-on to the treatment of CAH. The more radical suggestion made by this entanglement was that "sex" could not be reduced to a binary form because virulent metabolic plasticity constantly interfered with its stability.

And where is the intersex child's personhood in all of this? Metabolic plasticity is not a straightforward concept through which to extract a sense of agency. As Hannah Landecker has explained, metabolism is best understood as "a third concept" upending the distinction between organism and environment.[38] Whereas a model based on an organism/environment split would see Wilkins as intervening from without to induce specific orthopedic effects on sodium retention and sex, that is not what happened in the clinic, as the limited success of patient charts as a technology shows. The possibility of cultivating "resonance" between salt and sex points to a third concept of metabolism where both organism *and* environment, body *and* medical technology, are affecting and being affected simultaneously. This overwhelmingly lively plasticity carries no inherent political or social significance. The child's life is immanently at risk, but successful treatment also included a rigid binary cultivation of the sexed body. This is a kind of plasticity that remains underappreciated by feminist, intersex, and trans studies. If we continue to think of intersex medical history as one of an imposition of sex and gender norms on the organism entirely *from the outside*, then cortisone would be a mere instrument. It turns out, however, that the real gender trouble has less to do with the categories of sex and gender than with their living residence in the child's body and the partially autonomous nonhuman agency expressed in embodied plasticity, one that was quite successful in forestalling the question of genital surgeries, but at great cost to the child's health. If the actual children whom Wilkins saw at the Harriet Lane Home seem even more distanced from the medical narrative in this chapter than in the previous one, it is because they were extremely instrumentalized, rendered not only silent but often kept entirely uninformed about what was being done to them by doctors. Yet even in this highly disenfranchised clinical setting, their own plasticity continued to assert its own agency, albeit one that hardly acted in the children's interests.

The reason that Wilkins was willing to cling to binary sex in cases of salt-losing CAH, I argue, even when that could put the life of the patient at risk, is that the binary imperative was a racialized phenotype. The crucial detail was scrupulously recorded by Wilkins in a 1952 article he published in *Pediatrics*: each of the patients upon whom he experimented to produce the protocol for salt-losing CAH was "a white female" or "a white infant."[39] That whiteness names an investment in a racial normativity that had previously been articulated as eugenic stock during Young's surgical paradigm. As the transition to the postwar era heralded the end of an explicitly eugenic language of race improvement and extermination in the life sciences, the eugenic preoccupations that had typified endocrinology during the interwar period rhetorically faded. It would be a mistake, however, to assume that the eugenic *techniques* underwriting modern endocrinology similarly ended in the 1950s. On the contrary, the experimental use of cortisone illustrates continuity in practice. Wilkins aimed to resolve a metabolic condition that would simultaneously normalize the growth rate, metabolism, *and* sex of the body, directing it toward a binary phenotype that was merged with the resolution of the salt-losing crisis. The whiteness of these children was so valuable as a racial formation that it allowed Wilkins to justify putting children's lives at risk to achieve a binary sex as *humane* practice, presaging Morland's argument about Money.

Stated somewhat differently, the precise measurement and manipulation of plasticity proved impossible for Wilkins. Salt-losing CAH is a strong example of how plasticity, having tipped on its own agential force toward being inimical to the life of the child, tended to disobey the endocrinologist's technical or discursive prowess as much as it simultaneously enabled it. That partial autonomy was, again paradoxically, also the material means by which Wilkins was able to partially manipulate metabolism through synthetic hormones, changing the sex of the body and designating femininity, not masculinity, as the proper phenotype for children assigned as female at birth with CAH. Wilkins's persistence in the face of a lack of resonance between sex and salt describes his investment in an abstract racial formation of sex—the shadowy second meaning of the phrase "a *white* female" left behind in his published work. Wilkins made a risky choice in trying to make such powerful forms of embodied plasticity fit into phenotypic models of a sex binary, for there was no way to extinguish the constant threat of a loss of resonance that his patient charts record. And while the invention of gender was meant to save the sex binary from imminent conceptual collapse, Money's reliance on Wilkins's work with CAH preserved that instability and threat of collapse inside the new category.

Gender as Plasticity's Analogue

When Wilkins hired Money at the outset of the 1950s to work with fellow psychologists Joan and John Hampson, they built the theory of gender upon what they took as a coherent outcome of Wilkins's work with corti-sone and other hormone therapies: that children's plasticity was incredibly receptive to medical intervention early in life through coordinated hormone therapy and plastic surgery. In other words, they bought into the metonymic slide from medically significant conditions to arbitrary binary phenotypes. The theory of gender was a new interpretation of long-standing clinical research into children with a field of overlapping development and sexual "disorders," increasingly refined hormonal syntheses aimed at harmonizing and normalizing specific metabolic and sexual processes and normalizing plastic surgeries on the genitals.[40] As a psychologist, Money was neither trained nor permitted to direct hormonal or surgical intervention, so he made theoretical and diagnostic inferences from the available clinical data produced by his colleagues. Those practicing endocrinologists, psychia-trists, and surgeons, in turn, informed their clinical practice with Money's theories.

Money and the Hampsons saw upward of sixty "hermaphroditic patients," both children and adults, before publishing several articles in the *Bulletin of the Johns Hopkins Hospital* in 1955 in which they outlined the medical concept of gender.[41] Articulating their specific interest in "cases of contradiction between gonadal sex and sex of rearing," they published a table in the first article that mapped those characteristics through "endog-enous hormonal sex," "type of hermaphroditism," and what they now called the "gender role" of their patients.[42] To explain this new category, they wrote: "The term gender role is used to signify all those things that a per-son says or does to disclose himself or herself as having the status of boy or man, girl or woman, respectively. It includes, but is not restricted to sex-uality in the sense of eroticism."[43] This statement was repeated more or less verbatim in the subsequent articles they published that year. More important was their finding that "gonadal structure per se proved a most unreliable prognosticator of a person's gender role and orientation as man or woman; assigned sex proved an extremely reliable one."[44] While their col-leagues Young and Wilkins had long distrusted the gonadal model because it held no predictive value, Money and the Hampsons felt that the sex in which a child was raised *did* play a determining (but not deterministic) role.

The immediate goal of the 1955 articles, then, was to overturn the gonad-ocentric paradigm and to save the sex binary from conceptual collapse caused by the indeterminacy introduced by plasticity.[45] New research on chromosomes had excited researchers hopeful of a genetic determination of sex—but had fallen apart just as quickly as chromosome tests became available. It turned out that XX and XY were unreliable sources of meaning and that there were also many more chromosomal combinations in humans that cast doubt on the presumed binary logic of the system.[46] By the time Money and the Hampsons began their research, it was also well established that the gonads did not "direct" the sex hormone circulation of the body in a causal sense. An ovary or testis might be present but not secrete any meaningful estrogen or testosterone. Or, it might secrete both, but one or both would not be processed by the rest of the body. The body was also capable of converting one hormone into the other. Estrogens and androgens did not really have "feminine" or "masculine" meanings at all. Or, as in cases of CAH, other glands such as the adrenals might cause sexual effects.[47]

Facing the looming conceptual crisis of binary sex, gender made a key difference. Money and the Hampsons suppressed the concept of intersex as a "mix" of two sexes so that they could eliminate the concept of natural human bisexuality that had dominated the life sciences for a century. The concept of gender referred to a psychosocial dimension *of* sex, rather than a separable ontological entity. Gender role was introduced as one of many components of sex that, they explained, clinicians could look to in cases of intersex children for guidance on sex assignment: chromosomal makeup, gonads, "external genital morphology," "hormonal sex," the sex assigned to the child at birth, and "the gender role established and ingrained through years of living in a sex already assigned."[48] Money and the Hampsons were very careful to insist that there is no ontological reason to assume any of these components exerts a deterministic role in sexual differentiation. Rather, their argument was drawn from clinical observation and practical efficacy: first, chromosomes have essentially *no* predictive value; and second, the gonads are equally weak. Indeed, even relative hormone levels of testosterone and estrogen in infancy or early childhood are poor predictors of eventual somatic and psychological development, given what the researchers described as "the frequent difficulty of predicting hormonal sex before puberty and of the possibility of corrective hormonal intervention."[49] Unable to offer a deterministic framework for sexual differentiation, Money and the Hampsons strategically changed the context of the debate. Henceforth, their question had to do not with the ontology of sex but exclusively with "the life adjustments of the patients in our series"—how normal they *felt* or how well they adapted *socially*.[50] With

that twist, a gender role that contradicted the visible body could be identified as pathological *because it might lead to social stigma or psychological
distress*—the phobic origins of the concept of dysphoria.

The twist is well known to feminist, queer, trans, and intersex critics,
for it consists of the arbitrary production of medical abnormality out of
social norms, rather than endogenous risk to the life of an intersex person.
What has not been as well noticed is the part played here by a discourse
of plasticity. Like Wilkins before them, Money and the Hampsons had to
consent to the partial biological autonomy of the child's plastic body in order
to normalize it. Plasticity was the vehicle that would guarantee that intersex children's bodies could be made to fit the assigned gender role that they
argued was so predictive. Arguing that "gonadal structure per se proved a
most unreliable prognosticator of a person's gender role and orientation as
man or woman," they claimed instead that "assigned sex proved an extremely
reliable one" because the body's alterability could be psychologically inter-
nalized by the child.[51] The most controversial and often critiqued argument of Money's theory of gender is that choosing a sex that matched *or
could be matched* to the external genitals, assigning it to the child, and rearing
with minimal doubt could "ensure" a concordant gender role. This point
has often been described as an extreme form of behavioralism, if not a per-
versely fundamentalist kind of social constructivism, but those interpreta-
tions miss how much Money and the Hampsons relied on an analogy to
material, biological plasticity whose implications they could not control.[52]
Like Wilkins, they proposed to chase after and optimize sex in the body
to the greatest possible technical extent by consenting to the agency of its
plasticity. Their advice to clinicians presented with intersex newborns or
infants makes this clear:

> It should be the aim of the obstetrician and pediatrician to settle
> the sex of an hermaphroditic baby, once and for all, within the first
> few weeks of life, before the establishment of a gender role gets
> far advanced. . . . It is our recommendation that, in assigning the
> sex in these ambiguous instances, consideration be given first to
> the appearance and morphology of the external genitals. If the
> external organs are so predominately male, or so predominately
> female that no amount of surgical reconstruction will convert them
> to serviceably and erotically sensitive organs of the other sex, then
> the sex of assignment should be dictated by the external genitals

alone. All further surgical and hormonal endeavor should be
directed towards maintaining the person in that sex. . . . If the
external genital anatomy of a neonate is thoroughly ambiguous and
the possibilities of surgical reconstruction are equally promising in
either direction, then gonadal and hormonal considerations may
be more heavily weighted.[53]

Clinicians are directed to assay the relative plasticity of the child's growing body and to assign sex on the basis of whatever the body seems most
receptive to forming, as well as what the clinical team is capable of doing
through surgery and hormones. At the time that Money and the Hampsons were conducting their research, clitoridectomy and vaginoplasty were
much more effective procedures for producing normative-looking genitals
than surgeries for hypospadiac phalluses or phalloplasty. Money and the
Hampsons often felt that choosing to assign an intersex baby to the female
sex because it would be "easier" to create female external genitalia was a
self-evidently better option than raising a child as a boy with a small penis.[54]
While this is an incredibly arbitrary and normalizing contention, it is also
a technical and discursive concession to the plastic agencies of the body.
Sex reassignment could not override and neutralize all intersex vitality to
impose a binary. Sex reassignment paradoxically relied on intersex plasticity to accomplish transformations in the body through hormonal and surgical intervention that also met their limit in that embodied plasticity's
agency. The profound limitation Wilkins encountered in trying to make
salt and sex resonate was not resolved by the introduction of gender. If
anything, it was merely deferred under the cover of "social stigma" and
"adjustment."

How could gender simultaneously be based in an analogy with biological plasticity and yet seek to extinguish the theory of natural bisexuality
and mixed sex? The crucial difference was made by child development.
From their first published paper in 1955, Money and the Hampsons deployed
an analogy to language acquisition as a form of developmental plasticity to
secure their argument about how gender was formed. While continuing to
defer the question of gender's etiology, they explained that "a person's gender role as boy or girl, man or woman, is built up cumulatively through the
life experiences he encounters and through the life experiences he trans-
acts."[55] Since the precise nature of such transactions is unknowable, they
went on to say that "gender role may be likened to a native language. Once

ingrained, a person's native language may fall into disuse and be supplanted by another, but it is never entirely eradicated. So also a gender role may be changed or, resembling native bilingualism may be ambiguous, but it may also become so deeply ingrained that not even flagrant contradictions of body functioning and morphology may displace it."[56]

The analogy to language suggests that plasticity is forceful and unstable early on in human life but has a definite window, after which it is meant to recede. Child development as a temporal form restricts plasticity to a profoundly conservative narrative, domesticating it in the service of a newly rigid sex binary. Money and the Hampsons argued that cases involving "older infants and children" are therefore "the most problematic and difficult problems of sex assignment encountered," not because older children might be able to consciously resist or contest their medicalization better than infants but because their plasticity was fast receding.[57] As with any analogy in medical science, there was a major imprecision to this argument. They conceded that it "is not possible to state a fixed age at which gender awareness becomes established" but then went on to argue in their next breath that such awareness takes place "somewhere around eighteen months" of age.[58] Money would repeat the same general line for the rest of his career, adjusting the age parameters every so often but without being able to substantiate the claim. Of course, he precisely did *not* need to prove the point, for it was the imprecision of the analogy that animated its clinical operation.

Gender allowed Money and the Hampsons to undo the idea that humans were naturally bisexual or sexually indeterminate. Instead, though children were born exceptionally plastic, that plasticity now needed to grow in a developmental direction, *either* male or female, *to prevent social stigma*. The sex binary, which had nearly fallen apart in medicine over the previous fifty years, had new life breathed into it by gender, justified not on an ontological basis but by a developmental matrix. Masculinity and femininity were recodified as the only two phenotypes into which a child could grow. Medicine's task became to normalize the development of intersex or gender nonconforming children so that they would grow up to be *either* a woman or a man, and nothing else.[59]

This shift entailed the effective end of an older discourse on "hermaphroditism," which, despite its viciously dehumanizing connotations of natural monstrosity and its racist associations with evolutionist primitivism, had also incorporated a radical threat to the sexed order of things. If intersex bodies were of nature, then perhaps there was nothing natural about the sex binary. Perhaps the sex binary was a massive misrecognition of biology. Or as many interwar endocrinologists had believed, perhaps all humans were, to a certain degree, normally intersex, so that masculinity and femininity were mere tendencies, rather than absolute forms, and human life existed along a range of benign variation, including trans life.

Money and the Hampsons, who were quite anxious about the risks in making such a profound shift, let it find form in the problem of counseling child patients and their parents:

> Ninety-nine times out of a hundred, the public construes an hermaphrodite as being half boy, half girl. The parents of an hermaphrodite should be disabused of this conception immediately. They should be given, instead, the concept that their child is a boy or a girl, one or the other, *whose sex organs did not get completely differentiated or finished*. A few simple embryological sketches showing the original hermaphroditism of all human embryos in the undifferentiated phase, and the late stage at which external genital similarity of males and females is still apparent, are of inestimable help in conveying the enlightened concept of *genital unfinishedness*.[60]

There are echoes here of the previous medicalizations of intersex children, going as far back as Young's surgical approach, which was organized by the developmental age of his patients. The difference is that gender significantly consolidated the theory that bisexuality was a single, temporary stage in development, "the undifferentiated phase" that was normal so long as it did not persist too long. Money therefore counseled clinicians to quash any notion of mixed masculinity and femininity in the minds of parents of intersex children and to replace it with the idea that the child's development was incomplete, that "genital unfinishedness" was a pathology that could, paradoxically, be corrected through hormones and surgery because of the very same plasticity that had resulted in the original condition. Intersex embodiment was redefined as a developmental condition where sex was no longer mixed but unfinished. While the difference made by development was powerful, however, as a metaphor for children's growth, it went too far, leaving itself vulnerable to the material resistance from embodied plasticity that had frustrated Wilkins.

From Intersex to Gender:
The Metonymy of Plasticity and Phenotype

There was an important series of metonymic slides in the 1940s and 1950s from the child's generally plastic body, including sex, to the specifically intersex body and back to the new universalizing scale of gender. Indeed, so effective was such metonymy that it would soon enable a further slide from a clinical theory of gender developed for intersex children to a clinical theory of transsexuality. With the availability of potent new hormones, the transformation of the sexed body during development promised itself anew to endocrinology in a way that made such slides attractive to clinicians like Wilkins, Money, and the Hampsons. As poor as the ground for those movements may have been epistemologically—they would be rather easy to deconstruct their reliance on the discourse of development to justify arbitrary binary models couched in genital appearance—to dismiss them on those grounds would ignore how, as Donna Haraway counsels, it was precisely because there was a poor metaphorical fit at hand that the slide materially effected a new treatment protocol that "worked" in practice—at least for the most part.[61]

Plasticity filled the metonymic gap in Wilkins's work between medically significant conditions associated with CAH, such as cardiac complications, cancer risk, metabolic crisis, and benign variations in genitalia, and bodily morphology, which carried no health risks. Cortisone had effects on both, after all. Money followed his lead, attempting to domesticate the agency of children's plasticity even further by reading it through a developmental framework that gave it a pretext for being forced into binary form. In so doing, he also carried forward Wilkins's racialized sense of plasticity as an abstract whiteness that necessitated altering the body without consent and in nontherapeutic ways in the name of a universalizing humanity— this is where Morland's concept of plasticity-as-humanism came from at Hopkins. That plastic meant "white" *made gender work* as an experimental technique for sex assignment. The folding of binary sex normalization into conditions that also included life-threatening and other metabolic irregularities marks the place where the plasticity of the endocrine body is both activated *and* racialized. The line between medical necessity—for instance, preventing death from salt loss or preventing the potentially carcinogenic and cardiac side effects of high amounts of androgen—and the aesthetic normalization of the body and genitals necessarily blurs at the level of technique. This proved significant to gender's clinical efficacy. Money, like Wilkins, justified interventions into the intersex child's body on the grounds of a humanism that read those children's bodies, both abstractly and visibly, as belonging to a whiteness that could not coexist with nonbinary phenotypes. Instead of cardiac risk or cancer, Money used the language of social stigma and adjustment to cover over the arbitrariness of deciding on sex and gender without the consent of the child. Nonbinary children *needed* to be forcibly normalized because their whiteness precluded the social stigma they might otherwise endure.

Although it was not really new, this racialization of plasticity in gender was in a way *more* pernicious in the postwar era than it had been previously because the abandonment of explicitly eugenic science and medicine was also an alibi for a very difficult-to-see racial normativity. It makes sense to say that in its invention gender *was* a form of race. The morphology of the sexed and gendered body *was* a racial formation in Money's schema of development. Put more simply, gender was a phenotype, much as sex had been during the preceding fifty years. By neutralizing the theory of natural human bisexuality, however, gender was a much more rigid phenotype than sex had been, obviating any claim that the human body could be naturally mixed in masculinity and femininity or that it might grow into nonbinary forms naturally.

This is also where Paul B. Preciado's careful attention to the invention of gender in *Testo Junkie* falls dramatically short. In contextualizing Money and his contemporaries in the Cold War and capitalist milieus of postwar American imperialism, technoscientific ideology, and emergent modes of capitalist subjectification, Preciado agrees that gender marked a decisive moment in the twentieth century. "If the concept of gender has introduced a rift," he has written, "the precise reason is that it represents the first self-conscious moment within the epistemology of sexual difference."[62] In other words, "With the notion of gender, the medical discourse is unveiling its arbitrary foundation and its constructivist character, and at the same time opening the way for new forms of resistance and political activism."[63] In neglecting the racialization of gender as phenotype, however, Preciado's calls for "an array of politics of physical experimentation and semiotechnology" in the vein of "practices of autointoxication" or an "auto-experimental form of do-it-yourself bioterrorism of gender" misfires.[64] Deinstitutionalizing the techniques of sex and gender's medicalization in and of itself did not break with the racially normative logic of the alterability of sex and gender as human phenotypes. Access to the tools of a dissident endocrinology was always stratified by race and class, for one thing. At a more abstract level, the gender-hacking body Preciado calls for would also be racialized white in its uncritical affirmation of plasticity's capacity for creative transformation and reinvention. Making use of the same techniques as the medical system, albeit without the endorsement of doctors, did not undermine the racialized economy of plasticity concretized in the 1950s, for it misrecognized the degree to which instability and indeterminacy were incorporated into the clinical invention of gender. What's more, just like Wilkins and Money, Preciado makes the risky assumption that gender's embodied plasticity is actually available for political work, that it has no agency of its own to resist or ignore its technical cultivation.

For that reason it is doubtful that children could even include themselves in such a micropolitics, for their dehumanization by medicine as living laboratories has so severely impaired the exercise of their personhood that it underwrites the model of political agency that *Testo Junkie* promotes. Preciado makes much of the case of "Agnes," a transgender girl who stole estrogen tablets from her mother starting at the age of thirteen and was able to convince doctors at the University of California, Los Angeles, in the late 1950s that she was intersex in order to get access to sex reassignment surgery. For Preciado, Agnes represents "*copyleft gender politics*" where new possibilities for sexed and gendered life were built through "leakage points in the state's control of fluxes."[65] Yet I would argue that such leakages in control are better understood as already incorporated into the medicalization of sex and gender through the operationalization of plasticity in the clinic. Wilkins conceded as much in his difficult attempts to treat salt-losing CAH, and the concession to plasticity's unruliness was codified by Money and the Hampsons in their redefinition of it as temporary and developmental. Plasticity was never meant to be completely controlled; it was always meant to leak out of its institutionalization. That is precisely the work that racial normativity accomplishes for medicine; moments of partial failure actually regenerate the clinical apparatus and make the human form continually available for further alteration. Agnes may have been able to manipulate her doctors and psychiatrists, but the availability of estrogen pills in her white, middle-class home in 1950s Los Angeles was an integral part of why she was of such interest to doctors. Though she may have subverted discourses of gender and sex, she hardly occupied a subversive position within the racialized politics of plasticity.

Could Agnes have broken free from the instrumentalizing interest in her white body that brought so many children like her into clinics? She returns again in chapter 4, which considers these questions anew in the emergence of the new field of transsexual medicine in the United States. At the moment of the invention of gender, however, the reigning mood at Hopkins was to disregard and minimize anything resembling claims to personhood, autonomy, or self-knowledge from children. While many intersex infants were too young to speak or be aware of the therapies administered and procedures performed on them without consent (and many were never told what had been done to their bodies), some children were old enough to talk back to the staff at the Harriet Lane Home.[66] In one of their 1955 papers, Money and the Hampsons narrate the case of a child first admitted at age three and a half. Identifying as a boy, he was diagnosed with "hyperadrenocortical female pseudohermaphroditism." Although at birth doctors felt "uncertain" about the baby's sex, they decided several days later to advise the parents that their child was male. At the Harriet Lane Home, he presented a challenge for Money, the Hampsons, and their staff, who were of the opinion that he should be raised a girl instead. As Money reported,

> As soon as he recognized my face as unfamiliar, he approached me, saying over and over again: "Got to call my Mommy." There was a look of stark terror about him, and a note of frantic urgency in his voice. He did not object to a genital examination, but kept perseverating, uneasily: "The nurse cut my wee-wee." I could not find much logical coherence between this and other reiterated sentences, and could not understand some of his baby-talk pronunciations. I was left wondering whether the child has some kind of cerebral defect.[67]

This, recall, Money was saying of a three-year-old. He ordered an IQ test, which came back with "dull normal level" results (hardly a smoking gun). Money went on to say that "with familiarity, the child's speech became easier to understand."[68] The case summary emphasizes the repetition of the phrases "The nurse cut on my wee-wee. The nurse hurt me. Cut on my wee-wee" and the recurring call to see his mother.[69] Money dismissed the constant concern, retorting that, "in *a typically childish way*, he had grossly misconstrued his surgical experiences to signify that his penis was being mutilated and perhaps might suffer the fate he conceived had befallen his sister's genitals" (i.e., her lack of a penis).[70] Money's rhetoric stood on a rather obtuse adult innocence, as if it had never occurred to him that a three-year-old might express anger and fear at the nontherapeutic surgical alteration of his body without his permission. Money even went as far as to say that "in an older person, this kind of reiterated illogical thinking would be identified as delusional and psychopathological. . . . It is not so completely benign, however, that one cannot afford to treat it casually and with indifference. The longer such misconceptions stay unrectified, *they become increasingly ineradicable.*"[71]

The echo in this interpretation of his theory of gender through the phrase "increasingly ineradicable" is unmistakable. Money labored intensively in the case summary to neutralize the meaning of this intersex child's speech, to render it irrational. If they did not act soon, the child's elected gender role, which was at odds with Money's, would become ineradicable. This time, at least, Money was not to have his way. Despite the child's body being considered by doctors to be "female" in all ways except cortisol overproduction, Money finally conceded that, "for this child, the risk of a sex change ending in psychiatric disaster was judged too great to justify the change."[72] This child, who identified as a boy, was permitted to remain a boy. The possible damage wrought by his severe anxiety over being hospitalized and the power of adults to mutilate his body, of course, had already been done.

Money's developmental wager on plasticity did not eliminate its capacity for embodied resistance. While he may have succeeded in suppressing this boy's speech, his decision not to try reassigning him as a girl is an admission that he could not secure biological consent from this child's body. Plasticity may have been prized discursively for a capacity to take on new forms, but it also expressed its own embodied capacity to grow into forms that disobeyed medical technique and discourse, and Money knew that as well as any of his colleagues. Despite the shifts from the era of Young's surgical procedures to the era of synthetic hormones, Money's theory still almost crumbled in the face of this three-year-old, who seemed to agree with his body's expressive masculine form. The thin scrim of developmental discourse, which had no real referent in the body, allowed Money to escape the collapse of his paradigm, as he could simply argue that this boy's gender identity had already consolidated, that he was too old and no longer plastic enough to be raised as a girl. The self-consciousness weakness of that argument is evident in Money's viciously ignorant dismissal of the boy's speech, the one thing Money *thought* he could control. The clinical scene is shadowed by the knowledge that embodied plasticity, while floating the entire medicalization of sex and gender, also contained the capacity to refuse Money's coercion.

Countless children, like this intersex boy, were forced into serving as living laboratories for the invention of gender. The fact that in less than a decade Money would help found the first gender clinic at a university hospital to provide transition and gender confirmation surgery to trans people is evidence of just how much these children informed the emergent discourse of transsexuality. The invention of gender also signaled a moment of discursive closure, not only because the sex binary was conceptually reinforced but because the loss of the discourse of hermaphroditism included the loss of a certain ambiguity and overlap between trans and intersex life that had proved so profitable during the first half of the century.[73] While clinicians like Young and the psychiatrist Thomas Rennie had exercised a gatekeeping role around trans and intersex patient overlap as early as the 1930s, by the 1950s the medical parameters had narrowed much more profoundly, even as the possibility for trans medicine grew exponentially.

Set in the broader context of this book, where the 1940s and 1950s serve as a bridge between the first and the second half of the trans twentieth century, I am also arguing that the emergence of gender was responsible for the attempted reduction of transition to a binary model. If in the early twentieth century there were multiple definitions of transness that circulated between the lay and the medical domains, the postwar concept of transsexuality tried to double down on binary transition as the only acceptable model because the concept of gender greatly reinforced the binary coherence of sex. The irony is that the very medical paradigm that would finally permit institutional medical transition and gender reassignment in the United States on a large scale would also dramatically curtail the types of trans people eligible for such treatment and the forms of medical support that they would be allowed to access. Money's developmental argument helped to implant at the core of transsexual medicine the idea that the only acceptable transition was from one visibly binary sex to another, installing passing as a medical goal. Nonbinary and "intermediary" forms of social and embodied life that had characterized trans life in its interaction with medicine over the previous five decades were deeply restricted now that binary masculinity and femininity had been reinforced as developmental phenotypes for all human beings. While these restrictions had been under construction for several decades, the concept of gender gave them a vicious clinical force that disqualified less medicalized or nonmedicalized forms of trans and intersex life that had retained some autonomy from the clinic in the early twentieth century.

But Money, like Wilkins and Young, ultimately risked too much on the premise that he could direct plasticity into predictable binary forms, and the next two chapters show how the imposition of binary transition by the medical model of transsexuality was unable to extinguish the multiple definitions of transness that had flourished in the early twentieth century, particularly in the case of children. Plasticity and development's multiple itineraries continued to antagonize clinical practice well into the postwar era. While the resistance of a three-year-old who challenged Money on his medical authority and the violent effects of such normative logics were dismissed by him as so much childishness, transgender children who had to fight their way into clinics in the 1960s would take up their embodied plasticity in creative and unpredictable ways.

CHAPTER 4

From Johns Hopkins to the Midwest

Transgender Childhood in the 1960s

T HE OPENING OF THE GENDER IDENTITY CLINIC at the Johns Hopkins Hospital was framed as a watershed moment for the new field of transsexual medicine at the time of its announcement, in November 1966. Fearing that it would in fact be *too* momentous an event for a controversial field, the Gender Identity Committee that oversaw the clinic, composed of senior figures in obstetrics and gynecology, psychiatry, pediatrics, and plastic surgery, including Lawson Wilkins and John Money, had actually never intended to go public. They had come close to exposure once after the clinic's first patient, a black trans woman referred from New York by Harry Benjamin, received a cash offer from the Baltimore *Afro-American* to cover her story.[1] The doctors managed to discourage her from doing the article, and her gender confirmation surgery was undertaken in relative secret. A few months later, however, the *New York Daily News* described a "stunning girl who admits she was male less than a year ago and that she underwent a sex change operation at, of all places, Johns Hopkins Hospital in Baltimore."[2] When the article prompted a phone call to the clinic from a *New York Times* reporter, the Committee decided to hold a press conference to get in front of the story.[3]

At the press conference, the Committee explained that the clinic had been created "to deal with the problems of the transsexual, physically normal people who are psychologically the opposite sex," and that it had "been in operation de facto for one year," though only the one person so far had advanced to the surgery stage.[4] Other patients were working their way through the clinic's incremental process, which included extensive medical and psychiatric examination, hormone therapy, and a pilot requirement of living publicly in one's gender identity for at least a year before surgery.[5] Money served as something like the intermediary between the clinic and Harry Benjamin's practice in New York, which referred most of the first patients who had not already been to Hopkins. The funding for the clinic was also, like Benjamin's, underwritten by the Erickson Educational Foundation, a philanthropic organization funded by the oil magnate and trans man Reed Erickson and dedicated to trans causes.[6] While before the press conference the clinic had received around 100 requests from people in the know seeking transition and surgery, after going public the number of requests skyrocketed, with more than 1,500 reaching Hopkins over the following two years.[7]

Dedicated exclusively to a trans clientele, the Hopkins program positioned itself as a brand-new type of clinic in the United States and is described as such in most transgender histories.[8] What its doctors did *not* disclose at that press conference, however, greatly revises the way we understand trans life in the 1960s. In 1964, a year before the clinic was established in secret, Money and several of his colleagues had been aggressively lobbying to take on as a full-time patient someone they had recently diagnosed as transsexual. In January 1965 they succeeded: the Criminal Court for Baltimore City, where the prospective patient was on trial for burglary, issued a court order for "surgical sex repair" at Hopkins in lieu of incarceration.[9] The judge was convinced by Money and his peers that the defendant's criminal record was really a side effect of a misunderstood medical condition, "transsexualism," and that surgery would break a spell of delinquency, arrest, and state institutionalization that stretched back some five years. The patient, "G.L.," was transferred from jail to a ward at Hopkins to await surgery. At the time, however, G.L. was only seventeen years old; their[10] mother had to consent to the judge's order and sign the medical consent form for the surgery. Psychiatrists at Hopkins had been in contact with G.L. since age thirteen, when G.L. was referred to the hospital by school officials for delinquent behavior.[11] G.L.'s case history indicates that the first official gender confirmation surgery for a trans patient at Hopkins was actually arranged for a child. Or rather, it should have been. Conservative forces in the psychiatric faculty at Hopkins succeeded in delaying the surgery date several times, and in the interval G.L. ran away from the ward, never to return.

What does it mean that this "watershed" moment for transsexual medicine is shadowed by the absent presence of a trans child a year earlier? The 1960s were a decade of proliferation and early consolidation for transsexual medicine, as Benjamin, Money, and other, lesser-known doctors greatly elaborated its nosology and basic protocols and began a sustained public relations campaign with the help of trans people to establish its legitimacy.

Some doctors also began providing gender confirmation surgery with regularity across the United States for the first time. During the same period, trans activism took on a more public and combative role. The Compton's Cafeteria Riot, for instance, happened in San Francisco only a few months before the press conference at Hopkins.[12] Yet the scrutiny applied to this decade has not considered the ways in which children understood themselves to be transsexual too, let alone were able to seek out and be recognized by doctors. Some trans children, like G.L., found doctors who were willing to oversee hormone treatment, public transition, and even gender confirmation surgery under the pretense that it would constitute an experimental test case. For other children, by contrast, doctors were more interested in trying to *extinguish* transsexuality during childhood, now theorized as the developmental period of its onset. These latter clinics tended to favor psychotherapy or psychoanalysis over endocrine therapy, although when the psychological approach consistently failed it was often followed, if reluctantly, by hormones.

What both clinical approaches have in common is that the plastic body of the child had become so naturalized that it served as the foundation upon which medical and psychological interest in self-identified trans children became meaningful. Children were of immense importance to the first full decade of transsexual medicine because they incarnated the alterability of the biological body in development, promising the future growth of the field of medicine in every sense of the word. That the part children played in this decade has been completely overlooked only underlines the immense purchase of the racial plasticity of the trans child's body in the postwar era. Children were meant to recede into the background of the gender identity clinic, to remain the developmental and plastic bedrock upon which doctors conducted their work, even though plasticity itself was in reality far from a passive force. Trans children, too, were far from passive and compliant with this project.

G.L.'s life was forcibly rendered into discourse by the language of law and medicine, leaving nothing else behind in the archive, particularly in the way of their own self-knowledge, voice, or perspective on their arrest, trial, and time spent at Hopkins. However, some trans children in the 1960s punctuated their increasing objectification and instrumentalization, if only momentarily. At the same time that doctors were cataloguing and theorizing the childhood onset of transsexuality, the instability of plasticity emerged especially "sideways"[13] in the accounts trans children gave of themselves.

Particularly in their letters to doctors, children demonstrated that the biological body manifested as a problem of form, where the potential meanings of "growth" were disrespectful of the developmental medical model. Forms of growth not quite (binary) gendered yet not teleological gathered in these letters, suggesting some of the ways in which trans children engaged their own lives on terms not wholly captured by medicine, however fragile and short-lived. In reconstructing children's role in the emergence of transsexuality, the *weakness* of medicine's pretension to have played a causal role in defining trans life is found in the ghostly surrounds of official discourse. Yet the undermining of transsexuality's rationality through the vibrancy, latency, and laterality of trans children also meets a second kind of boundary. A decidedly visual and visceral form of antiblackness constituted a much starker line between those trans children who were able to write into the formal problem of their bodies and those black trans and trans children of color whose traces of life during the decade are left behind in the more destructive context of institutions of confinement and deprivation such as the psychiatric ward. This chapter follows the trans child's body across the clinic, the written letter, and the psychiatric ward to limn some of the fragile apertures and harsh closures of the 1960s.

The Formation of Transsexual Medicine

Hopkins may have been the first American hospital to offer gender confirmation surgery for transgender patients in a formal clinic, but its opening was prefaced by some fifty years of work with intersex and trans people. The techniques of hormonal transition and surgeries, as the preceding chapters have explored, had been well established for some time. Still, until the 1960s it was incredibly difficult and rare to find a venue in which to perform surgery without a recognized endocrine or genital "abnormality" (categories from which transsexuality was excluded because the biological body was judged "normal"). Rather than naming some technical or paradigm shift in the 1960s that would account for the transformation of American medical norms and the consolidation of a field of transsexual medicine, I argue that much of the key change in attitude among professionals came from their increasing experience working *with* trans patients and members of the community who strongly advocated for themselves. It was patients who convinced doctors to take their self-knowledge and requests more seriously, although this task was much harder for children. While hormones

were not very controversial, before G.L. trans patients of all ages were sty-
mied in their efforts to access surgery.

When the Brady Urological Institute at Hopkins finally became willing to diagnose patients with "transvestism" and, soon thereafter, "transsexualism," in the mid- to late 1950s, a shift in attitude slowly took root
among those doctors who would later form the Gender Identity Clinic.[14]
In 1959 Milton Edgerton, a prominent figure in the Plastic Surgery Department, brought a private client of his to the Institute. A trans woman from
New York in her late thirties, "Lane's" recorded complaint on admission
came in the form of an unambiguous, direct quote: "I would like to be converted from male into female as completely as possible." Edgerton reported
that since the age of eighteen, when she left her hometown in Missouri,
Lane had "dressed and lived in the role of a woman in society," building a
successful career as a dancer.[15] She had lived with a man for eight years, to
the point that Edgerton referred in his notes to their "marriage," although
the relationship had broken off a few years prior. In 1955 Lane had found a
doctor in New York who referred her to a colleague willing to provide
breast augmentation surgery. Edgerton remarked that "she selected the
woman physician because it seemed to her that a woman should just know
more about a woman's body than a male surgeon might." Unfortunately,
the "ivalon mammoplasty," which was a brand-new procedure, led to a complication in one breast, requiring that the implant be removed and put back
in. Now that the issue was resolved, however, Lane reported feeling much
happier. Edgerton asked her how her friends would describe her after surgery. "She states that they tell her that she is much more 'interesting,'" he
recorded, "there is now a gleam in her eyes, that she is 'much more fun to
be with.' The patient verifies that these reflect her internal feelings and she
says, 'in fact, I am quite a different person.'"[16]

Edgerton's use of Lane's preferred pronouns in her medical records represents a significant departure from decades of a detached, disregarding
view practiced by most medical professionals with trans patients. It seems
that Lane had made something of an advocate out of Edgerton by the time
he arranged for her to visit the Institute. "The patient would suggest to
me that she is quite determined and consistent in her desire to remain as
a female in her role in society," he explains. "She has arranged with considerable competence to support herself and to avoid serious emotional
depression with a very difficult adjustment problem in the past 20 years."
As a plastic surgeon, Edgerton hedged that "it would be difficult for me to

pass on the psychological indications for this surgery," but he nonetheless argued quite strongly that "the patient could withstand the surgical procedures." Although he did "not believe this operation has been performed in previous cases reported in medical literature," referring to the United States, Edgerton began to outline his plan for how, "if we elect to go ahead with this surgery," there would be a team of endocrinologists at the Brady Institute with whom he would like to work, and he summarized the technique of vaginoplasty he would like to undertake. "We explained to the patient that we would not undertake surgery without the full consent and cooperation of the psychiatric and medical physicians who have seen her," he concluded.[17]

This last caveat proved to be insurmountable. Lane was interviewed by two psychologists, John Hampson (who worked on Money's psychohormonal team) and John Shaffer. The latter "spent some eight hours with the patient, evaluating the patient's psychological state by various personality surgery and project tests." Lane then met with the psychiatrist Eugene Meyer, who penned a report to Edgerton. "The operation requested by this patient is an unusual one," he suggested at the outset. Meyer was impressed that many of Lane's colleagues and friends did not know she was a trans woman and that "questioning elicits no 'break' in patient's female self concept." Other than some depression stemming from the breakup of her longterm relationship, Meyer emphasized in his evaluation the absence of any psychological distress, psychosis, or "schizophrenic trends." Indeed, he went so far as to say that "I have no evidence that the patient's personality, level of anxiety or state of psychic organization is such as to definitely contraindicate any operative procedure."[18]

Writing to Edgerton alone, Meyer was quite candid. "My initial reaction to this proposal and to serious contemplation of its implementation by surgery was a distinctly negative one. My first reasoning was that anyone contemplating and seeking such an operation, by definition, had to be mentally unbalanced to a major degree and, therefore, any operation could only supplement and deepen neurotic or psychotic trends." In an uncharacteristic moment of honesty for a psychiatrist, however, he went on to say: "After seeing the patient and talking with Drs. Hampson and Shaffer, this first perception or view has altered." Admitting the lack of local precedent, at least in his mind, for "such an unusual and rare operation," as well as vague "legal aspects," Meyer nevertheless concluded that "it is conceivable, although it defies most deeply ingrained assumptions, that the operation contemplated could result in a measure of psychologic [sic] relief. . . . It seems to me that the decision must be made in light of these facts." However, Lane's medical file ends after this letter. Although the precise reason is not archived, it is mostly likely that the willingness of Meyer to sign off on the psychiatric rationale and of Edgerton to undertake surgery was met with a firm refusal from the senior staff at the Brady Institute or elsewhere at Hopkins. Still, in convincing the two of them to endorse her goals, Lane exemplifies the real difference trans people were making in their concerted efforts to challenge medical professionals to listen to them and fulfill their requests.[19]

Interestingly, Money's name is conspicuously absent from Lane's records. It seems during the 1950s that he played a fairly aggressive gatekeeping role at the Institute, attempting to dismiss trans patients when they came looking for support and access to surgery. In 1954, when a retired trans woman from Ohio came to Baltimore, Money wrote her a lengthy letter. "The main body of this letter," he explained to his colleagues in a separate report, "is used in reply to all homosexuals and transvestites who write seeking information about treatment."[20] The text is quite difficult to interpret. It makes several claims that appear outright disingenuous coming from Money, given his simultaneous work on the sex reassignment of intersex children and the new theory of gender he was preparing to publicize. To a certain extent, the letter suggests a rhetorical strategy at a very conservative medical institution, where Money would have to work carefully and behind the scenes for more than a decade before getting his first approval for surgery, for G.L. At the same time, the letter also testifies to the harsh clinical reality of the decade during which transsexual medicine emerged. Doctors were perfectly willing to diagnose, evaluate, and study trans patients in detail for the benefit of their own research before brusquely rejecting their actual requests.

Money began by drawing a hard line between "two quite distinct types of sexual disorder," intersex embodiment ("Physical disorders in which the sexual organs are improperly formed . . . and other sexual features of the body do not develop properly at the end of childhood) and "nonphysical disorders, like homosexuality and transvestism, in which there are peculiarities in the growth and development . . . all of which are subject to learning, especially in the earliest period of childhood." While the separation of intersex and trans categories had been growing at Hopkins since at least the 1930s, Money's further distinction between intersex cases, which were "physical," and trans cases, which were "nonphysical" and "subject to learning," anticipated the new framework of transsexuality. Breaking with the model of the early twentieth century, he stated that "there is not a fragment of medical evidence to suggest that these disorders are caused by abnormalities of the hormone-producing glands"—although, as we will see, some of Money's peers disagreed with him on this point.[21]

Despite the early outline of a differential transsexual diagnostic model, Money's main point teetered on the disingenuous. "Changes of sex, about which you asked," he wrote, "in this country are not performed on physically normal people like yourself." This was not inaccurate, on the whole, since no U.S. hospital had as yet officially sanctioned surgery. His substantiation of that point, that "it is impossible to undo the work of nature," however, ignored even his own research projects at Hopkins. Anticipating a central transphobic argument from the political right and trans exclusionary feminists, Money claimed that "a man cannot be turned into a woman. It is possible to remove all the male sexual organs surgically, but it is not possible to supply all the female reproductive organs, so that the patient ends up neither female nor male." Similarly, he contended that "it is possible to give hormones so that the breasts will grow on either males or females, but in a male the beard continues to require shaving and the voice remains as masculine as ever." Much of this characterization of transition and surgery was simply medically inaccurate, and it's likely that many of the patients to whom Money sent this letter knew that.[22]

Anticipating that this argument would read as ridiculous, Money added a second, "the psychological one," although this stood on even less solid ground in light of his ongoing research on gender. "According to all the available medical evidence," he explained, "it is impossible for a person to change all the habits of a lifetime as a male—habits of thought, of feeling and of action—simply because he gets hormones and undergoes surgery." Again anticipating trans exclusionary feminist arguments, he claimed, "You may wear women's clothes but, in spite of your conviction of yourself, you will never think and feel like a woman, through and through." The contrivance on display in this letter was reinforced by its ending, which backtracked to a fair degree, no doubt in recognition that these arguments were unlikely to convince any trans patient who made the effort to seek out the Brady Institute. Money advised the trans woman to whom he was writing to "continue with this judicious combination of expressing yourself at some times, and of holding yourself in check at others." This was in spite of the fact that the immense emotional strain of being able to live as a woman only part time had caused her to experience periodic blackouts, one of the reasons that she had come to Hopkins in the first place. Unable to restrain his desire to study trans life even when he simultaneously refused to consider the situated perspective of a trans person, Money closed the letter by asking that she keep in touch. "Please feel free to write again," he said, apparently without irony, "if you think that we at the Johns Hopkins Hospital can be of further assistance."[23]

These abrupt blockades of access to medical care were not unique to Hopkins, either. Even when doctors at other institutions officially arranged surgery for trans patients, last-minute legal interventions from local hospital boards frequently prevented procedures from being carried out. When the former GI Christine Jorgensen returned to the United States from Denmark in 1953 to a massive media storm, her narrative of traveling to Europe to obtain surgery was instantly iconic in part because it was relatively accurate. From the early 1950s to the mid-1960s, Benjamin kept track of the places to which his patients who had the means traveled in hopes of undergoing "the conversion operation" and prominently among them figured Denmark, Italy, Morocco, and Mexico. In a few cases, some trans women were successful in having surgery performed ad hoc in the United States, but only after undertaking the dangerous step of self-castration to prompt emergency intervention. In 1965, when the Hopkins gender clinic opened, a few rare surgeries had been performed in New York City, San Francisco, Houston, and Memphis.[24] The only serious attempt at regularly undertaking gender confirmation surgery for trans patients prior to the opening of the Hopkins clinic was likely Elmer Belt's private urology practice in Los Angeles in the late 1950s, but by 1962 he gave up without having completed a single procedure, facing too much opposition and obstruction from local hospital boards.[25]

In 1958 "Agnes" saw the psychiatrist and psychoanalyst Robert Stoller at the nearby University of California, Los Angeles, Medical Center. Assigned a boy at birth, Agnes knew from a young age that she was a girl and was now, reaching adulthood, searching for a doctor to obtain access to gender confirmation surgery. When Stoller and his colleagues examined Agnes, they found her to be by their standards a "normal," if "feminine"-looking, "male," with one glaring exception: her gonads produced an incredibly high level of estrogen, no doubt a large part of the reason for her feminine appearance. Such a starkly biological suggestion of transsexuality had never been

observed, and the case greatly excited Stoller as the beginning of a definitive endocrine theory that would legitimate and clarify the new field
of medicine.[26] After later undergoing surgery, however, Agnes returned to
UCLA for a follow-up interview during which she confessed that she had
actually started taking her mother's estrogen pills at age thirteen in hopes
of changing her body.[27] She had not previously disclosed this to her doctors,
and it turned out that her estrogen-producing "testes" had never really
existed. Benjamin, who had been following the case, was deeply disappointed but continued to hold out for a biological explanation for transsexuality. In the mid-1960s he latched onto new neuroendocrine research
on the relationship of the gonads to the hypothalamus, hoping for a possible brain-based hormonal explanation.[28] Importantly, these initial forays
into the gonads and the brain served to reinforce a developmental framing of transsexuality's onset. Agnes's careful manipulation of her doctors
is also one evocative example of how trans children attempted to work
within the severe constraints of a model that took great interest in their plastic bodies but offered them no voice or autonomy in making medical decisions. That Agnes was also a middle-class, white trans child whose mother
had a seemingly massive supply of oral estrogen tablets, however, is a second key detail about how the new category of transsexuality was racialized
in the 1960s.

While the straightforwardly biological explanation for transsexuality
Benjamin hoped for never materialized, he still contributed greatly to the
consolidation of the field from the early 1950s to the late 1960s. Five decades
after Magnus Hirschfeld's work on transvestism, the word "transsexual" was
first employed in English by the sexologist David O. Cauldwell in a 1949
article to describe a patient who desired to change sex but otherwise was
considered to be biologically "normal."[29] Louise Lawrence, a well-connected
trans woman in the San Francisco Bay Area who was helping Benjamin contact similar people at the turn of the 1950s, introduced him to Cauldwell's
work, from which he adopted the term "transsexuality."[30] Still, Benjamin
also felt attached to the taxonomy and approach inherited from his old
friend Hirschfeld. Benjamin's informal experience with trans patients at the
turn of the 1950s, adding to his preexisting reputation as a leading endocrinologist bridging the American and the European traditions, amounted to
a certain instant renown—not to mention his willingness to serve as a
congenial patriarchal figure. In 1953 he met Christine Jorgensen, recently
returned from Denmark. [31] Benjamin took her on as a patient in his private

practice, and they began strategizing about what to do with the countless letters written to Jorgensen seeking support in obtaining health care and gender confirmation surgery. As was so frequently the case for Benjamin, the help and labor of well-connected trans community members like Jorgensen and Lawrence made his clinical research possible.[32] And yet while doctors were far from the only labor force behind the discourse on transsexuality, they received nearly all of the credit and recognition.

In 1953 Benjamin put together a symposium on transsexuality, which took place at the New York Academy of Medicine. In several articles that followed from its proceedings he outlined the new diagnostic category. Reflecting his ties to the pre–World War II era of endocrine and sex research, he proposed that "it is well known that sex is never one hundred per cent 'male' or 'female.' It is a blend of a complex variety of male-female components." The medical management of "'intersexes' of varying character, degree and intensity," moreover, "makes 'sex' a rather flexible concept." The ultimate point of this work was to reject transsexuality as psychosis and instead propose a psychosomatic outline of a condition coherent enough to merit hormone treatment and gender confirmation surgery. Reaffirming the centrality of a developmental, biological etiology to all sexual morphologies of the body, Benjamin opined that "the genetic and/or endocrine constitution (often a psychosexual *infantilism*) has to provide a 'fertile soil' on which the 'basic conflict' must grow" into transsexuality. In theorizing such a biological basis for a condition primarily expressed psychologically, he added, rhetorically, "Has not [Eugen] Steinach shown us in his highly suggestive experiments how feminized male guinea pigs . . . *behaved* like females[?]"[33]

In 1964 the Harry Benjamin Foundation was established through a three-year grant from the Erickson Educational Foundation (EEF); indeed, without the financial backing of Erickson, a trans man, it is unlikely that transsexual medicine would have grown and professionalized in the 1960s.[34] Benjamin used the opportunity to formalize his working relationships with most of the other prominent researchers and doctors in the field, building a national advisory board with several connections to Europe.[35] A smaller, dedicated group of researchers who were able to make the regular trip to New York convened at trustee meetings at which patients were presented and discussed across disciplines and institutions. When the Hopkins Gender Identity Clinic started to take shape the following year, it was integrated into the work of the Foundation, with a similar overture made toward the

Stanford gender clinic that soon followed. Yet the funding flow from the EEF was transient, and Benjamin had an extremely querulous relationship with his wealthy benefactor, Erickson. By 1967, as the initial grant period was drawing to a close, Benjamin's Foundation was practically bankrupt and was therefore forced to cease formal operations.[36] Nevertheless, during its existence the Foundation served as a key vehicle for connecting and promoting the research that was the basis for transsexual medicine at otherwise disparate locations across the country.

Benjamin also decided to write a book that could appeal to sympathetic but uninformed doctors, as well as prospective or current trans patients eager for more information and a scientific authority. When he sat down to write *The Transsexual Phenomenon* in 1964, Benjamin had records on hand from 189 trans patients at his private endocrine clinic. He began by running a series of data analyses on them that provide some insight into how children fit into the first few years of his transsexual practice and the Foundation. His youngest recorded patient at the time was seventeen, and there were a half-dozen other teenagers under the age of medical consent in his roster, there presumably with the consent of their parents.[37] Benjamin was very interested in the childhoods of his patients for elaborating the onset of transsexuality, or what he had speculatively called "psychosexual infantilism" in 1953. To that end, he examined his patient data to see the "first evidence" of their sense of gender identity. Nearly all his patient records returned answers such as "Always" or "As long as remembers." He also noted the age of onset of puberty and various kinds of "Evidence of Childhood Conditioning" that might explain his patients' cross-sex identifications.[38]

The Transsexual Phenomenon that resulted is a roaming, undisciplined text that attempts to introduce a range of skeptical or curious readers to a new field of medicine draped in rhetorical mystique, while mounting a polemic in favor of legitimizing gender confirmation surgery. Benjamin's mostly pedagogical mode of address covers a range of subjects, couching transsexuality in a Steinach-derived theory of human bisexuality and plasticity, adjusted to the postwar era. With a nod to Money's work from the 1950s, in particular, Benjamin explained that "'gender' is the nonsexual side of sex," which is to say the psychological manifestation of what, trained in the German tradition of medicine and biology, he had long just called "sex." More important than nomenclature, according to Benjamin, was the fact that "the advancement of biologic and especially of genetic studies" has eliminated any "absolute division" of the sexes. In his estimation, "The dominant status of the genital organs for the determination of one's sex has been shaken, at least in the world of science."[39] Benjamin summarized "up to ten or more separate concepts and manifestations of sex" that compose each individual, positing that the exact balance of genetic and environmental factors remains unknown, asking readers to "keep an open mind."[40] Nevertheless, true to his field, he still emphasized that masculinity and femininity are "to a large extent" results of "the *endocrine sex*," which, as he impressed upon readers, is "mixed" in every person "to an even greater extent" than any other factor. "Therefore," Benjamin concluded with his characteristic confidence, "we are all 'intersexes,' anatomically as well as endocrinologically."[41]

This broadly intersex explanation for sex in general and transsexuality in particular may seem somewhat counterintuitive in view of Benjamin's goal of legitimizing a new field of medical specialization. In claiming that biology teaches that we are all a mix of male and female, he teetered on the edge of the radical claim that transsexuality is unexceptional and potentially a universal tendency of sexed life—something like a morphological counterpart to Gayle Rubin's proposal of "benign sexual variation" as a model for thinking about sexual practices and cultures.[42] The implication was hardly one that Benjamin endorsed, and the rest of *The Transsexual Phenomenon* veers into an armchair-slumming account of perversion and tragedy restricted to a small minority of the population, as if to violently undo the prospect.

Still, the plastic value of biology and the endocrine body were both such that Benjamin felt convinced that the treatment of transsexuality as a "mental state" required not psychotherapy but hormones and surgery.[43] The lack of specificity in defining transsexuality in relation to intersex conditions constitutes an epistemological problem that *The Transsexual Phenomenon*, like the new field of medicine to which it contributed, could not resolve—it had been growing, after all, since the early twentieth century. "To avoid misunderstanding," Benjamin clarified at one point that transsexuality "has nothing to do with hermaphroditism," but without a substantive explanation as to why.[44] His insistence on the naturalness of life's bisexuality could not contain the cross-contamination between the two ostensibly abnormal categories (transsexuality and intersex) and the ostensibly normal category (a cisgender body, which, as Benjamin had already established, does not even exist in reality). Only the developmental timescale of biology and childhood is able to bring order to this matrix of sex and gender by making intersex and transsexuality two "underdeveloped" forms of human life, as he put it, incomplete versions of male or female human form requiring medical intervention to achieve normal articulation.[45] The child, in other words, intervenes once again to organize the field of sex and gender along a teleological progression from an original bisexuality to a mature masculinity or femininity. The arbitrariness of that teleology, though, haunts *The Transsexual Phenomenon*, as it had Hugh Hampton Young, Wilkins, and Money before him.

Benjamin also faced the nosological challenge of distinguishing the new category "transsexualism" from "transvestism." The latter, which for Hirschfeld at the turn of the twentieth century encompassed both erotic cross-dressing and living in a sex different from the one assigned at birth, could not easily be left behind, not in the least because many patients were not especially invested in drawing a distinction or adopting the new medical category. Louise Lawrence, for instance, was happy to call herself a transvestite in the late 1950s, and while she lived full time as a woman, she felt no need for hormone therapy or surgery, observing that "the 'Christine Jorgensen' trend" was a generational shift at best, rather than a medical truth, or a passing fad, at worst.[46] To manage the varying degrees of biological or cultural tint to transvestism and transsexuality, Benjamin concocted a Sexual Orientation Scale (S.O.S.) with seven degrees of cross-dressing and/or the desire to change sex, hopeful that it would work well enough descriptively to encompass most of his patients.[47] Only the most "extreme" cases on his scale—that is, a "seven"—would qualify in his mind for gender confirmation surgery.

Benjamin also had to distinguish transsexuality from homosexuality, still laminated onto sex and gender through the historical residue of the nineteenth-century discourse of inversion. Indeed, he lamented in *The Transsexual Phenomenon* that Americans insisted that the terminology of homosexuality refer to the realm of gender identity even though the German idiom of "intersexuality," in his estimation, is more tolerant of the biological and psychological intricacy demonstrated by human life.[48] Nevertheless, Benjamin also staked a relatively unambiguous claim to analytical separation of gender from object choice, one that would become integral to the medical gatekeeping around transsexuality: "The sex relations of the male homosexual are those of a man with man. The sex relations of a male transsexual are those of a woman with a man, hindered only by the anatomical structures that an operation has to alter."[49]

Benjamin's interest in the trans childhoods of his adult patients is evident in his observation early on in *The Transsexual Phenomenon* that "true transsexuals," in his experience, "invariably date the beginning of their deviation to earliest childhood." "While it is quite possible that such statements may merely express the wish that it be so," Benjamin emphasized that "transvestic tendencies, in the great majority of all cases, were noted in the first five or six years of the child's life."[50] The developmental framing he borrowed from Money's new concept of gender, according to which any natural bisexuality at birth must grow into either a masculine or a feminine form by adulthood, made the child a necessary core of Benjamin's category of transsexuality. Although he could never satisfactorily prove his speculations about its neuroendocrine basis, the scientific and medical consensus on the incredibly plasticity of children's bodies and minds carried enough force to travel with his research and writing in the 1960s. Benjamin's clinical research on trans children also remained largely theoretical and retrospective, since he saw only a handful of teenage patients at his practice on the Upper West Side of Manhattan prior to the 1970s. It was on the other side of the country that one clinic began taking on many trans children of all ages and, in so doing, found quickly that plasticity was much more autonomous than the new discourse of transsexual medicine desired it to be.

Childhood Transition in the 1960s:
UCLA's Gender Identity Research Clinic

The Department of Psychiatry at the University of California, Los Angeles, founded a Gender Identity Research Clinic in 1962. Since this clinic never offered gender confirmation surgery or explicitly suggested it was created for trans patients, it has generally not been considered to "precede" the Hopkins clinic, despite having opened earlier. With funding from the National Institute of Mental Health (NIMH), it lasted into the 1970s, although by then its work with young children had come under heavy fire, mainly from gay activists who protested psychotherapeutic attempts at eliminating effeminacy or proto-homosexuality in young children.[51] At the time of the clinic's founding, a memo circulated by the Department of Psychiatry explained that it would "study and provide treatment for intersexed patients," but this was probably a strategic misdirection. Despite stressing that "we are not at this time offering diagnostic treatment services for anatomically and endocrinologically normal homosexuals, transvestites, or other sexually perverse patients," such patients *precisely* became the main focus of the clinic.[52] The historical porosity of intersex and trans life inherited from the early twentieth century still provided enough cover for an interdisciplinary organization that saw a wide range of trans and gay patients, including many children as young as three to five years old. Not offering surgery, UCLA perhaps made itself more accessible to a range of patients who did not necessarily fit the new diagnostic archetype of trans-sexuality and helped it secure direct funding from the university and from NIMH, which was exceedingly rare during this decade. The clinic's archi-tects were also more interested in psychology and psychoanalysis than any of their contemporaries, especially Benjamin and Money. The psychiatrists, psychologists, and psychoanalysts who ran the clinic during the 1960s were generally skeptical of the prevailing obsession with endocrinology in diagnosing and treating transsexuality. They felt that psychotherapeutic approaches had not been exhausted and that children, in particular, repre-sented a unique opportunity for such treatments. However, through their opposition the clinicians at UCLA were just as entangled with the prob-lem of the plastic body as were their colleagues on the East Coast.

Robert Stoller, who directed the clinic for much of the 1960s, is emblem-atic of this psychological take on the plasticity of gender. Trained as both a psychiatrist and a psychoanalyst, he directed the clinic with Richard Green, who had studied under Money in medical school. From UCLA, Stoller developed a distinct critique of Money's vision of gender identity and sex assignment, one that did not quite oppose psychology to biology but at least argued that the former could be used more profitably to overcome any variance in the latter—in many ways an inversion of Benjamin's para-digm. As the 1960s wore on and the hope of an endocrine explanation for transsexuality continued to evade researchers—notably in the high-profile case of Agnes, who had apparently made a resentful enemy out of Stoller by outwitting him—UCLA became a home to work that was both hos-tile to and suspicious of trans children, while ironically going much further with hormone treatment and transition for children than the ostensibly welcoming clinics on the East Coast.

Stoller's account of the psychodynamic etiology of transsexuality dur-ing childhood was similar to arguments made by psychoanalysts about the genesis of homosexuality in the 1950s. He argued that too much closeness between an infant assigned male at birth and its mother at a developmentally sensitive moment precipitated an originary identification with femininity in the baby. That first identification, given time, would eventually grow into adult transsexuality. Whether or not milder versions of the same process explained homosexuality or effeminacy was a question that Stoller tried clarify, with as little success as Benjamin had had. In making this argument, Stoller's work on transsexuality assigned to itself the ambitious task of rewriting Freud's theory of infantile sexual development: basically, a debiologizing reading of sexuation. "What Freud thought was an elemental quality, 'masculine protest' or 'repudiation of femininity' in men," Stoller explained, "rather than reflecting a biological force, is a quite non-biological defensive maneuver against an earlier stage: closeness and *primitive identification with the mother*. Comparably in females earlier than penis envy in little girls is a stage of *primary femininity*. The biological lies deeper still."[53] This theory of "too much mother," while barely distinct from contemporaneous models of the psychogenesis of homosexuality, drew its impetus instead from Money's imprinting theory of gender identity, analogized to language. In the archetypical case of the transsexual, Stoller saw the mother's imprinting of femininity onto the child through too much closeness as the pathological assumption of gender identity during a crucial infantile stage of development.

Unlike his psychoanalytic peers, Stoller saw no conflict at the core of transsexuality but rather a pathological primary identification. In his contemptuously titled book *The Transsexual Experiment*, published in the 1970s and based on his research at UCLA, he explained the distinction this way: "I see male transsexualism [sic] as an identity *per se*, not primarily as the surface manifestation of a never-ending unconscious struggle to preserve identity. To me, transsexualism is the expression of the subject's 'true self' (Winnicott's term)."[54] Rather than transsexuality being the symptom of a deeper conflict in gender and personality, Stoller repurposed it as the pathological *absence* of a conflict between normatively antagonistic masculinity and femininity. Through this move, Stoller located himself squarely within the developmental paradigm of sex and gender, for the acquisition of that Winnicottian "true self" marked a threshold after which a transsexual identity was effectively unalterable by therapy. The psychic plasticity of gender had by then closed, an assumption drawn by analogy from biological theories of sexual differentiation, as much as Stoller claimed to present an alternative to biological approaches.

Despite his open and virulent pathologization of trans people, Stoller was ironically willing to reluctantly endorse the pursuit of transition for patients who had crossed that threshold. For those young enough not to have reached that developmental stage, however, Stoller felt that a transsexual identification and resulting identity could be preempted, if not aggressively eradicated, by sustained psychodynamic therapy. "It seems impossible to treat the adult transsexual successfully," he suggested in *The Transsexual Experiment.* "Even at age 6 or 7, our work is formidable."[55] This intensified emphasis on the childhood onset of gender identity magnified the importance of children to the medicalization of transsexuality during the 1960s perhaps even more than Benjamin would have sought. As Stoller put it bluntly: "Treatment of the transsexual boy may be the only way to prevent adult transsexualism."[56] Trans children, however, were rarely as obliging as Stoller imagined.

Unsurprisingly, given the rigid reading of sexual difference in Freud upon which this theory relied, therapy for trans girls essentially consisted of attempting to induce an Oedipal complex through the transferential interventions of a male therapist.[57] Given the phallocentric presumptions of "male transsexuality" and "too much mother" that lay at the heart of Stoller's model, he also had very little to say about the trans-masculine experience, save for a rather clumsy chapter in *The Transsexual Experiment* in which he inverted the terms of his theory of trans-feminine patients. Yet the hard-line quality of his published work was not reflected in Stoller's clinical practice, not to mention the work of his colleagues at UCLA's gender clinic. Many so-called effeminate boys *were* brought in by highly anxious, overwhelmingly white, and middle-class parents for consultation and psychotherapy. In these cases, which became the subject of outrage for gay activists, the prescription often mimicked the stark terms of *The Transsexual Experiment, at least at first.* Green worked with many of these children and their parents, and a transcript from one consultation undertaken in 1969 suggests the pervasive social anxiety over white masculinity and the developmental basis of gender identity that drove this aspect of the clinic's work:

DR. G.: How did you hear about my work here? Were you referred?
MR.: We read it in the L.A. times. She [the mother] had asked our own family doctor about some of these mannerisms of his and suggested that we wait until 5 years of age.
MRS.: He said at this time it's hard to tell whether its [sic] pathological.
DR. G.: Tell me this now. How far, how long ago did you first have these concerns that there was something effeminate about him?

MRS.: I'd say in the past year we were beginning to become concerned about it.

MR.: We read an article in Newsweek Magazine where it talked about homosexuality. One thing it sort of summarized was that one thing they noticed about all of them and that was that boys are quite a bit criers and that got us to thinking because boy, we've got a crier on our hands.[58]

This clinical scene reflects the project of trying to prevent the development of gay men by aggressively subjecting effeminate boys to normalizing therapy. Green's role in this business is brilliantly taken to task by Eve Kosofsky Sedgwick in her foundational essay "How to Bring Your Kids Up Gay."[59] Yet in the medicalization of effeminacy, queer theory has overlooked just how many other children were diagnosed immediately as *transsexual*, eventually receiving support from doctors and psychologists in transitioning during their childhood despite the reigning pathogenic discourse. Ultimately, it mattered quite little beyond theory for the faculty involved in UCLA's gender clinic whether femininity in children assigned as boys at birth was interpreted as proto-homosexuality or transsexuality, as was the case more broadly for researchers who undertook similar work in the 1960s.[60] The common problem of developmental timing drove consultation and treatment. Not that the gender clinic faculty involved were uninterested in the intellectual problem; the psychiatrist Alan Rutterberg, who began receiving referrals through the clinic in 1964, stressed the importance of making a diagnostic distinction between childhood homosexuality and transsexuality in a conference paper he gave in the late 1960s. In describing to his audience one of his five-year-old patients, whom he had diagnosed as transsexual, he found it "fascinating" that "the psychiatric literature is almost devoid of any description of the particular entity." In case his audience was not following him, he continued: "I want to make it clear that I am not referring to the well-elucidated category of effeminate little boys or boys with transient cross-gender identifications, familiar to child psychiatrists. What I wish to describe is a little boy whose feminine identification was so strong, secure, and consistent as to justify the use of the term transsexual to describe him."[61] And yet in this very case, as Ruttenberg noted, the five-year-old had first been brought in by parents worried their child would grow up to be "a full-blown homosexual."[62] The categorical trouble encountered by Hugh Hampton Young in the 1930s remained, to be sure, but it was underwritten by a deeper consensus over gender and sexuality as developmentally organized phenomena.

Lawrence Newman, another psychiatrist affiliated with the UCLA gender clinic, tried to synthesize these tensions by drawing on Money's theory of gender acquisition. The earlier "studies of hermaphroditic children," he explained, had established "that the way a child is reared during his first two to three years of life will determine *thereafter* whether he feels himself to be a male or a female." On that basis, Newman wagered, turning to his own colleague, "Stoller has demonstrated a specific combination of family circumstances which lead to the development of profound femininity in boys."[63] Where Money advocated for endocrine therapy and surgery, however, Newman agreed with Stoller that psychotherapy should be pursued intensely with children. He sketched the problem thus:

> If we define a successful treatment of transsexualism as one which
> would make the transsexual give up his cross-gender orientation
> and become comfortable with his physical sex, a treatment, for
> example, which would replace the male transsexual's femininity
> with masculinity, *we must acknowledge that nothing approaching this
> exists*. If profound cross-gender orientation is detected early in life,
> no later than by age five or six and intensive individual therapy for
> the child and counseling for the family instituted on a regular basis,
> reversal of gender orientation is possible. With feminine boys the
> treatment is based upon interfering with the child's feminine
> fantasies, reassuring him that he is a boy and will not grow up to
> be a girl, while at the same time, helping him to see that being a
> male has many rewards.[64]

In his clinical work with both trans boys and girls at UCLA, however, Newman failed to follow his own words and often ended up overseeing transitions for his child patients, precisely because such "intensive individual therapy for the child and counseling for the family" had absolutely no anti-trans effect. He tended to see the onset of adolescence as the practical threshold at which there was no point in pursuing psychotherapy anymore to change a patient's gender identity. "Georgina," one of the trans girls he saw regularly in the 1960s, therefore began to live full time as a girl when she turned fifteen. With Newman's guidance as supervising psychiatrist, as well as the permission of her parents and school officials, she was able to transfer to a new school in the Los Angeles area, legally change her name, and complete high school as Georgina, while continuing to visit UCLA for estrogen therapy. "Much later," Newman recollects, she secured gender confirmation surgery.[65]

In spite of the hostility inherent in Newman and his colleagues' approach at the discursive level, they regularly oversaw transition and hormone therapy for trans children, relying on the developmental model of the child in which psychological plasticity comes to a close after a certain time. The memoranda of the weekly "Saturday Clinic Conferences," which served as the primary way for faculty to share research and clients across disciplines, record many snapshots of the wide variety of trans children who passed through the clinic's doors. In fact, many children and their parents were *literally* brought in front of the assembled clinic staff at those Saturday morning meetings, presented by their attending physician or therapist and subject to observation by the rest of the faculty. Some of the earliest memoranda from 1963 and 1964 mention "a five-year-old transvestite" and "a 15-year-old transvestite-transsexual" who were scheduled to take part in a Saturday conference.[66] Others from the later years of its operation, 1969–1970, scheduled visits for "an adolescent female-to-male transsexual who insists on androgen treatment and completing high school as a boy," "a 13 year old female-to-male transsexual," "a 12 year old 'pre-transsexual' boy," and "a nine-year-old girl with transsexual tendencies."[67] As the wide variations in age and terminology over the decade suggest, there was no single organizing rubric for trans children at UCLA. Nor were meticulous records kept on just how many children were seen by everyone involved in the interdisciplinary clinic.

The discursive centrality of the child's plastic body to transsexual medicine, as established by Benjamin and then inverted by Stoller and his UCLA peers, found itself mired in the clinical reality of treating children. The desire to fully instrumentalize the trans child's body for normalization or the eradication of trans life was forced to confront the partial autonomy of plasticity and the resistance to such capture. For that reason, a paradoxical situation emerged in the 1960s whereby those clinics discursively the most receptive to trans children, such as Benjamin's and Hopkins, offered the least in the way of practical transition, while those that were discursively the most hostile, such as UCLA, oversaw the most thorough hormonal and public transitions. The remarkable achievements of trans children and their families at UCLA, in the face of intense institutional transphobia, however, probably have more to do with their tenacity and with the overriding value of children's bodies to transsexual medicine than with any spirit of openness and dignity on the part of clinicians. The doctors at UCLA were generally beneath compassion in their day-to-day work. Stoller's intake notes on a 1963 consultation with a five-year-old possibly trans child, for instance, end on a chilling but typical punctuation: "I would not want him for my son."[68]

Writing the Body as a Problem of Form

The unprecedented discursive and clinical extension of transsexual medicine in the 1960s relied at every turn on the child's plastic body to picture the onset of transsexuality and to imagine technical approaches to treatment and therapy in developmental terms, both psychological and hormonal. As UCLA's reluctant, if not overtly hostile, approach demonstrates, trans children were not taken seriously as subjects or participants in this endeavor, nor were they accorded any autonomy or voice by medical practitioners. However, the overriding value of trans children as plastic bodies also created an alluring, if fragile, aperture for those children to attempt to cultivate different relationships with doctors and medical science that did not reduce them yet again to the animate substrate of medical technique. One of the only traces left behind by trans children in the 1960s where they do not materialize through a discourse spoken by others is in their handwritten letters to doctors. Here, although the idioms and grammar of transsexuality necessarily remain in play to secure legitimacy and attention, the trans child's body also moves ever so slightly sideways out of the rigid constraints of medical discourse, taking incipient shape as a problem of form that will not be confined, even if it never achieves the stability or intelligibility that might warrant well-worn terms like resistance.

Benjamin's New York practice, particularly after he collaborated with Jorgensen, received a huge number of letters from trans writers, among whom were children as young as thirteen. When articles on transsexuality appeared in newspapers or the popular press across the country, Benjamin's name was surpassed in the number of mentions perhaps only by Jorgensen's. Indeed, the two often appeared one after the other at the end of articles to direct curious readers toward the "experts." With so little medical literature in print, even before *The Transsexual Phenomenon* came out in 1966 Benjamin's name was frequently attached to anything ostensibly medical written about transsexuality.[69] Perhaps just as important was the trading of his address between trans adults or children, including through correspondence networks like Lawrence's or more informal pen-pal relationships.[70] Benjamin also maintained a friendship with the author of the popular "Dear Abby" advice column, ready to field letters from trans writers.[71] When Jorgensen's autobiography appeared, in 1967, it contained passages from Benjamin's work and an introduction he authored to authenticate her explanation of the medical side of transsexuality. Consequently, some children decided to write him after reading her book and either not receiving a response from Jorgensen or feeling too nervous about reaching out to a celebrity.[72]

However they found Benjamin, nearly all of the children who sought his help or advice stressed first and foremost that they knew what transsexuality was and that the term accurately described them. One trans girl, a high school junior from California, put it this way: "For approximately 5 years the wish to become a female has [been] and still is with me. This wish is very strong in me. . . . When I read your book my hopes raised to their highest level."[73] Many offered unsolicited variations on the soon to be standard autobiographical frame: "I have felt for a long time like a girl trapped in a boy's body, trying to get out."[74]

Puberty was often a trigger for seeking out a doctor's opinion. One seventeen-year-old trans girl wrote Benjamin of a "further need for urgency in my case," related to her rapidly increasing height. Already six feet one inch tall, she surmised that "I think it will be great [to be] that size as a girl," but that "the problem is that I'm still growing" and "life as a 6'5" girl would be terrible." Seemingly well versed in the logic of endocrine therapies, she added: "I understand that growth can be stopped with hormones. In that case, my treatment and growth can be controlled simultaneously. *This can only be done if I start now.*"[75] A sixteen-year-old trans girl from upstate New York likewise explained to Benjamin that androgen was something like an alien presence within her body, that she had become "extremely frustrated and humiliated by the hair that's getting thicker and darker on my body, by my voice that's getting deeper with every word I say; with my rough, acned skin. With every new day that androgen runs through my veins, I get more miserable. It has to stop! Androgen just isn't me; estrogen *is!*"[76]

In hopes of fitting the diagnostic model of which Benjamin was one of the principle architects, many children were quick to assure him that they were not homosexual and that they wanted nothing to do with what one seventeen-year-old trans girl called "the gay life." Though she had tried living as a feminine gay boy for several years, this girl explained to Benjamin that "last month" she "was in a bar and talking to another female impersonator, [and] she told me she was a transvestite. I asked her what it meant, she said it meant she didn't want sex with men or women until after she'd had a sex change. I gave this matter a lot of thought and it seemed to have put a whole new light on my life."⁷⁷ Indeed, convincing doctors, as well as parents, teachers, and other adults, to accept their claims to transsexuality frequently occupied the lion's share of children's letters. And in letters like this they reflected the growing abandonment of an older, sexual inversion model in favor of a 1960s form of sexual and gender *identities*.

Benjamin and his colleagues' replies were so standard and repetitive that Virginia Allan, the practice's secretary, would often write back on her own if they were unavailable or out of town—or if repeated letters from a single child had begun to annoy the doctors. A typical reply outlines a three-part argument. "You are very young yet and must give yourself a chance to mature," Benjamin wrote. "In 2 or 3 years, life may look differently to you." Of course some children, undeterred by the developmental rhetoric, would keep writing for the duration of those two or three years, and so Benjamin continued: "If you feel very bad, you should take your parents into your confidence. They are probably your best friends." Finally, he added, "You should also consider talking to your family doctor, or to an understanding psychiatrist."⁷⁸ Beyond this form letter, many responses from the practice included reprints of Benjamin's articles or a suggestion to purchase a copy of *The Transsexual Phenomenon*. Otherwise, replies from Benjamin and his colleagues were curt and generally dismissive, using the alibi of the medical age of consent and, in a strange rhetorical twist for Benjamin, the developmental language of the unfinished body of the child to shut down inquiries.

Many children expressed their frustration with the standard reply, the medical age of consent, and the unwillingness of doctors to see them, prescribe hormones, or authorize gender confirmation surgery. One trans girl from San Diego wrote Benjamin after the Gender Identity Clinic at Hopkins told her to come back at age twenty-one. "Perhaps I am young," she conceded, but continued, "I've felt this way all my life and I've tried other ways of living my life and now I know that by [*sic*] having the operation would be the best thing for me. This isn't something I have thought up over night. I only hope you'll give me a chance."⁷⁹ A sixteen-year-old trans girl explained it in more general terms to Benjamin: "And those who dismiss it as adolescency [sic] don't know what they're talking about. I've felt like this for 16 years, long before adolescency. It's just now I'm becoming increasingly aware of myself, both [physically] and psychologically."[80] When Benjamin replied to her ongoing letters with the routine plea to wait several years, she grew impatient and turned the developmental discourse of transsexuality back on him: "I don't want to wait until I'm growing old. I want to be a girl on the way to my old age. *I want to be a girl now so that I can grow up the rest of the way as a normal girl.*"[81]

While in their letters children tended to work carefully to stick to the parameters of transsexuality, hoping that their investment in medical narratives would be returned with help, the childish form of their writing and their lack of adult expertise with specialist language sometimes cracked the discursive veneer. Alongside their writerly genius are flashes of fascinating digression, as when a fourteen-year-old from Ohio who had received Benjamin's address from a fellow trans girl she knew began reciting all of her friends at school in an oddly repetitive list: "I would rather have a girl for a best friend than a boy. A lot of the girls like me. Sharon, Cindy, Patty, Linda, Colleen, Connie, Patty, Linda, Dixie, Sherry, Toni, Yvonne, Dianna, Cindy, Sheila, and Debbie, but the one I like most is Paula. She's fab! Only a few of the boys like me. Some of them are just jealous because I'm smarter than them."[82] This trans girl's pen pal, who lived in a different part of the state, turned out to be one of the most prolific letter writers to Benjamin's practice in the 1960s. For her, the trans body's growth wrote itself into the surrounds of her ostensibly "medical" letters, recording an interval of growth that began to spread out laterally from the rigid developmental narratives that otherwise confined her to the gatekeeping medical model of transsexuality.

It was not Benjamin but his colleague at his practice, Leo Wollman, who started to receive letters from this young trans girl in rural Ohio in 1968. Writing under a pseudonym, "Vicki"[83] introduced herself as "a 14 year old boy who wants nothing more out of life than to be a girl." While she had already come out to her father, "he is not understanding" and had withheld his consent for her to see a doctor in Columbus. In her first letter she asked Wollman to write back to try to convince her father to let her see the doctor—or perhaps, she wondered, could he just mail her a prescription for estrogen? Vicki also narrated an overview of her day-to-day life, mentioning that she was afraid at school "because the kids are cruel," that her grades had been slipping, that she had to be on a diet because of weight gain from emotional eating stemming from deep depression, and that she had tried to commit suicide at least once.[84]

Virginia Allan prepared a standard response for Wollman, which boiled down to one dismissive line: "Be patient, finish your education, and see how you feel once you are matured."[85] Undeterred, Vicki continued to write every few weeks to New York with various questions over the next two years: "Is it possible for you to get some kind of permit to let me wear women's clothes?" "Could you give me a prescription for something for my nerves?" Could she eat hormone cream to simulate the effects of estrogen therapy?[86] At the same time, she kept Wollman apprised of her life. After coming out to her best friend at school in a written letter, she was publicly humiliated when the note was then passed around the class. "I was never so embarrassed in my entire life," she wrote. Her peers were vicious: "They're always hitting me and yelling at me. My arms are black and blue and I can't help but not do anything." Wollman, who continued to let the secretary reply on his behalf, showed little interest in Vicki's reports.[87]

In the spring of 1969, Vicki sent exciting news: "Finally, my father said I could have the sex change." With that permission, she continued: "Here is what I want to you to do because I have tried but get too embarrassed. Please write him a letter telling why sex changes are preformed [sic] and that they (me) do not have to be hermaphodites [sic]."[88] It is possible that Vicki had made up the story about her having her father's permission in order to try to finally coax a useful reply that she could use to convince her father that she was trans, or maybe it was true. Either way, Wollman never wrote the letter and in fact soon left the office to resume a general practice in Brooklyn. Vicki continued to write to Benjamin. By the summer of 1969 she had moved in with her cousin in Columbus and went out in public as a sixteen-year-old girl. By her estimation, "people have never questioned me. I've been in ladies restrooms, been whistled at, and even been helped with my coat." She also felt certain that her father would now finally pay for her to see a doctor in Columbus. "The next letter I write," she added enthusiastically, "will either be telling you I get the operation or that I was turned down." To that end, she appended a further set of questions about trans children: "Who was the youngest female to become male? Who was the youngest [sic] male to become a female? Can sex-changes have children? What does it take to be a true transexual [sic]? Who was the first sex change? When was the first sex-change preformed [sic]? Do you make all your patients having a sex-change live one year in their new sex before surgery?"[89]

Vicki's letters, at first glance, present a field of tensions indicative of the opening and closure provided by the plastic body for a trans child in the 1960s. She was able to articulate her thoughts, albeit awkwardly and with an at times childish flair, through the medical discourse of transsexuality to relate to doctors as authorities who, if only she could convince them of her need, might grant her access to hormones and other supports. Wollman, however, used developmental discourse to reject her from her very first letter, as did Benjamin, touting the medical age of consent and the ostensible unfinishedness of the biological body at fourteen to counsel her to defer her hopes and needs. Where Vicki read the interval of childhood as a source of tremendous pain, Wollman and Benjamin preferred that she force herself to grow up before transitioning. In this version of their back and forth there was not much to say that was extra-discursive; the narrow intellectual value of Vicki's transsexual body to medicine was probably the only reason that Benjamin's practice would correspond with nonpatients like her over several years.

Yet if growing up, for Vicki, turned around the problem of whether she would become the girl and woman she knew herself to be, in her letters there were unanticipated lateral modes through which her trans body articulated itself without totalizing capture by the medical model. Possessed by what Kathryn Bond Stockton might call her childlike "passion for signification,"[90] Vicki wrote about herself and her body, whether wittingly or not, as a problem of form intrinsic to growth and plasticity. What emerged infrastructurally in her letters was a thick web of references to fat and weight—a preoccupation with the kind of nonteleological growth and latency that fatness incorporates. *Beside* how Vicki's body was part of a medical discourse that instrumentalized her growing body along a hormonal and gendered axis, in the thickness of her writing her body also became a richly formal problem in its wayward growth into fatness instead of socially recognized femininity (or, for that matter, masculinity). In *The Queer Child*, Stockton coined the term "sideways growth" to describe such unanticipated situations powerfully peculiar to "the publicly impossible child whose identity *is* a deferral," unable to be articulated during childhood and so forced to find almost unintelligible, shadowy outlets.[91] Stockton explored these circumstances as they are intensely present for "the ghostly gay child," a kind of child not meant to exist in the twentieth century and who therefore can be birthed only retroactively from adulthood.[92] These sideways growths lurking underneath normative timescales and models, instances where "the child who by reigning cultural definitions can't 'grow up' grows to the side of cultural ideals," also work well to describe the twentieth century *trans* child.[93] The problematic, normative conceit that opened this book—that there somehow were no trans children in the past—doubles in its local manifestation here by Wollman's refusal to recognize Vicki as a trans girl in the present tense of her childhood. In Vicki's case, however, what we find in her letters is less a lateral move away from the reproductive time that *The Queer Child* tracks than a volatile, fleshy scale of growth without teleological form: fat. In the interval of a refused but dwindling childhood, the way her body signified between fat and feminine leads us into "moving suspensions and shadows of growth" that "circumvent" both the childhood teleology of development and the burgeoning discourse of transsexuality in the 1960s.[94]

In Vicki's letters her fat incarnates the undecidable place where the desirable plasticity of the developmental gendered body that makes her intelligible to doctors as a possible transsexual dissolves into the unwillingness of biological form to obey the rigid confines of medicine, normative childhood, and the gender binary. Where development scripted a trajectory that moved in one direction, multiple modes of growth overran that neatness and spread the meaning of Vicki's trans childhood into nonteleological forms that show up only briefly in her letters. In other words, if Wollman refused to help her grow up into femininity, then in the interval her latency, animated by the pain and depression of virulent transphobia, was growing fat. These letters, whether wittingly or not, illuminate some of the ways in which being asked to wait to transition falls upon its own developmental premise: Vicki's body did not stop growing just because she did not yet have permission to grow feminine. Crucially, the forms into which she grew also partially disobeyed what either Wollman or Vicki intended.

In her first letter, Vicki described her body in detail in terms of shape and weight: "Well to begin with I'm 5'10." My hands and body (hips & waist) are not shaped like other boys. My fingers are slim, and soft like the girls at school. My waist is curvy so last night I took my measurements and the results were 40–33–40, and I weigh 168. The dietician said I should weigh 135–40."[95] The indecision between growing fat and growing feminine is already present in this introduction, with Vicki suggesting that her fingers and waist were naturally more like a girl's than a boy's but that her curviness had also been diagnosed as pathological growth by her doctor, hardly feminine at all but also a symptom of the psychosomatic effects of transphobia. Or was that feminine curviness being sanctioned—misrecognized, really—as fat by her dietician in order to undermine Vicki's sense of being a girl? It is hard to say with any certainty. "I started eating last year or so because I found relief in the refrigerator but found out it only added to my unhappiness," she continued. "Now I'm on a diet and have already lost 10 pounds." In this first letter Vicki also asked Wollman for a prescription for estrogen, among whose effects are weight gain and a redistribution of fat that might be at odds with weight-loss goals. Her living body was forced to grow in the shadow of a possible paradox of emotional eating, dieting, hormones, and transsexual diagnosis. Without having to say as much, Vicki seemed to be working to accommodate those tensions. Enclosed with this letter were two small photographs of herself, ostensibly dressed in boy's clothes, to help illustrate the matter of her dilemma in stark visual terms. In a close-up shot, her face is weathered by visible pain and exhaustion that make her look much older than fourteen. In a wide-angle shot take in front of her house, Vicki is facing away from the camera but turns her head back to look at the viewer, as if she is both surprised by and guardedly expectant of connection.[96]

When Wollman replied that Vicki should wait until she reached the age of majority to begin taking estrogen, his attempt to dismiss her instituted a crucial deferral, an interval in which waiting was nonetheless an aperture for growing, paradoxically in both a hopeful and a toxic sense.[97] "Well since nothing can be done until I'm 21," Vicki replied, "I'll just have to try and wait."[98] In that interval, the fat body continued to surface in her writing, usually orthogonal to "the point" of her letters but perhaps for that reason all the more formally important. She asked, for instance, for a note from Wollman that would get her excused from gym class, where her peers were so cruel and violent that her body became paralyzed—"I can't help but not do anything," she explained.[99] The strangely increasing paralysis of her growing, condensed into moments of conflict in spaces like the gym—growing possibly fatter or thinner but not more feminine in the eyes of others—was so extreme in magnitude that it both kept her alive and yet also inexorably poisoned the quality of her life, almost to the breaking point. "I think about running away," she confided, "but I can't. I've tried killing myself but *nothing happens*—at the very worse I just get sick."[100] After a year passed since she first "found out about a sex change," Vicki remarked, "I don't know how I've managed to live thru it."[101] In the interval she had not stopped growing, which would perhaps have been more desirable, for continuing to grow had been a disappointment to everyone who held uneven jurisdiction over her life: her doctor, her father, Wollman, and herself.

Elsewhere, Vicki began to wonder about some of the many paradoxes of eating and its relation to growing: would it simply make her grow fatter, or could it help her grow more feminine, too? "I read where someone was eating hormone cream and what it did to them," she mentioned in May 1969. "Well, I have found a place where I can get it. It said that person was eating 2 ounces of 10,000 units of estrogen (a month). So I figured that I will only be able to eat ½ oz. of 40,000 units of estrogen. I am still hoping it comes, because I sent for it 11 days ago, and it was in New Jersey."[102] Perhaps the suggestion of her actually eating hormones was too much, for Benjamin, who was now writing back after Wollman had left his practice, broke from his usual form response to say in no uncertain terms that she must not eat any hormone cream.[103] What about the possibility of eating hormones to feminize roused Benjamin out of his silence?

Perhaps he was even unaware of the prompt, for, in another way, the doctor's responses only to the most dramatic shocks or punctuations in Vicki's letters seem to reflect a rhetorical strategy that allowed him to miss the substance of her writing: the thick surround to the content of her letters, mostly latent and affective, sometimes breaking ever so slightly into signification. Never did the doctors want to address the plasticity of Vicki's fat or recognize that it was addressing them. Her last letters in 1970, for instance, revolved around finally securing access to estrogen through a doctor in Columbus. Now sixteen years old, Vicki expressed great optimism about her future, but the fatty tissue of the body saturated the space surrounding her signifiers in her final entry in the archival record: "And I wanted to know if [the hormone] estiryl will make my breasts large enough without implants. Because I don't want implants unless necessary."[104] After years spent trying to control, decrease, or slow down the plastic growth of her body, to stop it from getting fatter while waiting for it to be given permission to grow into a form recognized as feminine, Vicki seemed to ask that her breasts grow into their own, *on their own*, without implants.

While it would certainly be possible to read Vicki's writing as symptomatic of straightforwardly emotional pain, such structures reveal next to nothing about her situated knowledge as a trans girl in deferral. How can we explain, after all, that doctors who in principle had nothing to offer still corresponded with her for two years? The initiative and boldness that Vicki expressed by going toe-to-toe with the leading figures of transsexual medicine deserve to be underlined. It was no small feat to carry on about diagnosis, hormones, and breast development with two endocrinologists. Perhaps part of that discursive work for Vicki was refining a way of talking about herself, so that when she found a doctor in Columbus she was better able to negotiate with the clinic for what she needed. Still, is the virtuosic practice of medical expertise by a trans child really an account of "agency"? The extreme limitations of the medical model could not be more apparent in the constant refrain of "no" coming from Wollman and Benjamin, the force that stretched the interval in which Vicki continued to grow, fat but not feminine, at such a high cost—her frequent references to suicide attempts being only the sharpest example.

There is no scene of resistance in the writing of trans children. However, the plastic body, which admits no material distinction among growing up, growing fat, and growing feminine, did accommodate strange moments of partial signification for children like Vicki, organic detours where the indecision at the core of growth was a formal interruption of the rigid schema underwriting child development and transsexuality. What modes of autonomy or nonteleological vitality were occasioned or could have been cultivated by Vicki had those forms not been so quickly extinguished by medicine at every turn remain difficult to see, but only because children are forced into the position of lacking of access to any language besides adult signification. So long as that remains the case, the forms occasioned in trans children's bodies and letters in the 1960s will remain, like Vicki's, whispers filling the space between the signifiers of medical discourse.

The Psychiatric Ward, or, a Black Trans Girl's 1960s

Vicki's access to a writerly voice that, in its encounter with a medical discourse, generated formal problems that crept away from the limits of transsexuality, also relied on her plastic whiteness in a way that stood in stark contrast to the positioning of black trans and trans children of color in the archive. There are very few of them, as middle-class, white children disproportionately made it into gender identity clinics and private endocrinology offices given the degree to which plasticity had become synonymous with whiteness. The trans child with the largest collection of documents

I found in the archive was actually a black girl from New Jersey. Yet the volume of discourse surrounding her life was not enabling but devastatingly obfuscating. A thick stack of psychiatric papers describe in a different form of shadowy language the life of a girl institutionalized for decades under the flimsiest of schizophrenic diagnoses. Growing up in a poor, black neighborhood of Trenton, she was committed to a psychiatric institution through the foster care system, which had taken custody of her years earlier because of her mother's unsupported disability. For the next fifteen years psychiatrists took her profession of gender identity as evidence of "delusion," "mental retardation," and "sexual perversion," signing off annually on her continued confinement. The paper trail of her institutionalization made it into the archive in which I was looking only because in 1978 Jeanne Hoff, a psychiatrist and trans woman who took over Benjamin's practice after his retirement, petitioned to have her released. After interviewing the woman, who was now thirty years old, Hoff rebuked all of her transphobic diagnoses in a powerful letter: "Through all the florid language of the [psychiatric] reports there is an unmistakable moralistic disapproval of her effeminacy and homosexuality but not the slightest hint that the diagnosis of transsexualism was suspected, even though it was quite evident from the details provided.... She should be placed in the community, preferably living by herself" and "she should be permitted to explore the various problems that arise from cross-gender living, hormonal therapy, and surgical gender reassignment."[105]

For this black trans girl, the 1960s were a radically different decade from the one examined in the rest of this chapter. The state and medical institutions, having long colluded to confine and detain black people from their bodies and dispossess them of their personhood, took up her gender as evidence of insanity in order to suspend her childhood altogether, forcing her to "grow up" on a psychiatric ward. While this book argues for understanding the racialization of sex and gender through the equation of plasticity and whiteness, race here makes a second kind of crucial and highly visible difference. The racial innocence withheld from black children in the United States in order to justify forms of ongoing dispossession manifested as a withholding of the narrow parameters of the new discourse of transsexuality from black children.[106] Only through an errand of mercy by a trans-affirmative psychiatrist did the files created by this girl's institutionalization make it into an archive of transgender history. Many other trans children of color of the 1960s remain invisible. In the gulf that separates G.L., who was forced into the new model of transsexuality; Georgina, who was able and willing to transition as a teenager against the inclination of her doctors; Vicki, who was made to wait in an interval of growth; and this unnamed black trans girl, who had her childhood suspended by the state, we find a set of fractures birthed into the category of transsexuality from its very emergence.

CHAPTER 5

Transgender Boyhood, Race, and Puberty
in the 1970s

I N THE SUMMER OF 1973, John Money received a letter from a doctor
in upstate New York looking for advice. Having been "recently referred
a 15 year old girl *[sic]*, an exceptionally bright, articulate, well-read (perhaps unfortunately) youngster whom I have only seen twice thus far," the
doctor sought Money's counsel because "the data thus far strongly suggests that a diagnosis of transsexualism will eventually be made." While the
doctor was not himself trained in transsexual medicine, "at the risk of my
sounding grandiose or naïve" he explained that over the past several weeks
he had "read to the best I can ascertain everything written in English on
the subject until 1970." With the surfeit of new medical knowledge fresh in
his mind, he articulated his primary concerns: that "the process of diagnosis, evaluation, and management is a long and costly one," that the family
of the fifteen-year-old trans boy had "limited" financial resources, and that
he therefore wanted to "make certain that they incur no extra steps and
costs due to unnecessary duplication" of tests or exams. Since there was no
gender identity clinic in this particular city upstate, he made his primary
request: "I would very much appreciate drawing from your experience for
a suggestion as to when would be a good time to make a referral to your
clinic for evaluation."[1]

   In his reply, written a week later, Money articulated his now standard diagnostic and treatment protocol for transsexuality, calibrated for a
trans-masculine child. He more or less dismissed the doctor's worry about
the importance of a gynecological and endocrine exam to make a diagnosis of transsexuality. "If the findings are routine" in the former, "as I suspect
they will be," he wrote, "then there will be no need for special endocrine
examination." Similarly, he explained that "psychologic testing may prove
to be of ancillary interest in the establishment of the diagnosis, but is not a
sine qua non." Simply put, "one does not establish the diagnosis on the basis
of psychologic tests." Instead, Money counseled the doctor to interview

"corroborative informants" who knew the boy well but who, unlike his parents, were not too close to the subject to give presumably honest answers about his gender identity. "I consider it diagnostically almost indispensable," he emphasized, "especially in the case of a 15 year old child." Having dismissed the doctor's initial concerns, Money outlined the core of his diagnostic model. In his mind "the one test of signal importance in the diagnosis of transexualism is what I have called the two year real life test." During the two years in which this trans boy would live full time in his gender identity, Money explained, he would prove that he could "rehabilitate" himself "in the sex of reassignment." Success during those two years grounded eligibility for surgery. "In the case of female to male transexualism," he explained, "the final irrevocable step is hysterectomy and ovariectomy."[2] Because of its self-consciously limited results, Money did not recommend pursuing phalloplasty.[3]

Until this point, Money's letter is rather unremarkable. It rehearses what had, by the 1970s, become a general model of assessment and increasingly rigid gatekeeping to restrict access to transition and surgery to only those individuals who could "prove" both their adhesion to the "wrong body" model and their desire to pursue passing as the primary goal of transition. Yet here Money began to digress from the generic narrative for trans adults, returning to the child at hand, a fifteen-year-old boy. "I am willing to consent to mastectomy much earlier" than other surgical procedures, Money explained to his correspondent, "because it does make occupational adjustment as a male much easier." What's more, he continued, "it is not too difficult to do a breast implant, should there be a change of heart at any time in the future." Similarly, he went on, "I definitely go along with the idea of early treatment with male sex hormones." Many effects of androgens could be later reversed if need be, he explained. Only a change in voice was "irreversible and permanent," but even that could "be modulated in a soft and husky way, so as not to be too obvious and noticeable." Having made a case for hormone therapy and top surgery during childhood on the basis of its practical, biological reversibility, Money digressed into a point much broader in scope:

> Now that the legal age of voting and adulthood has gone down
> from 21 to 18 in over half of the states, I do not see any special reason
> to fix the age of 21, instead of 18, as the age of personal consent for
> transexual reassignment surgery. The most important thing to me

is the evidence that the person has lived in the sex of anticipated reassignment for two years, has been treated by society as a member of that sex, and has personally experienced and adjusted to the challenge of living in that sex.[4]

In sum, Money concluded, "I think you will find it very worthwhile to work with this patient." He advised the doctor not to refer the child anywhere just yet but instead to allow him to live full time as a boy immediately, start on hormones, and pursue top surgery. If in two years he "has succeeded in living the life of a boy," then Money suggested that the referral for gender confirmation surgery be to his clinic at the Johns Hopkins Hospital— provided that parental consent was obtained.[5]

While historiographically remarkable for queer and transgender studies, as we will see shortly, Money's reply to this doctor in upstate New York was also importantly *typical* for the 1970s. The growth of transsexual medicine at university research clinics in the 1960s had cemented a basic, if controversial, academic and professional standing for the field. In addition to Money's home clinic at Hopkins and the UCLA gender clinic discussed in the previous chapter, major gender clinics had been established by the University of Minnesota, Northwestern University in Chicago, the University of Washington–Seattle, and, perhaps most famously, Stanford University.[6] With funding from the Erickson Educational Foundation, Money and Richard Green had also edited a landmark volume *Transsexualism and Sex Reassignment* in 1969, bringing together more than twenty-five clinicians and researchers to codify the emergent norms of the field.[7] And, as Joanne Meyerowitz has argued, in the 1970s the United States saw a quantitative increase in transition and gender confirmation surgery, primarily because private clinics also began to offer services *without* requiring the lengthy two-year assessment that Money and his peers had used to try to limit access to medical resources. If adults were willing to pay and had enough money, it was somewhat easier for them to get access to hormones and surgery during this decade than the previous one.[8]

Given the central role that children had played in the consolidation of the field's diagnostic and treatment protocols since its founding, it is not surprising that in the 1970s trans children continued to participate in the broader trends of the decade. Many transitioned under the supervision of doctors, living out and full time, taking hormones, changing their names, going to school and, more commonly than in the 1960s, securing access to surgeries during childhood. Yet this chapter begins with Money's letter in particular because it addresses a trans *boy's* childhood and transition. While this book has argued, through and through, for the importance of insisting that transgender children do have a history that stretches across the twentieth century, there is in this chapter an added dimension to that insistence. Whether or not trans women's disproportionate visibility for much of the history of the twentieth century is a distorted effect of the obsessive focus on their bodies by medical science or a concomitant conceptual and clinical disinterest in trans masculinity or some combination of both, the question is even more strained in the case of children.[9] A second, generational presumption oddly yet to be challenged comes into play: the sense that trans men (and boys) did not come of age demographically until the 1990s. It has been too easily assumed that, prior to that decade, many people who might have at a later time identified as transgender or transitioned to some degree were instead butch lesbians.

This chapter explores trans boyhood in the 1970s to investigate the generational and historiographical assumptions of the so-called border wars and the misplaced preeminence of the *Diagnostic and Statistical Manual* in queer theory and transgender studies narratives about gender nonconformity and childhood. I suggest that both fields have gotten much of this time period and its aftermath wrong, mainly by overemphasizing generic medical discourse at the cost of specific histories of the clinic, which often outright contradict the former. Not only were there many trans boys during the 1970s who are unrepresented in this scholarship and whose lives are more generally unknown, but also their childhoods and medicalized interactions with doctors both cut across the presumptions of the trans-masculine-butch-lesbian border wars and also presaged a certain contemporary discourse around puberty and the "reversibility" of childhood transition. In this final chapter of this book, what follows disassembles and reconstructs the immediate history that informs the contemporary medical model of transgender childhood by arguing for the specificity of trans boyhood prior to the cultural visibility of trans men in the 1990s. Much of the "debate" in the twenty-first century around the suppression of puberty and the "reversibility" of childhood transition looks less settled in the context of 1970s trans boyhood. Yet any desire to recuperate a coherent narrative or identity to trans boyhood also undoes itself when juxtaposed alongside the lives of black trans girls during the same decade. Proceeding through this impasse will take us, ultimately, to the tangled legacy of plasticity in pediatric trans medicine I discuss in the conclusion to this book. But first, to understand the importance of the 1970s, we must displace the prominence of the year 1980.

The Generational Politics of the Border Wars

The year 1980 marks a certain kind of retrenchment for access to transgender medicine in the United States with the codification of "Gender Identity Disorder" (GID) in the *Diagnostic and Statistical Manual* (*DSM*) of the American Psychiatric Association (APA). The gatekeeping model of medicine developed by Harry Benjamin, Money, and their colleagues eventually won out over the diffuse range of private clinics that offered surgery to those who could pay during the 1970s.[10] At the same time, while there had been numerous uncoordinated attempts since the 1960s to cover the costs of transition through state medical programs or private health insurance, the codification of GID provided a very difficult but important opening toward insurance coverage for trans medicine, one still extremely tenuous today.[11] Yet the *DSM* has also been leveraged to mark an oddly uninterrogated set of historiographical and narrative divergences in queer and transgender studies: a split between (homo)sexuality and trans embodiment and between trans masculinity and trans femininity. Both divisions ought to be much more troubled by the experiences of trans children.

From the outset of *Histories of the Transgender Child* I have argued that the prevailing narrative today about transgender children is that they are of the present and the future—that they have no past. If there is in any way an implicit historiography of trans children, though, it takes its cue from the changes made to the *DSM-III* released in 1980. David Valentine argues in *Imagining Transgender* that the 1970s witnessed the consolidation of a major categorical split between homosexuality, which, as gay politics took shape, increasingly defined itself as gender-normative, and transsexuality, which was not allowed to be sexual at all but increasingly relied on asexual "wrong body" narratives. For Valentine, the declassification of homosexuality by the APA in 1973 and the introduction of GID in 1980 mark the decisive events in that process: "By the time the *DSM-III* was published in 1980 . . . a new diagnostic category had been established—Gender Identity Disorder (GID). GID created a diagnostic place for people who had not previously been explicitly recognized as such in the pages of the *DSM*, transsexuals and others who engaged in *visibly* gender-variant behaviors and who had previously been understood at least partially through the categories of homosexuality and transvestism."[12] Valentine adds, however, that this cleaving of sexuality-as-object-choice from gender-as-identity desired by gay activists is also the accumulated effect of a century's worth of strain on the nineteenth-century discourse of "inversion," which mixed object choice and self-presentation in an all-encompassing category of "sex."[13] It would be accurate to say that lesbian and gay politics more or less acquiesced in the 1970s to a sexological model through the removal of homosexuality from the *DSM* and the splitting of gay and lesbian from trans politics.[14]

In her monumental 1991 essay "How to Bring Your Kids Up Gay," Eve Sedgwick made a striking claim about an effect of this shift. The 1973 decision to delete homosexuality from the *DSM* was in practice severely undercut by the introduction in the subsequent *DSM-III* of GID. Reading psychoanalytic and psychotherapeutic work in light of the bait and switch, Sedgwick underlined the stark effect of "the theoretical move of distinguishing gender from sexuality." Far from eliminating homosexuality as a treatable condition, "the *de*pathologiziation of an atypical object-choice can be yoked to the *new* pathologization of an atypical gender identification."[15] In other words, the result of the change in *DSM* from 1973 to 1980 is that "while denaturalizing sexual object-choice, it radically *re*naturalizes gender."[16] And it is the child who has to pay to price. The material cost of the turn, for Sedgwick, is possibly the very life of the effeminate boy, who is utterly cast aside by the mainstream gay and lesbian politics that sought demedicalization through gender normativity, while being left newly vulnerable to the psychiatric profession's displaced desire to eradicate all gay people by preventing their development during childhood. In such a situation, Sedgwick argues persuasively, the effeminate boy becomes "the haunting abject" of the epistemic shift from 1973 to 1980.[17] Even an ostensibly gay-affirmative therapeutic discourse could still participate in the genocidal impulse to eradicate homosexuality by leveraging GID to treat sexual object choice by proxy, through childhood gender.

Yet there is still another ghostly child here, one that neither Valentine nor Sedgwick detects. There is a way one could read the introduction of GID as a proxy for pathologizing homosexuality in proto-gay boys while also excluding the many trans children who were also interpellated by the new classification. That is clearly not Sedgwick's intention, but in the wake of "How to Bring Your Kids Up Gay," the trans child, unlike the effeminate boy, has received no attention in queer theory. This reading of the *DSM* lends credence to the idea that there were, somehow, no trans children at that moment. Only when the psychiatric treatment of proto-gay boys for effeminacy becomes politically intolerable in the 2000s would the label "GID" be applied to transgender children instead—yet another displacement of the residual energy of inversion. As gay children were folded into the state as protectable under certain (highly racialized) circumstances, transgender children became the new focus of pathologizing discourse. Or so the story might go.

To be clear, this extrapolation does not exist per se in queer theory. It remains only an implicit takeaway from work on the *DSM* and gender nonconformity. It *does*, however, exist in media coverage of the "first" transgender children of the mid-2000s on, which refers again and again to fear in parents that their child might be lesbian or gay before they learn of the "new" categories of gender identity and dysphoria now being used to describe transgender children.[18] A strange recapitulation of the analytic separation of sexuality from gender reoccurs, despite Sedgwick's careful mining of the epistemic instability that entangles them. Transgender is made the historical and medical successor of homosexuality. Or, more precisely, the transgender child is made the implicit successor of the proto-gay child. What's more, given the anxious obsession of therapists with effeminacy and femininity in "boys," there is little space to see the *trans* boys who interacted with some of the very same clinicians critiqued in "How to Bring Your Kids Up Gay."[19] The ghostly effect Sedgwick illuminates in the case of the effeminate boy replicates itself again by implying that transgender childhood, not to mention boyhood, could not become a concern until after 1980.

The broadest point here is that using the *DSM* as the starting point for a history of trans children is mostly useless. This book has, therefore, proceeded otherwise, since many of trans children's twentieth-century histories took place long before the codification of GID. The sense that transgender is a successor category to homosexuality in childhood is not supported by the history of the clinic. Over the arc of *Histories of the Transgender Child*, for instance, children's transness has already appeared through multiple discursive domains that undercut succession narratives, including intersex, sexual inversion, homosexuality, and transvestism. This chapter, while focusing on a decade in which the intense emphasis on binary transition seemed to preclude the persistence of multiple definitions of trans childhood, shows that in fact the continued indeterminacy of the concept of plasticity created a series of fault lines of race and gender inside the concept of transsexuality, so that childhood transness retained its multiplicity.

The actual experiences and identities of trans and queer children themselves, as opposed to the discourses mobilized to speak about them, are
much more difficult to assay. Nevertheless, in this chapter the 1970s offer a
very different way into the "border wars" between butch lesbian and trans
masculinities that turn upon this problem of succession.

In *Female Masculinity*, Jack Halberstam carefully investigated the so-
called border wars between butch lesbians and trans men, contextualizing
them, like Valentine, in a longer history of sexology where the aftershocks
of the medical model of inversion led to ongoing political and identitarian
friction. I am less interested in questions of subjectivity and identity than
in Halberstam's implicit periodization of trans masculinity and butch masculinity, which reinforces the sense of historical succession inadvertently
established in the uptake of Sedgwick's essay. In an important moment
in the book's chapter on the border wars, Halberstam writes: "The border
wars between transgender butches and FTMS presume that masculinity is
a limited resource. Or else we see masculinity as a set of protocols that
should be agreed on in advance. Masculinity, of course, is what we make of
it; it has important relations to maleness, *increasingly interesting relations to
transsexual maleness, and a historical debt to lesbian butchness.*"[20]

Taking a very long historical view, say, to the early twentieth century
and working-class lesbian social words in the United States, it *is* plausible
to claim that butchness produces a historical debt for trans masculinity. Or,
even earlier, there is the controversial claiming of Stephen Gordon's character in *The Well of Loneliness* as a lesbian, an invert, or trans.[21] As the second chapter of this book explores, the earliest, pre-transsexuality medical
procedures for changing sex included transitions from feminine to masculine. Although the discourses of homosexuality, inversion, and lesbianism
frequently overlapped and haunted the surrounds of early twentieth-century
masculine lives, by at least the 1920s and 1930s there were public trans men
like Michael Dillon, Alan Hart, and Bernard.[22] In any case, Halberstam in
Female Masculinity in the 1990s took a much more recent view on "the public emergence of the female-to-male transsexual (FTM) in the last decade
or so."[23] It is this slide from a rise in public visibility to an implicit historical argument of precedence and succession between butch masculinity and
trans masculinity, one that seems to have been left largely unchallenged in
the wake of *Female Masculinity* and other early texts on the border wars,
that quickly becomes unfamiliar with the introduction of the archive of
trans boyhood in the 1970s.[24] For the 1970s were not a decade that defined

nonnormative masculinity exclusively in terms of lesbian life in advance of a category of trans masculinity that had yet to come of age. Rather, for many trans children, boyhood, even in its medicalization, undoes the historiographical presumptions on which the preeminent place of the *DSM* and the border wars both rely. What becomes less clear, without the narrative certainty provided by the uptake of Sedgwick's, Valentine's, and Halberstam's work, however, is how to proceed if that boyhood ignites no epistemological clarity of its own. And the racialization of gender that this work in queer and trans studies has overlooked introduces a further problem for efforts to recuperate a clear trans masculine subject out of this decade.

Trans Boys In and Outside the Clinic

It is difficult to say how much "easier" it became for children to seek out doctors in the decade that Meyerowitz characterizes as "the liberal moment,"[25] but the overall climate seems to have become more hospitable in the 1970s than it had been in the 1960s. Money's sense that the lowering of the voting age heralded something of the spirit of the era seems to have held more broadly. While the clinic in which he worked at Hopkins was actually shut down in 1979 after years of infighting among faculty, others, both private and public, expanded during the decade.[26] Harry Benjamin, now in his eighties, also retired at the end of the decade, while Charles Ihlenfeld and Leo Wollman, his copractitioners, left the practice, too. By the end of the 1970s the office was taken over by Jeanne Hoff, a psychiatrist and trans woman who brought a new approach to the clinic that was in part informed by her own experience being subject to medicine.

The medicalization of trans masculine bodies in the 1970s was still widely regarded by its gatekeepers as lagging behind the curve of trans femininity. While Money's rehearsal of his generic approach in the letter that opened this chapter reflects the general consensus of the field, there had been relatively little change in its medical content since the 1950s. In that decade Elmer Belt, a surgeon in Los Angeles who attempted to provide gender confirmation surgery to his trans clients before being shut down by local medical boards, had been interested in pursuing transition and surgery for trans men. Belt corresponded at the time with Benjamin to strategize about the possibilities. Benjamin mentioned having once met Harold Gillies, the plastic surgeon who would become canonized for his work on phalloplasty, in London, but Benjamin remained unsure whether the procedure Gillies had developed was worth recommending to clients. Belt in fact already had a client who was interested and who had found a way to get top surgery from a different surgeon in Los Angeles. "Fortunately or unfortunately," Belt explained, this person had a cystic ovary that made it possible to also justify hysterectomy as medically necessary, opening the door in his mind to adding phalloplasty to the list of procedures he would undertake.[27] While Belt was ultimately unsuccessful, the relative feasibility of top and bottom surgery at the end of the 1950s did not change a great deal in the two subsequent decades. While the architects of transsexual medicine, such as Benjamin and Money, had seen trans men as patients since the very beginning of their clinical research, they continued, like most practitioners, to give massively more emphasis to trans women. One of the distorting effects of this asymmetry between trans masculinity and trans femininity is that the medical archive repeats a certain disqualification of trans masculine transition as somehow less complete, judging it against the standard of trans femininity's protocols.[28]

It was in the broader context of this medical distortion effect around trans masculinity that trans boys came into contact with doctors in the 1970s. From all over the United States, children took up the pen and wrote directly to clinicians. One fifteen-year-old from Tennessee wrote to Ihlenfeld, who was still part of Benjamin's practice in New York City, in 1975. "I need your help bad," he explained, for "the pressures of every day life and school are really getting to me and I don't know which way to turn." He had already written to the Erickson Education Foundation "several times," which was how he had obtained Ihlenfeld's address. "I found hope and new [sic] I wasn't going crazy when I read an article about transsexuals and the sex change operation." Having unsuccessfully visited his family doctor and a psychiatrist, the latter of whom "ran [a] test on my mind," the letter writer felt stuck. "I don't know what to do next. I need to make my life as normal as possible . . . sometimes I get so depressed I just don't get where [sic] I live or not but I'm still hanging on coz I'm gonna get help." At this point he reiterated, "I'm a girl physiacaily [sic] but I'm a boy in my mind and soul. . . . I've read you have dealt with cases of people like me."[29]

In his reply, Ihlenfeld did not simply dismiss the letter, as Benjamin's office had routinely done in the 1960s with similar inquiries. "Although you are very young," Ihlenfeld nonetheless suggested "that you write to Ira M. Dushoff, M.D.," providing an address in Jacksonville, Florida, before adding: "Of course, no ethical physician will treat you without the consent and cooperation of your parents."[30] Why, exactly, did Ihlenfeld recommend this trans boy to someone in Florida when he had written from Tennessee? Several years earlier, Dushoff had founded a private clinic, the Gender Identity Association, which operated without the constraints (or the resources) of a university research clinic or a state-funded institution. Despite the private status, Dushoff worked quite actively with clinicians at major university clinics and frequently spoke at conferences, colloquia, and other events in the field of transsexual medicine in the 1970s, suggesting why Ihlenfeld would have felt comfortable making a referral in a letter.[31] It is possible that Ihlenfeld felt that the trans boy who had written him would have better luck accessing hormones or surgery options at a clinic formed in many ways with that privatized goal in mind, especially if parental support was insecure.

If trans boys from the New York City area wrote for advice, Benjamin's practice now frequently encouraged them to come in for a consultation, with or without the permission of their parents (although without parental consent Benjamin would go no further).[32] When a seventeen-year-old from New Jersey wrote to Ihlenfeld in the summer of 1976, he said that he felt that his parents should not hold him back from medical transition. At this point he was already living as a boy "all the time, with the exception of school hours only." Although he resided with his parents, he clarified that "I support myself." As for his parents, they "consider me as a 'failure,' a 'freak of society,' and a 'poor investment.'" After "a good deal of reading about my problem," he found that experts "all seem to agree that the effects of hormone treatment, with the exception of the deepening of the voice, are reversible when the dosage is stopped. Under these circumstances, I feel that minors ought to be able to receive treatment without parental consent." The uncanny closeness between his rhetorical form and Money's letter that opened this chapter suggests, indeed, that this seventeen-year-old had probably been reading his work closely and drawing on it. The new idiom of the "reversibility" of hormone therapy in the plastic body of the developing child emboldened him to argue, somewhat paradoxically, that, as "a responsible, mature person," he was ready "to begin this much needed change" without the consent of his parents. "While flatly refusing to help me," he explained, his parents "also state that they would not hinder me either."[33]

Although legally the barrier of parental consent remained effectively insurmountable, the practice's secretary, Virginia Allen, wrote back to invite the seventeen-year-old to contact her for an appointment. On the carbon copy of this reply she annotated a few subsequent developments, noting that she had spoken to him the following week by phone and explained the clinic's "fees" and "expectations" and "our routines." She added: "Will call back.[34]" Later that fall he came in to the office, accompanied by his mother, for an appointment with Agnes Nagy, who had recently replaced Ihlenfeld. It seems that this was his only visit to Benjamin's clinic, however. When Jeanne Hoff reviewed Benjamin's files after taking over the practice years later, she merely noted that the seventeen-year-old reported during that appointment that his family doctor did not believe he was actually trans, but she did not speculate about whether that had anything to do with why he did not continue seeing Nagy or whether the mother's opinion and consent had changed.[35]

Medical figures like Money and Benjamin, who by this time commanded a considerable reputation for expertise, also received many inquiries from other clinicians who worked with children who either identified as or were being diagnosed as transsexual. By the 1970s Money's voluminous correspondence in particular was preoccupied with a range of inquiries from doctors and other providers around the country and internationally who wanted to establish their own gender clinics and offer medical transition and reassignment and who generally felt that his experience would be of benefit to their work.[36] Still more wrote to Money about specific clients, often their first to raise the category of transsexuality. One therapist with a sixteen-year-old trans boy "who is contemplating surgery for sex change" sought Money's published work in order both to refine his approach and to have something to give to his client to read.[37] One clinical psychologist in Arizona who had already read *Transsexualism and Sex Reassignment* was looking for "more up-to-date references" in order to work with another sixteen-year-old trans boy. He also inquired as to whether Money knew "of any medical facility in the Southwest that performs female to male reassignment, should my patient pursue surgery," but it seems that Money did not reply, and his secretary instead sent reprints of some of his recent publications.[38]

While rarely clear in such letters, it seems likely that many of these trans boys had begun seeing therapists with the consent of their parents—indeed, many may have actually been dragged into therapy by parents uncomfortable with or hostile to their gender identity. Yet other trans children came into contact with medicine through more disciplinary institutions that had first detained them. Mental health wards and juvenile court or probation systems were two of the most common alternate routes into medicalization, and in many jurisdictions these institutions effectively blurred into one another. One resident psychiatrist at an inpatient facility in Connecticut who wrote to Money was quite vague about how the seventeen-year-old trans boy under his supervision had been committed, referring to "both the desire for sexual transformation and a multitude of behavioral problems" present at admission. In this case, however, while the "behavioral problems" had more or less "become non-existent" since the patient's admission to the hospital, "the wish for sexual change remained unchanged and intact," apparently convincing the psychiatrist of the validity of this boy's desire to transition. Now that he was considering discharging the boy sometime in the next several months the psychiatrist was concerned that "the parents are unaccepting" and believed that it was "doubtful whether they would agree or authorize any medical procedure." Looking for advice on "follow-up care" for the child while he was still in high school, "especially for a minor without parental authorization," Money forwarded the letter to John Meyer, a colleague in psychiatry at Johns Hopkins.[39] In his reply, Meyer agreed that there was a "general lack of out-patient facilities that deal with this type of issue" and that finishing high school should be of equal priority with transition. While Meyer felt that a seventeen-year-old would be quite welcome to pursue outpatient treatment at the Sexual Behaviors Consultation Unit within the psychiatric division of Hopkins, perhaps combined with attendance at a local boarding school, he stressed that he was also "certain that it would require both parental authorization and parental support since the patient is a minor child."[40]

The willingness, however reluctant, of these clinicians to advocate for their trans masculine clients is itself partially a distorted effect of the archive. Only those persuaded by the claim of gender identity of their clients and the viability of the category of transsexuality would have bothered to write to someone like Money. Still, the ways that trans masculinity was even partially legitimized puts a great deal of pressure on the notion that butch lesbian identity was the obvious category in this era. A social worker at a psychiatric hospital in Missouri, for instance, wrote to the Social Service Department of the Johns Hopkins Hospital about "a very intelligent 17 year old female transsexual who, by definition, wishes to live and be accepted as a member of the sex opposite to her biological sex." This trans boy had been hospitalized twice in six weeks; first for suicidality and then "to begin hormonal treatment until 21; i.e., surgical care if indicated." The social worker wanted advice on "the social problems that arise" from childhood transition.

Successful and consistent binding, for one, presented a challenge. "We are also concerned about helping her [sic] enter college as a boy," she added. At the moment he was finishing high school by correspondence from the hospital, and the school itself was "unaware of the actual problem." The social worker expected that with college, by contrast, they could "send in all application materials and the doctor will write the dean of students after acceptance."[41]

The Department of Social Work at Hopkins forwarded this letter to Money, who wrote back to generally affirm the plan proposed. Once again he argued for top surgery during childhood, writing: "I think it is unjustifiable to be obliged to fiddle-faddle with chest binding when mastectomy would achieve so much more for this patient who is already embarked on hormonal masculinization."[42] The quick shift in this trans boy's hospitalization from suicide watch to hormone therapy, as well as the possibility of top surgery, reflects the degree to which trans boyhood was an established, if only because deeply medicalized in this instance, category in the 1970s. The lack of references to the specter of "homosexuality" or lesbian identity in these documents suggests that even if the generational claim that butch masculinity was more widespread than trans masculinity during this decade holds outside the class and race demographics of the medical context, there was nevertheless an established community of trans boys who attempted to negotiate the incredible authority of medicine to affirm their sense of self and embodiment without encountering the frictions of a "border war." Yet the increasing reach of medicalization into trans boyhood was neither uniform nor as unproblematic as the case of this boy in Missouri might suggest. As more trans boys transitioned and more trans children in general accessed surgery in the 1970s, the racialized plasticity of the child's growing body upon which medical science had long relied yet again shifted in form. Here the desire to affirm trans boyhood to overturn the generational narrative of the border wars encounters a series of important complications.

Reversibility and the Racialization of Puberty

The clinical affordances of the 1970s actualized the now well-established developmental logic of transsexual medicine to an unprecedented extent. Some children were able to undergo gender confirmation surgery before reaching the age of majority, something that, other than in the unique case of "G.L" at Johns Hopkins in 1964, had more or less been removed from consideration by the gatekeeping function of clinicians. The case of trans boys is more complex, however, because of the asymmetry through which bottom surgery was not granted the same status for boys and girls. Given Money's insistence that top surgery for trans boys *was* highly advisable but also not yet widely accepted, it is difficult to assess how many trans boys who encountered doctors during the 1970s accessed forms of surgery, rather than being limited to hormone therapy. The relative symbolic weight given to surgery for trans girls and women in this moment makes the fact of trans girls securing access during childhood quite remarkable, too. Of course, this growth in access was hardly an index of emancipation, medical or otherwise. What's more, the changes to the *DSM* in 1980 would more or less close the window to childhood surgeries, making the situation short lived. And the window itself was founded on a renewed racialization of puberty and plasticity through the incipient concept of "reversibility." The latter move would persist well past the decade, founding the diagnostic and treatment matrix in which we still live today.

The archive of 1970s medicine contains scattered references to trans children undergoing gender confirmation surgery during childhood, but always after puberty had set in. There was also a constant and high degree of self-awareness on the part of adults about the potential controversy of granting children access to surgery. In a letter addressed to Money that lacks a clear context, an adult from New Jersey recounts the story of a friend's trans daughter, who was able to access surgery in 1976. "Two weeks ago I met a girl of sixteen, who three weeks ago was a boy of sixteen," explains the letter writer, who consciously or not followed the common rhetorical framework attached to transition found in journalistic accounts.[43] This trans child had apparently begun hormone therapy at fourteen and switched school districts to begin attending as a girl with the support of both her parents and the principal. "This went on until two or three weeks ago," continued the letter, until it was explained to friends at school that she "was going into the hospital over Christmas for some surgery on her ovaries and may miss a week or two in January." The surgery had to take place in New York City, with a certain "Dr. Granato," for "the last analyst they visited in N.J. said 'how dare you question me! I am a psychiatrist!,'" rejecting the request for a referral. The anecdotal story concludes with the recollection that the girl's father was surprised by "the understanding he received from school officials but not from the medical profession in N.J."[44]

Granato, it seems, was able to provide surgery to trans children in the New York City area on more than one occasion in the 1970s, perhaps having cultivated a reputation for access at a moment when surgery during childhood was still on the whole quite rare.[45] However, even if New York was in some ways at the forefront in offering availability and access, this does not mean that other clinicians around the United States were uninterested or unmotivated to arrange surgeries for children. Indeed, some wrote to high-profile institutions like Johns Hopkins to see whether they could refer clients under eighteen for surgery because there was a lack of local facilities.[46] Or, in the case of a fifteen-year-old trans girl who had been seen at a psychiatric clinic in Arkansas, the attending doctor wrote to Money directly because the situation had provoked too much anxiety among staff for the patient to pursue surgery any further, in spite of parental consent. "Our local Obstetrics and Gynecology people are unwilling to consider working with the case," he explained, "because of his [sic] minority—fearing possible lawsuits when the patient becomes 21."[47] Unfortunately for both of these children, Hopkins itself had an extremely strict policy of not allowing anyone under twenty-one into its program, and so it remains unclear whether either of them was able to find access to surgery during childhood.

The fact that some trans children did access surgery, including not just trans boys seeking top surgery but also trans girls, did not go unnoticed. The periodical *Sexuality* commissioned Ihlenfeld to write a general article titled "The Transexual" for a 1972 issue. It seems that the original article was never published and that its story of a trans child was replaced in the final issue with a more generic story about a trans adult. The reasons for the switch are unclear, although it is difficult not to wonder whether a story about a child was rejected for being too controversial. In the unpublished draft, Ihlenfeld recounted the story of "Joanna," who arrived at Benjamin's practice with her mother at the age of seventeen. Joanna had first seen a psychiatrist when she was twelve, although it was not clear then to adults what her femininity meant. At age fourteen she went to another psychiatrist and said that she felt herself to be a girl, not a boy; however, in an example of one of the harshest psychiatric reactions of the era, she was diagnosed not as transsexual but schizophrenic. After Joanna was hospitalized twice on that faulty premise, for a total of six months, her mother read an article about transsexuality in a magazine that mentioned Benjamin and decided to pursue that avenue instead.[48] "The first thing we did for [Joanna]," Ihlenfeld narrated, "was to begin female hormone treatments. After nine months, [Joanna's] breasts began to develop as an adolescent girl's."[49] A month later Ihlenfeld and Benjamin referred Joanna to a psychiatrist who could grant a referral to surgery. "It has been established that most of us by the time we're four have a clear sex identification," Ihlenfeld interjected, ostensibly for the benefit of the readership of *Sexuality*.[50] Joanna obtained gender confirmation surgeries at age seventeen. Ihlenfeld seemed quite self-conscious about that narrative, despite how generic it was for the era. "Not all transexuals undergo surgery so soon after diagnosis," he hedged. Indeed, "Dr. John Money, an authority on transexualism feels that a transexual should live at least two years as a woman" first. "Joanna's case is unusual," he concluded, "in that most transexuals do not get help so young. We can't treat patients under twenty-one without their parents permission, and very seldom do these people have parents as understanding as Joanna's."[51]

This draft article distinguished no single deciding factor that explains why surgery became more accessible to some children, like Joanna, in the 1970s, while for others the roadblocks were too numerous or onerous. Still, an emergent logic around development and puberty among clinicians from the prior decade was also coming to maturity in a way that increasingly justified surgery for teenagers, albeit at a high cost to younger children. Chapter 4 examines the University of California, Los Angeles's Gender Identity Clinic, where children ranging from three to eighteen years old were seen by an interdisciplinary team of psychologists, psychoanalysts, psychiatrists, endocrinologists, gynecologists, and surgeons beginning in 1962. The gap between the published work of the major figures at that clinic and their actual clinical approach to trans children is taken up in that chapter in detail. What is pertinent again here is that the clinic's director, Robert Stoller, in particular, advocated using psychotherapeutic and analytic techniques with young trans children to *prevent* the development of trans identity by adulthood. Yet because such psychotherapeutic attempts were useless, in reality most clinicians at UCLA, including Stoller, also reluctantly allowed their child patients to transition as teenagers—that is, once puberty had begun. As the 1960s wore on, the basis of this discrepancy at UCLA came to settle on the proposition that there was no biological or psychological use in trying to preempt the onset of transsexuality after puberty had begun. Stoller, who more than others held to the transphobic hope of intervening psychotherapeutically in childhood to eradicate trans life altogether, conceded that "it seems impossible to treat the adult transsexual successfully" (where "success" meant to erase their sense of self), but then "even at age 6 or 7, our work is formidable."[52] For Stoller, transgender childhood was the decisive test case for his transphobic psychiatry and psychoanalysis. Either transsexuality could be "treated" psychologically during early childhood to the point of being eliminated or else there was no use pursuing any further psychotherapeutic approaches at all. Although Benjamin was less overtly hostile to the viability of trans identity, in a letter to a fellow doctor in 1971 he nonetheless referred to the work of "Stoller and Green of U.C.L.A.," according to whom "young transsexual children may indeed by helped by psychotherapy," whereas "it is useless in the true transsexual adult."[53] This emergent sense that something decisive about the intractability of transsexuality could be said to come into effect during childhood had become a topic of intense interest for clinicians by the 1970s.

The threshold meant to manage the difference between the malleability of childhood and the futility of anti-trans intervention in adulthood was, precisely, puberty. For a 1979 issue of the newsletter *Transition*, published by the trans organization Confide, contributor Garrett Oppenheim interviewed Ihlenfeld on the subject. The resulting article's title, "Ihlenfeld Cautions on Hormones," indexes the double bind of the expansion of medicalization in the 1970s for transgender childhood. As access to transition grew, the developmental and disenfranchising premises upon which it rested also intensified, rigidly constraining the forms that access could take. The article, which styled itself as a general Q&A with a well-known practitioner, essentially became an interview about the centrality of the child to transsexual medicine. Asked what causes transsexuality, Ihlenfeld first admitted that medical science had no answer and that Stoller's version of its ostensible psychogenesis was not convincing. He then launched into a digression on children and biology, which Oppenheim recounted thus:

> "Still, there must be *something* inborn [about transsexuality],"
> Ihlenfeld conceded, "because when two children are reared in the
> same family, only one of them is likely to become a transsexual." . . .
> For reasons such as these, Ihlenfeld is against giving hormones to
> persons under the age of 18; in fact, he prefers that they be at least
> 20 or 21 years old before they start on this route. "I did have one
> patient who had surgery at 17 and is doing well," he said. "But in
> general, identity is still fluid in adolescence. There's a chance that
> gender feelings still might change."[54]

The internal inconsistency of Ihlenfeld's reflection could hope to save itself only through its developmental logic. If the trans child is fundamentally plastic (a quality here expressed as a "fluid identity"), then a transphobic treatment aimed at eradicating trans identity might find purchase at an early enough age, molding the child to cisgender ends. For Ihlenfeld, this plastic possibility for normalization justified the refusal of hormones to anyone under eighteen that Oppenheim reported. Yet at the same time the reference to *"something* inborn" is not just a fantasized biologism but rather a recognition that the plasticity of childhood does not neatly resolve along the lines that Ihlenfeld initially describes. As we already saw, Ihlenfeld's own clinic most certainly *did* prescribe hormones to trans children under eighteen, so his public stance on the "caution" necessary in connection with the use of hormones in *Transition* was contradicted by his own medical practice. That he refers to "one patient who had surgery at 17 and is doing well" in fact puts that contradiction on display for readers. The presumed plasticity of the trans child, the plasticity that floats the entire field of transsexual medicine, ends up underwriting two opposite outcomes in the same paragraph. It suggests that transsexuality can be preempted, while it also suggests that the plastic body takes on too much of its own agency during puberty to accept the reversal of trans embodiment and identity. The article continues by noting that "Ihlenfeld cites the works of Dr. Richard Green [at UCLA], who has attempted to identify potential transsexuals before puberty and to alter their gender identity. *But it's difficult to identify transsexuals when they are children,* he added."[55]

The operative phrase in this otherwise cluttered interview is "before puberty." The sense that puberty marks a threshold after which transsexuality cannot be eradicated by doctors or psychiatrists backed both the expansion in access to transition during adolescence in the 1970s and a renewed push toward rigid gatekeeping that included Ihlenfeld's claim that younger children might be excluded from access to hormones, never mind surgery. In many ways, this contradictory state was the predictable outcome of the developmentalization of plasticity since the early twentieth century. Since endocrinology had established that plasticity materially exhibited no natural inclination toward any particular sexed form or gendered meaning, the teleology of development had been mobilized to give it a significance and reliability that it had never really demonstrated. The metaphor of the child's developing body was meant to domesticate plasticity, but it could never accomplish that task because of its partial misfit with the phenomenon it was supposed to describe. Interestingly, then, in the very same issue of *Transition* the "Legal Poser" section, which hosted anonymous letters looking for legal advice and provided replies from a lawyer, ran a column titled "Hormones at Age 17?" The letter was from "a 17-year-old transsexual residing in New York State" who was "eager to start my hormone therapy as soon as possible." The writer explained that "my psychiatrist agrees that I should eventually go through a sex change, but my parents are dead set against it. Friends tell me that doctors are allowed to treat minors confidentially, without their parents' knowledge or consent." Wondering if that could "apply in my case," the writer concluded by asking, "How long must I wait before I can start hormone treatments without my parents' being able to stop me?"[56]

Richard D. Levidow, described by *Transition* as "widely known as a champion of legal rights for transsexuals," provided the reply to this letter. The outlook was grim: "It will be difficult, if not impossible, for a 17-year-old—who is legally an 'infant' in New York State—to receive hormone therapy without his parents' consent," he explained. Any doctor who prescribed hormones in the scenario the anonymous writer had described "would be placing himself in considerable legal jeopardy." Having shot down the idea of treatment without parental consent, Levidow added that "when the patient is legally 'emancipated'—usually at age 18—he [*sic*] will then be in a position to commence hormone therapy if his psychiatrist and his medical doctor believe this would be beneficial to him."[57] Whether or not the slight ambiguity of emancipation taking place "*usually* at age 18" was meant to open the door to a way of getting around parental consent, Levidow's response was on the whole emphatically negative.[58] Between Ihlenfeld and Levidow, the message to the readers of *Transition* was that both medicine and law were unanimous in barring transgender children from hormone therapy.

At the same time that psychiatrists, endocrinologists, and doctors were overseeing more hormonal and surgical transitions for trans children than ever before, they also undertook a rhetorical campaign to split the category of transsexuality through the threshold of puberty, attempting to disqualify younger children and keep the door open to the erasure of trans identity altogether by once again banking on the plasticity of the child's growing body. Only now, plasticity was understood to undergo an important change in form during adolescence, becoming less receptive to cultivation by medical science and more unruly in puberty before it began to recede altogether. Lawrence Newman, a psychiatrist at UCLA who in the 1960s began reluctantly letting children under his care transition, put it quite plainly in an article for *Medical Insight* magazine in 1970: "Because *transsexualism cannot be cured after puberty,* it is imperative that the disorder be identified at an earlier stage when curative treatment is possible."[59] Again, the instability of this insistence is important, for while the child's plasticity might offer the suggestion of eradicating transsexuality before it had consolidated, it at the same time implied equally that *all children* were to some degree *normally* unfixed in their gender identity, casting doubt on the overall legitimacy of the gender binary. Here, the specter of the overlap between gender-as-identity and sexuality-as-object-choice reenters the frame. "The future transsexual is a very feminine little boy who prefers to wear girls' clothing," Newman explained. This child "prefers girls as friends and avoids boys and roughhouse play, loves to take care of dolls and do housework, and—most malignantly—will on occasion say that he wishes to grow up to become a woman."[60] The ascending litany of symptoms is unexpectedly fragile, for only the "most malignant" of them is drawn from the diagnostic model for transsexuality (and occurs only "on occasion"), while the others could just as easily have applied to the pathologization of proto-gay children. Newman seemed bothered by the implication and tried to explain it away by specifying that "all children enjoy imitating the opposite sex on occasion; *the issue here is the intensity of the cross-gender interests.*"[61] Rendering childhood cases of transsexuality a more intense version of either proto-gay or entirely normal childhood development was a poor form of resolution. Newman therefore reinforced the sense that transgender children ultimately incorporate a moment of psychic and biological malleability in distinct contrast to "the older transsexual whose gender misidentification has become *irreversible,*" justifying intervention on the violent basis of the possible extinction of trans life altogether.[62]

Puberty signaled the end of a certain normal reversibility of sex and gender, at once a form of developmentally diminishing biological plasticity that could be receptive to hormones and also the expression of a psychological fluidity irresistible to psychiatrists and analysts such as those who ran the clinic at UCLA. The pernicious quality of the discourse of reversibility is that it could at one and the same time enable Money to advocate for hormone therapy and top surgery for trans boys while also letting Ihlenfeld and Newman imagine reversing transgender identity and embodiment out of existence. What's more, the new emphasis on puberty and the reversibility of childhood sex and gender marks an entangled change in their racialization. The plasticity of sex had since the late nineteenth century been racialized in a normative sense as a synonym for a eugenic form, an alterability stored latently in the human, open to cultivation in a project of species improvement. The invention of gender in the 1950s smuggled that eugenic principle into the postwar era, sublimating it even further into the abstraction of the endocrine body. Now the temporal form of that racial normativity, the cultivation of sex and gender into phenotypic ideals of male and female, took on a more distinctive contour in childhood. The morphology of the body and mind could be "reversed," to a certain extent, but only prior to puberty. The ideal human form was one that could move fluidly through sex phenotypes prior to adolescence, when the developmental teleology of gender identity would apparently become so fixed as to be indifferent to psychiatric intervention.

The significance of this refinement of plasticity into a partially reversible and puberty-bound phenomenon took place in the larger context of a renewed medicalization of puberty during the 1970s, one highly charged with racial meaning. Most prominently, the Tanner Scale of puberty development came into widespread usage. During the 1960s, James Tanner and W. A. Marshall had undertaken longitudinal studies of the bodies of girls and boys from childhood to adulthood, objectifying the timing and growth rates of genitals, height, weight, and secondary sex characteristics. In a 1969 study on girls and a 1970 study on boys, both published in *Archives of Disease in Childhood*, they rendered a statistical progression of "normal" developmental processes for puberty out of the aggregate anthropometric data they had produced.[63] Ostensibly, the resulting Tanner scale was meant to handle the overwhelming *variability* in child development. Yet in most ways their method was lifted without acknowledgment from turn-of-the-century eugenic anthropometry, producing an ascending teleological scale of normal phenotypes that had no basis in anything other than their interpretation of statistical compilation. The temporalization of a "normal" age range for pubertal development also enabled the uptake of a very old and persistent discourse on the hypersexualization of black women and Latinas, which from the 1970s on led to an obsessive focus on the supposedly "earlier" puberty of black and brown girls.[64]

While the racialization of puberty in the nascent era of reversibility signaled a continuing investment in an abstract, eugenic form of whiteness located in the flesh of the sexed body and the depths of the gendered psyche, it was also laminated onto other forms of racialization that were hypervisible, with devastating consequences for black trans children in particular. While the medical model continued to suture the category of transsexuality to a latent whiteness coeval with plasticity, with all of the gatekeeping and renewed surveillance that incurred for white trans children, black trans children found themselves in decidedly more precarious institutional situations. Black and brown trans children tended to be subjected to much harsher forms of confinement than transsexual medicalization, as well as to an utter dismissal and suspicion of their self-knowledge. Indeed, as had been the case in the 1960s, the fact of blackness often amounted to a disqualification from the discourse of transsexuality altogether. In 1970 the director of a juvenile mental health clinic at a hospital in Ohio wrote to Money about a fifteen-year-old patient. This trans girl, who was African American, had been admitted to the hospital's emergency room after "taking an overdose of 15–20 barbituric pills." After being stabilized, she was transferred to the juvenile psychiatric ward. "The patient was known to be an 'overt homosexual,'" according to the director, and the intake procedures aimed not merely to assess the causes of the suicide attempt but also to produce "advice as to post-hospitalization treatment plan for patient's problem in sexual identification." The director described the fifteen-year-old in physical detail, emphasizing "fine features" that were "markedly effeminate."[65] He also underlined her general depression while on the ward. Other than noting that she "spoke in black ethnic style, using as few words as possible and often employing slang words which required further elaboration and definition," the psychiatric evaluation that the director enclosed with his letter did not consider what it might mean to a black trans girl to be hospitalized.[66] For instance, she reported a great fear of being arrested and sent to jail, but this was dismissed as a delusional symptom, rather than an acute awareness of her vulnerability to state violence.

The ward's general suspicion of and disdain for this black trans girl is collected in the psychiatric evaluation's continual rejection of her claim to be a girl. The psychiatrist remarked that "He [sic] does not think the fact that 'wanting to be a girl' or his [sic] homosexual activities were a problem."[67] Yet her parents also reported that "by age of two [she] preferred wearing girls' clothing and participated in 'girl's play.'" Apparently she first told her mother at age thirteen that she "wished to be a girl." A year later she asked "to be admitted to the hospital." She came to the very same hospital in which she was now confined, where she and her mother met with a psychiatrist. She expressed then that she "wished at that time an oper-ation to become a girl," but apparently "no follow-up was carried out."[68] In 1970, when she was held on the ward after the suicide attempt, the eval-uation concluded with two diagnoses: "Depression with suicidal attempts" and "transexual behavior." In particular, "the physical changes of puberty" reportedly were causing "discord between the patient's internal view of him-self [sic] as feminine, and the reality of his perception by others as a male." In nearly every way this narrative was generically, emphatically trans for the era. Yet the psychiatrist immediately undercut his own diagnosis. "One might speculate," he wrote in the "Recommendations" section of his evalu-ation, "that only by becoming a girl literally could [name redacted] have piece of mind and resolving of internal conflicts." Rather than endorsing that possibility, however, he instead suggested that a "more thorough inves-tigation along these lines may be necessary" and advised that the director consult with Money.[69]

In a move that was stunningly unethical, Money wrote back to the director that "the best thing to do is to try and rehabilitate him as well as possible *as a homosexual*, even as a full time impersonating homosex-ual."[70] While Money promised to send information on estrogen therapy, this also brought a racist caveat. "The advantage of estrogen for the ex-tremely effeminate homosexual," Money wrote, "is it gives him the breasts he wants. *From my point of view, the great advantage is that it's also a func-tional castrating agent* which has a tranquilizing effect on behavior in gen-eral. It may indeed . . . temper behavior the patient has been showing."[71] Although this girl had been given a diagnosis of transsexuality and although the director had written to one of the most recognized clinicians involved in transsexual medicine, both the psychiatrist in Ohio and Money went on to disqualify her from the category altogether, turning to its latent over-lap with homosexuality-as-inversion to deny her self-knowledge that she was a girl *and* to open the door to hormones only in order to further the eugenic goal of sterilization as a form of racial hygiene.

The disqualification and dispossession of blackness that structured this girl's experience with medicine and confinement adds an important coun-ternarrative to the transgender boyhood of the 1970s that the first part of this chapter recounts. The deeply compromised project of medicalization was actually a relative privilege for those white children whose plastic bod-ies were desirable enough to be folded into the category of transsexual-ity by its gatekeeping clinicians. In marked contrast to the trans boyhood this chapter has explored, black trans girls were subject to massive scrutiny during this decade, often arrested or confined to mental health wards in questionable circumstances. Those cases where a juvenile probation or parole officer, attending psychiatrist, therapist, or social worker decided to write to a clinician like Money for advice were ironically perhaps the most humanely handled, not to mention those that could most easily make it into the archive of transsexual medicine.[72]

Despite this prevailing situation, small glimpses into the nonpathologized lives of these black trans girls outside confinement are also scattered across the bureaucratic paperwork that worked to maintain their detention. When a psychiatrist in Colorado wrote to a professor of pediatrics at Hopkins about a seventeen-year-old black trans girl he was seeing in his clinic, he mentioned in passing that she had plans, after graduating from high school, to attend "the Art Institute in San Francisco."[73] In a psychologist's letter to Money about a fifteen-year-old black trans girl he was counseling in Kentucky, interspersed with the generic evaluation narrative is a reference to her "long frosted hair (a la his [sic] heroine Stevie Nix [sic])."[74] In a psychological test that involved composing a story, she "told the story of Rhiannon, 'the schizophrenic Welsh Witch,' a character from a Fleetwood Mac album in which the refrain is 'Will you ever win,'" explained the psychologist. "The Rhiannon of [her] story is a young, beautiful devil worshipper who is lonely but wants to be loved for herself. She has many lovers but none who love her for herself, so she finally remains alone and learns not to care and 'thinks about what she thinks.'"[75] We are left to wonder whether she was able to find in her own life the same capacity that her imagined Rhiannon possessed, the ability to find within a situation of enforced vulnerability and confinement the space to "think about what she thinks" as an assertion of black trans personhood, of black trans girlhood.

The Queerness of Trans Childhood

Although trans boyhood was a distinct category of embodiment and medicalization in the 1970s, it cohabited with a range of different experiences that cut gendered, sexual, and racialized lines across trans childhood and the category "transsexuality." While in its most medicalized instances trans boyhood did not seem to interact much with the specter of lesbian masculinity, the hypervisible difference made by race and antiblackness does suggest that homosexuality continued to be leveraged against trans identity for many black trans children who encountered medical authorities, a form of trans erasure *through* gay visibility. At the same time, the renewed medicalization of puberty through an emergent discourse on the reversibility of sex prior to adolescence also tried to divide trans childhood not so much by masculinity or femininity as by phenotypes of age and development, making early childhood the anxious locus of continuing—and wildly unsuccessful—attempts to eradicate trans life as it grew in childhood. The aims of this chapter, then, are not only to invalidate the generational presumptions of the border wars, the relative invisibility of trans boyhood relative to trans girlhood, or the implicit historiography they have founded in queer theory and trans studies. More important, trans boyhood and its counterpoints insist that we ask different questions altogether about race, gender, sexuality, and childhood. The black trans girls whose experiences of the 1970s clashed so profoundly with the white trans boys of the same decade make clear that there is no reparative, general narrative of trans childhood from this moment to usurp those that have gone relatively unchallenged since the 1990s.

Part of what we have lost, having framed queer and trans childhood in the post-1980 terms of the separation of sexuality-as-object-choice from gender-as-identity, is the way that the child *should* pull us back into more troublesome territory. As Kathryn Bond Stockton has argued, the queerness of the concept of the child really ought to radically *undermine* the neatness of such divisions. Reflecting on what has changed since the 2009 publication of *The Queer Child*, Stockton considers the lessons we can take from the way that gay and trans children have rapidly grown in visibility in the twenty-first century. She asks how, in other words, to square that growth in self-proclaimed identity with her argument that the twentieth century was characterized by a *ghostliness* in the child concept incarnated by the case of the gay child and the problem of delay to which it was attached. In an illuminating note in this essay on "The Queer Child Now," Stockton textures the issue thus:

> Certainly, as I argue there [in *The Queer Child*], transgendered and gender-queer children have been subjected to harmful delays of unspeakable sorts—by parents, medical and psychiatric authorities and public discourse. The distinction of the ghostly gay child, and why it *figures* childhood delay, is its insistent and quite intense *sexualization* by authoritative forces and its own

sexual self-understandings. The sexual assumptions surrounding "gay" slide onto the "gay" child *as a concept* and thus have made its present-tense existence so precarious (since these assumptions are deemed so "adult"). Trans kids get sexualized in various ways, but often their sexual object choice is actually downplayed (harmfully, prejudicially)—even by allies—so as to focus on gender identity. The complex collision between "trans" and "gay" for many queer kids is beyond the scope of this present essay, though my current research takes it as a focus.[76]

If the gay child was the archetypally ghostly creature of the twentieth century, figuring the strangeness and impossible sexuality of delay in the child concept more broadly, then certainly the trans child was ghostly during that century too with reference to the developmental temporality of binary gender. That ghostliness was intensified by the problem of the desired separation of object choice from gender identity, the need to desexualize trans children in a way that ultimately made their existence in the twentieth century even less imaginable than it might have otherwise been. We are confronted by the deeply unsatisfying neatness of that split. The "complex collision between 'trans' and 'gay' for many queer kids" comes up just as soon as we would exorcise the ghosts of the past century (an exorcism distinct from the haunting situation of absence described by Sedgwick in "How to Bring Your Kids Up Gay"). Instead of generational splits or borders, there is an indeterminacy at play—the "queerness" of childhood Stockton names precisely evokes this—that threatens to undo the entire situation, bringing the narrative of the move from twentieth-century ghostly children to twenty-first-century out-and-proud children down upon itself. How, precisely, is a child to know where queerness as sexual-object-choice begins and transness as gender-identity ends? How can we claim to know, either?

For that matter, how could *any* authoritative discourse ever really know, especially medicine or psychology? This chapter adds historical texture to Stockton's argument. In relying so profoundly on childhood plasticity to ground its access to sex and gender, transsexual medicine worked itself into an impossible epistemological position. In the growing body of the child there could be no ultimate distinction between queerness-as-sexual-object-choice and trans-gender-as-identity because the child needed to remain the most indeterminate of forms in order to float the medical model. Indeed, identity was never the foothold of transsexual medicine, despite its obsession with the psyche and narratives of the self. Indeterminacy rather provided cover for the normalizing logic of transition and the transphobic desire to eradicate trans life psychotherapeutically before it grew up, casting some trans children as desexualized while willfully misreading others as gay to deny their transness. Yet the very same indeterminacy so cultivated by medicine also guaranteed that the growing separation of (trans) gender from (homo)sexuality that received such a boost by the end of the 1970s in the new edition of the *DSM* could never have any real traction in the body of the queer and trans child. Stockton sees the riddle here that medical science will not let itself see, that the border wars will not let us see, and that mainstream LGBT politics will not let itself see.

Taking a broader look than Stockton at the arc of the twentieth century tracked across this book, it is also important to emphasize that the 1970s do *not* show that the multiple definitions of transness that had flourished in the first half of the twentieth century had been replaced with a single, binary model. While from the 1920s to the 1940s, as chapter 2 argues, transness in childhood took on a range of divergent connotations, including intersex, inversion, homosexual, and transvestite meanings, that multiplicity of trans childhoods was not, finally, extinguished by the paradigm of transsexuality. On the contrary, the antiblack fractures of the discourse of transsexuality, read alongside the incorporation of a largely white trans boyhood and girlhood, underlines how multiple modes of trans childhood were still very much in operation in this era. The unifier among them was not binary gender but an investment in trans children's relative plasticity, in this case organized by gender (the asymmetry between top and bottom surgery for boys and girls) and race (the antiblack logic of medical gatekeeping). And while the comparison of trans boyhood and girlhood, for both black and white trans children, may on the surface seem to imply a kind of congealing of the category "trans" in this chapter into something more solid than it has signified earlier in this book, as if it had become more binary by this time, the point I am making is actually quite different. While insisting on the distinction of white trans *boyhood* or black trans *girlhood* might seem to imply that trans childhood was never nonbinary or that it reinforced the gender binary as such, that impression is an ideological conceit of the medical model in the postwar era, as chapter 3 shows. The instability of plasticity subtending that model reminds that the trans boys and girls who appear in the medical archive informing this chapter are far from representative of trans childhoods in this era. Indeed, they are, in this chapter perhaps more than others, highly *un*representative. The vast majority of trans children did not interact with the doctors or psychiatrists profiled in this chapter. Only those who were pulled into a relation (even one of rejection) with the discourse of transsexuality are visible in this archive. But the unrepresentative quality of this account is not a wholesale limitation on this chapter's argument. Much as I argued in the case of the trans child before transsexuality, the partiality and fragmentary quality of this archival account leads to a more important destabilizing point about trans childhoods.

As we move closer and closer to 1980 in this book, approaching the epistemological matrix of transgender medicine in which we live today, the 1970s ought to serve to undermine both the coherence of where we find ourselves and the sense that we are somehow in the midst of something new with trans children. The emergence of the discourse of reversibility and its concomitant racialization of puberty in this era is missing from the twenty-first-century "controversy" over puberty suppression therapy. At the same time, pushing plasticity's most available phase back to before puberty has also resulted in a situation today in which childhood transition has become linked for some clinicians to what Claudia Castañeda rightly identifies as a form of developmentalism that aims to eventually erase all visible trans difference. Some pediatric clinicians today promise a future where visible transgender difference will be preemptively eliminated by children's seamless and plastic transitions that begin before puberty sets in. The trans child today promises the future stealth adult of tomorrow.[77] The conclusion to this book takes up these questions further in light of the histories of trans children and plasticity that this book has tracked over twentieth century.

Establishing the existence of trans boyhood in the 1970s, then, turns out to be much less of an establishing gesture than we might have expected. It is important to challenge the generational narrative of the border wars and the overvaluation of the *DSM* in the historiography of gender identity, sexuality, and childhood, but that destabilizing project has no unified narrative or recuperated trans masculine subject to turn to as a replacement. The queerness and the transness of children under the developmental temporalities we have confined them to, as Stockton incisively reminds, simply will not harbor such stability. Despite itself, even trans medicine reveals that in its paradoxical attempts to cultivate children's racial plasticity. Recovering a trans masculine subject from the 1970s would serve only to cover over those stark forms of antiblack governance, medical objectification, disenfranchisement, and confinement to which some trans children were subjected in the 1970s.

And yet, here I also pause. There remains something insistent, urgent, and, indeed, spectral about trans boyhood in the 1970s that feels unfinished, even in the most medicalized precincts of the archive. In an elusive but important way, Jeanne Hoff's assumption of Harry Benjamin's clinic in 1979 indexes a moment of palpable transformation, when a trans psychiatrist was, perhaps for the first time, in charge of a practice for other trans people.[78] Hoff's careful and exhaustive work in reviewing all of Benjamin's files and trying to follow up with his existing clients, while simultaneously taking on new patients at her office on the Upper West Side of New York City, represents a shift that cannot be simply lumped in with the incredibly hostile and transphobic doctors and psychiatrists discussed in this chapter. Though the medical model was still based in gatekeeping and an unacknowledged racialization of gender, Hoff cared deeply about the well-being of her clients to a degree that is viscerally embedded in the archive she gifted to the Kinsey Institute. Her work demonstrates a level of empathy entirely absent from transsexual medicine since its advent—not to mention its predecessors in the early twentieth century—an ethic of care that, although greatly constrained by the material circumstances and history of psychiatry and endocrinology, was also entangled with her situated perspective as a trans woman. It is important to underline that Hoff represents yet another trans person who took an active and complicated role in medicine, rather than being its object.

Hoff worked with children, including trans boys. Because she took the time to interview them without only reducing what they said to standard diagnostic biographies, her notes offer comparatively richer glimpses into trans boyhood than those of her predecessors. When one trans man she was seeing mentioned that his catalyst for seeking support came at age seventeen, when he was praying in church and heard the voice of god telling him to become a man, Hoff did not pathologize the adolescent scene as evidence of an immature delusion, as so many other hostile clinicians did.[79] Indeed, Hoff included a level of self-reflexivity in her notes that stands in stark contrast with the overconfident, dispassionate, and dissociated view most doctors took. For example, while talking with a young trans woman for the first time about her life, she recorded, with a reflexive flair in parentheses:

"Got female hormones at age 15 from [a New York City] medical clinic (*by asking for them!*)."[80] Amid a mountain of paperwork for medical examination and initial diagnosis, Hoff recorded about a seventeen-year-old trans boy that "David Bowie is pt.s idol."[81] In an evaluative letter from the gynecologist to whom the boy was sent as part of the initial entry process for the office, the doctor mentioned that the boy had found his way to Hoff through an article about the trans tennis star Renée Richards, who was then in the news. The boy was currently at a high school for aspiring artists and performers after being socially ostracized and physically attacked during junior high,[82] the doctor added, and his mother "is very receptive" and "willing to pay her expenses" for access to medicine. Although the gynecologist did not use his pronouns in this letter, she too noted that "her present idol is David Bowie and in fact, she resembles him strongly. She deliberately styles her hair like him and was wearing a David Bowie T shirt the days I saw her."[83]

These small vignettes, while ephemeral, texture the ghostly surrounds of the trans child in the 1970s. Providing neither certainty on the relationship between gender and sexuality in the growing body of the child nor outright resistance to the authority of medical science and its racialization of gender development, they nevertheless interrupt, if only slightly, the otherwise orderly flow of medical discourse. And so it seems, however anecdotally, that even the 1980s at Hoff's clinic were not necessarily marked by as severe a retrenchment in access to medicine's resources for trans children as occurred elsewhere in the United States. One trans man, for instance, began seeing Hoff in 1980 at the twilight of his childhood, having just turned eighteen. At first he met with Hoff weekly while finishing high school and getting access to hormones and, later, top surgery. By 1985 the appointments had decreased to once per month, but he continued to see Hoff until 1988.[84] By then, he had enrolled as a medical student, and in 1999, although it had been more than a decade since his last appointment, he wrote to Hoff to tell her the good news that he was now a senior resident in internal medicine.[85] While providing no certainty on broader questions that the child fundamentally unsettles, this trans boy's trajectory out of childhood, out of the clinic, and into the practice of medicine himself underlines just how central trans children have been as complex participants in medicine—not exactly redemptive architects, to be sure, but never its silent objects.

How to Bring Your Kids Up Trans

T HE TWENTY-FIRST-CENTURY FIGURATION of the trans child as
futuristic does harm when its novelty erases the historical prece-
dents to the demands for recognition, dignity, and a livable life that are
being made by and on behalf of trans children today. This book has worked
directly against the conceit of the newness of trans childhood, not just to
point out that it is historically inaccurate but also to demonstrate that it
has politically infantilizing consequences for trans children, now deprived
of a century's worth of precedent that might enfranchise them. The political struggle for access to bathrooms, for instance, which connects public
accommodation, businesses, prisons, and schools, has become a signal case
of the limitations of trans childhood's dominant mode of futurity. A trans-
inclusive Title IX policy was first authored by the Department of Justice for
schools receiving federal funding in 2016, put on legal hold by the courts
later that year, and ultimately rescinded in August 2017. The media coverage of this process repeatedly framed the right to bathroom use as "a new
issue," further undermining the legitimacy of trans children's fight and cloak-
ing them with a libelous air of caution, as if the entire endeavor were experimental and risky.[1]

The *New York Times* rehearsed this emphasis on newness when the paper
called Gavin Grimm, a Virginia teenager who sued the Gloucester County
school board after it barred him from using the boys' bathroom, "the new
face of the transgender rights movement" for pursuing the lawsuit and organizing around school bathrooms.[2] While the legal battle under Title IX is
certainly new, casting Grimm as emblematic of a novel civil rights issue
misunderstands the temporal structure of his own case. It turns out that
Grimm *was* originally allowed to use the boys' bathroom with the permission of his school's administration for some time, without incident, until
parents of other children at the school politically mobilized against him,
no doubt hoping to take part in a larger legislative and political attack on

trans bathroom access that has grown in fervor in recent years. And as a journalistic exposé of the legal battle points out in passing, "School districts that dealt with the issue *for years* under the radar on a case by case basis are now trying to balance rules concerning transgender bathroom access with the privacy concerns of critics."[3] The true "newness" of bathroom policy, it turns out, has much less to do with trans children being unprecedented than it does with a highly contemporary form of anti-trans backlash that has taken the convergence of trans visibility and vulnerability as an opportunity. The putative rhetoric of "privacy concerns," "safety," and the egregiously weak proposition that genitals or binary "biological sex" can usefully direct policy are convenient displacements for naked political violence against trans life. Beholden to futurity's temporality of perpetual deferral, the trans child continues to be a figure through which anti-trans forces can focus their efforts to undermine any future at all for trans people, while simultaneously suggesting that they have no meaningful historical precedent.

If trans children cannot mortgage the future to pay for civil rights that they lack today, the past century might serve to deepen the public reality of their lives, challenging anti-trans forces. Think again of Val, whose trans childhood in the early twentieth century I discussed in chapter 2. When she began attending school in rural Wisconsin, around 1930, her parents made sure she was able to attend as a girl, even going so far as to ensure that "special arrangements for toilet, etc. were made."[4] Far from a new concern, then, the archive of the trans twentieth century shows us unambiguously a trans girl's use of the girls' bathroom at school almost nine decades ago. The historiographical basis of reactionary, transphobic politics, whether from Evangelical conservatives or trans-exclusionary feminists, both of whom presume that in some fabled past the gender and sex binary was an unproblematic institution that smoothly organized U.S. social life, is outright negated by Val's childhood. And while Grimm's legal case has made him a public face of a contemporary struggle, imagine how it might *strengthen* his position to be able to mobilize Val in his fight, pointing to a century-long precedent for bathroom access. What's more, the assumed cisness of children during that century means that alongside Val and the other trans children in this book were countless, unnamed others whose experience is still hidden from view.

Val existed. Gavin exists. Trans children are not new, and their lives cannot be deferred to a future by design not meant to arrive. Their vulnerability, whether political, social, or material, is a product not of their being children but rather of the historical infantilization they have been made to bear. Throughout the twentieth century this vulnerability was manufactured to a major extent by medicine, which reduced trans children to a problem of plasticity, rather than recognizing their personhood. While plasticity was also the reason for which trans children have been so central to the medicalization of sex and gender, the value they thereby accrued came at an incredibly high cost. For white trans children, being brought into the orbit of medicine involved being reduced to living laboratories, proxies for all kinds of theories and experimental medical techniques aimed at altering the sexed and gendered phenotypes of the human. For black trans and trans of color children, by contrast, the racialization of plasticity as white tended to disqualify them altogether from this medicalized framework on the presumption that they were less plastic and therefore less deserving of care, in many cases intensifying state systems of detention and incarceration that took hold of their lives instead. The discourse of plasticity has prescribed one narrow form of futurity through whiteness for trans children, while simultaneously denying any future at all to those who are structurally barred from its highly managed shelter.

The fractures wrought by reducing trans children to a reservoir of racial plasticity persist into the present day, as scholars' work on the contemporary pediatric endocrine clinic shows. Claudia Castañeda argues that it is precisely the liberal edge of pediatric trans medicine that leverages children for ends other than their own, promising through puberty suppression therapy a form of transition at an early age that is aimed *against* those trans people who transition as adults. In this developmental framework, visible trans difference produced by transitioning after puberty is increasingly cast as an atavistic relic, so that adult transitioning "becomes a kind of lesser version of transgender—because less completely trans-gendered in a bodily sense" than the child who pauses puberty.[5] While there is no inherent reason to confine puberty suppression therapy to this particular narrative, Sahar Sadjadi and Tey Meadow's important ethnographic work in the contemporary clinic shows how the desire and extreme pressure to find a biological etiology for trans life by locating gender's development "in the brain" has packaged profoundly normalizing rhetoric as scientific and progressive.[6] An early and gender normative transition has become valuable insofar as it uses children's exceptional plasticity to promise a future that erases trans visibility itself, a disturbing reconsolidation of the sex and gender binary that also evokes eugenic echoes of the "proper" racial phe-notypes of human sex from early twentieth-century endocrinology. Rather than resisting a binary system, in this case plasticity continues to reinforce and even strengthen it.

While the concept of plasticity today organizes trans medicine to lever-age trans children's supposed success against trans adults' supposedly tragic failure, Ann Travers's ethnographic work with a racially and economically diverse group of North American trans children also reminds that the metic-ulously medicalized narrative of trans childhood is massively *un*represen-tative, displacing low income, nonbinary, and trans children of color from ostensibly trans-affirmative discourse, when in reality they probably con-stitute by far the demographic majority of trans children.[7] Limiting the public framing of trans children to the medical establishment extends the general infantilization of these children by its discourse and rationality. If that is the case, then what does the history of racial plasticity tracked across this book suggest about the future of pediatric trans medicine? Can the con-cept of plasticity contribute to what Dean Spade and Eric A. Stanley call "gender self-determination" or what Paisley Currah calls "transgender rights without a theory of gender"?[8] *Histories of the Transgender Child* argues that it cannot, for plasticity is too entrenched as a vehicle for making trans chil-dren into figurative frameworks or etiologies for transness, if not gender itself.

The critique of racial plasticity as the unspoken ground of trans medi-cine—and, more broadly, of sex and gender as a living system whose admin-istration forms a key axis of modern biopolitical governmentality—is a vital starting point for rethinking and transforming pediatric medicine. That critique, which this book has undertaken for the twentieth century, confronts us with an array of immediate possibilities for reimagining the clinic, which would revolve around actually *listening* to what trans children say about themselves, grounding medical care in their desires, and aban-doning binary models of transition and dysphoria that continue to confine children to developmental teleologies ending in heterosexual masculinity or femininity. Rather than serving as a potential etiology for transgender diagnosis writ large or as living laboratories for harnessing plasticity, trans children need to have access to an enfranchised voice to articulate situ-ated knowledge to which medical practice is held accountable. As simple as it sounds, pediatric trans medicine would be radically transformed by actually *asking trans children what they want* and truly basing care on that knowledge. Giving up the etiological paradigm would disarm the transpho-bic pretenses in construing children's social transitions, puberty pauses, and hormonal prescriptions as dramas or crises. This reframing of trans pediatric medicine requires adult authorities to recognize that the very feeling that trans children's medical decisions require the conceit of panic and emergency is a way to disavow the fact that cisgender children never have to justify their gendered lives to this extent.

Dismantling the racialized, class-stratified structure of institutional U.S. medicine is a broader political project with high stakes for trans children, the vast majority of whom lack access to competent, responsible, and afford-able care in whatever form they might ideally ask for it. Removing infan-tilizing instruments like the medical age of consent would also enfranchise them to make self-determined decisions, particularly when being closeted or fearing reprisal and rejection from parents, guardians, and peers limits their ability to live a trans life. And decolonizing transgender childhood means both marking and working to displace the centering of whiteness in its expert and popular representation, producing and centering situated knowledge of black, indigenous, and trans of color childhoods. This book has provided only one example of how *all* Western biomedicine contin-ues to be eugenicist in practice, hoarding resources, stratifying quality of care, and normalizing the individual and population through highly granu-lar, racialized concepts of health that actively rely on a differential calculus of exhaustion, illness, and death for entire groups of people deemed unde-serving. The dethroning of institutional medicine and the transfer of the wealth and authority of insurance companies, pharmaceutical companies, doctors, and researchers into the hands of communities would go a long way toward ameliorating many of the most egregious forms of planned neglect that affect trans children (and adults), especially those of color.

While plasticity is a key concept through which to critically open up the underlying structures that produce these problems, it is far from an ideal political ground for imagining trans children and medicine differently. Plas-ticity has become so central to the flexible regime of neoliberal economies, where continuous adaptation and change is leveraged for near infinitesi-mal value extraction and the expansion of laboring to all productive bio-logical and cultural processes, that it cannot easily be adapted for different ends. Indeed, children in particular are quite easily folded back into labor and the extraction of value in ways that are ostensibly prohibited by law in new affective economies that are meant to supplement the diminishing returns of income inequality or biologically enhance children's development through medical means.⁹ What's more, the racialization of plasticity as white is by now so abstract and invidious that even projects like Paul B. Preciado's triumphalist call for an "auto-experimental form of do-it-yourself bio-terrorism of gender" and its dissident medical protocols, as I've suggested at several points in this book, are incapable of reckoning with the racial politics that float their model of voluntary, embodied political action.¹⁰

What plasticity *can* do is call upon us to reexamine whether it is worth holding onto the sex and gender binary at all. Another way to read the medical history that this book recounts is as a series of increasingly desperate attempts by doctors and scientists to save binary sex and gender from the threat of collapse that plasticity activated. Trans children have been forced to keep alive over the past century a tension between indeterminacy and form at the heart of plasticity, but this has always been a fragile and unfinished compromise, as numerous moments in this book show. The attendant point is that the transness of "trans childhood" changed across the twentieth century, as any social form would, rather than being defined by a binary. In the early twentieth century, as the concept of plasticity migrated into the medicalization of sex, childhood transness was articulated largely through a discourse of intersex embodiment and, to a lesser extent, the concepts of inversion and homosexuality. By the 1950s, as I argued in chapter 3, binary sex had so badly strained under the plastic framework that united these discourses and their inhabitation by trans adults and children that the category gender was invented to try to save it for the postwar era. Yet even the introduction of gender could only defer the paradox, rather than resolve it. By the 1960s and 1970s, as more and more children transitioned, it became clear that the developmental framing of core gender identity more often than not backfired upon the most transphobic clinicians at places like the University of California, Los Angeles, where failed attempts to eradicate trans identity in young children gave way to a consensus that teenagers could be allowed to transition and live as trans with support from doctors.

While this narrative of change over the twentieth century might seem on the surface to reinforce a succession from a pre- to posttranssexuality paradigm, in reality the only through line is the rich *variability* of trans childhood as a plastic state of being, in spite of its many colonizations by medicine. In chapter 2 I suggested that the ways that trans childhood was archived in the very early twentieth century multiplied definitions of transness out of the singular connotation of the postwar medical model. In the 1970s, as the final chapter showed, that multiplicity of transness had *not* actually been replaced by transsexuality's standardizing model of binary transition. The antiblack fractures of the discourse of transsexuality, which illustrated themselves in that decade through the rejection of black trans girls from the medical model in the very same moment that white trans boys and girls were being recognized as distinct constituencies, reminds that multiple modes of transness defined even the most intense domains of gatekeeping. While it may seem like the trans boys and girls in this book in the 1960s and 1970s, black and white, represent a more binary, congealed experience of transness than those from the 1930s or 1940s, my argument historicizes this easily made misreading. Any binary impression, to the extent that it exists, is in actuality an ideological effect of the incredibly limiting medical discourse of transsexuality, as well as the invention of gender, both which have been deeply invested in passing off the gender binary as much more natural than it has ever proved to be in medical practice or lived experience.

The arc of plasticity's indeterminacy from the first to the last chapter of this book is not offered as an adjudication of proper childhood transness, either. The resistance of embodied plasticity to binary categories was hardly the redemption of trans children, as the complex and elusive place it occupied their letters to doctors shows. In chapter 4 I argued that Vicki, whose rural trans girlhood in Ohio in the late 1960s was translated into a long series of letters to Harry Benjamin's office, invites us to recognize nonteleological forms of growth that move outward and away from what has typically been defined as binary "gender," or "growing up," into a tangled account of embodied knowledge about trans femininity, the limits of plasticity, and medical discourse that takes the form of fatness in her writing. The unanticipated significance of Vicki's letters communicates some of the ways that trans children grow beyond the narrow medical, social, and, above all, binary parameters to which adults have restricted them. In the interval generated by these deferrals, whether of medical support or recognition of her gender, Vicki experienced a profound indecision between growing feminine and growing fat. The palpable emotional pain and lack of autonomy expressed in her letters was, if anything, magnified by her embodied plasticity. As much as it resisted the medical model of gender, then, her embodied plasticity also resisted *her* efforts to find a livable life during childhood. For Vicki, the nonbinary tendencies of plasticity were not a source of resistive politics that made her life easier to live. On the contrary, the indeterminacy of her growth through childhood was a source of great pain.

Rather than calling for an affirmative politics of childhood plasticity aligned with gender self-determination, which is frankly hard to imagine, I argue instead for confronting the limits of plasticity in its irruptive tendency to refuse and disobey both medicine and the auspices of rational subjectivity, because that should lead us to question why we continue to focus our questioning of gender on trans children, rather than on the system of binary gender and cisgender embodiment. Plasticity is a good example of how under what Rebekah Sheldon terms "somatic capitalism" the extraction of value from children's biology encounters its own limit in the threat of "life's withdrawal," a runaway animacy activated at the point where *too* much life tips over into a rogue and inhuman force.[11] Biopolitics can alter life, but, as Sheldon points out, it cannot make life. For that reason the function of the figure of the child to reconsolidate humanness where the "wayward agency" of "life-itself" is the actual object of governmental technique produces an inevitable and uncontrollable surplus through its reliance on concepts like plasticity.[12] Sheldon points to how the figure of the child's living body unwittingly generates in the twenty-first century "a wayward and insurgent *zoē* as resistant to stewardship and the politics of care as it is to the mass-production processes premised on a pliable natural world."[13] This book points to the twentieth-century activation of children's plasticity in a similar vein, as the introduction of a biological problem that cannot ever be fully managed, one that makes plasticity resistant to any medical or political reclamation. If plasticity is unlikely to obey trans-affirmative politics any better than it has obeyed medical science, then it does provide a powerful example of why the desire to cling to binary sex and gender as natural forms is, ultimately, built upon a house of cards. If that is so, then it is all the more unacceptable to continue to ask trans children to serve as an etiology for transness, not to mention sex and gender more broadly, when cisgender children and the entire binary model of gender do not receive the same level of scrutiny.

With a sense of responsibility to Vicki's and so many other trans children's experience of medicine, I argue that plasticity is too combustible a concept to animate trans children in any way that does not also do them harm, for it ultimately reinforces the immense pressure they already bear to either prove an etiology for transgender embodiment or else serve by way of developmental suppression as a means to fulfill the genocidal fantasy that trans life not exist.[14] What's more, plasticity cannot easily serve to remedy its own historical damage because it has proven time and again to resist any and all attempts at stabilization. Rather, this book has striven above all to *set aside* altogether the question of trans children as an etiology for sex, gender, or transgender life. If that makes the definition of children's transness less easy to grasp, all the better, as perhaps this is an index of trans childhood losing its status as a stable singular concept and gaining its reality as an internally diverse field of experience. Plasticity *is* a useful lens through which to see that the very etiological impulse around trans children, the question of what constitutes their transness or how their transness would explain cis-sex and gender, is impossible to answer. Plasticity continually resists the stabilization that would be required of it to provide such a truth. Even when medicine succeeded in instrumentalizing trans children's bodies in the service of a normalizing binary medical model, neither that project nor the ostensibly binary trans identities of children in the postwar era overcame their indebtedness to a nonbinary, embodied plasticity. In reality, embodied plasticity has been a force doctors could count upon only to a limited extent, without ever controlling it. For that reason, plasticity at best reminds us that we need to dethrone singular definitions of transness, including trans childhood, and that the multiplication of what transness means is an urgent project for trans children's livelihoods, as trans children have been forced to give up the knowledge gained from their experiences to stand in for an explanation of trans life for more than a century. Trans children, especially black trans and trans children of color, have been forced to pay what amounts to perhaps the highest material price for the modern sex and gender binary. To begin to reckon with the immense damage that has caused would mean giving up the obsessive need to see trans children as representatives of something they are not, either indeterminate or binary creatures, and instead greet them as people whose transness is not up for investigation before they are listened to and recognized.

To conclude, *Histories of the Transgender Child* calls for an ethical aperture of relation, one oriented toward a different future for trans children that might still draw on the past but from a moment in the archive that does something utterly different from all of the doctors, parents, and other adults that have populated this book.

In the 1940s and 1950s, Louise Lawrence was an unrivaled (if under-recognized) expert on transvestism. Living in the San Francisco Bay Area, she carried on a carefully cultivated correspondence that became the central relay in a nationwide network of trans people in those decades, just before the rapid ascendancy of transsexuality. The people in her network wrote to one another for advice, to share their life experiences, to gossip, to organize, and for companionship.

Lawrence was also an archivist by felt necessity, carefully collecting and preserving her massive correspondence, compiling bibliographies and translations of titles on transvestism and transsexuality, and urging her peers not to destroy their letters, writings, or personal effects out of fear of exposure. Among the materials left behind after her death are a series of photo albums of mid-twentieth-century trans life, before the medical model of transsexuality overtook the spotlight and hoarded attention. Studio portraits of female impersonators from San Francisco's nightclubs fill many of the albums, and for the most part they depict an overwhelmingly white, urban social world. Nonetheless, they offer a rare visual record of a moment prior to the ascendance of transsexuality that would colonize and erase many of the heterogeneous social forms of trans life that predated it.[15]

One of Lawrence's albums contains everyday photos sent to her by correspondents from around the country. Most pages are covered by a few pictures of a trans person at home or at a social gathering, annotated in pen with the person's first name. One such entry is attributed to "B." There are several domestic photos of B comfortably at home as a woman, but the rest of her submission to Lawrence is a collection of small prints dated August 1956 and November 1957. She took the photos during two masquerade parades in Uniondale, a suburban hamlet on Long Island, New York. Evidently B knew Lawrence well enough to write witty captions on the backs of many of the photos, each signed affectionately "B." The series of about a dozen photos shows groups of children, none much older than ten or twelve, masquerading down the streets of Uniondale in a variety of costumes. What is notable is that most of the children are dressed as the "opposite sex." This kind of public spectacle was relatively commonplace in that era, drawing on an older tradition of "Mummer" parades from the late nineteenth century or the ragamuffin masquerades around Thanksgiving that were particular to the New York City area.[16] Several photos in a row profile the most flamboyantly cross-dressed masqueraders, who pose for the camera and show off their hair and makeup rather convincingly.

At the end of the series of photos is a small newspaper clipping commemorating the August 1956 parade, which was held to mark the end of

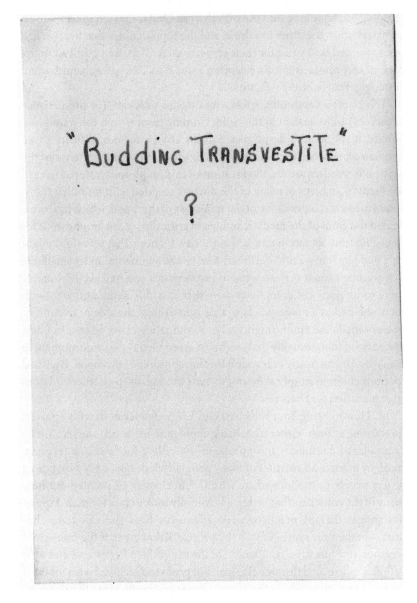

Figure 1. *"Budding Transvestite?" From the Collections of the Kinsey Institute, Indiana University. All rights reserved.*

the summer. Two children are pictured: one seated on a table, the other standing, each looking into the other's eyes. One is dressed in pants and a crewneck shirt, the other in a dress, and the caption notes that the two had been awarded best prize for their respective cross-dressed outfits. On the back of this photo is another caption from B to Lawrence, handwritten: "Budding Transvestite?" (Figure 1).[17]

The photo's captioning speaks to a desire to locate (in the parlance of this era) transvestism in the child. Coming from within the trans community, it speaks to a desire to see in the child a form of futurity based upon an *affirmative* place for trans life to grow. While the pretense of the caption is also humorous, the location of this photo today, stored next to the medical archives of many of the doctors credited with founding transsexual medicine, is evocative of the trajectory of this book, which has investigated the grain of the medical archive to critically lay the groundwork for diverging from its rationality and authority. B's hope that this child might be a *budding* transvestite performs a feat so monumental in its smallness that we might miss it if we were to brush past it too quickly. By *wanting* there to be trans children, by *desiring* that trans life should grow in children, she makes a powerful claim that runs against the tide of twentieth-century medicine and fittingly makes a competing claim against the new discourse of transsexuality that was being assembled at the same moment in the 1950s. Unlike nearly every adult that has appeared in this book, B wished for trans children simply *to be*, not to exist as a means to another end or as an explanation for transness.

In "How to Bring Your Kids Up Gay," Eve Sedgwick ends with a powerful warning against "either trivializing apologetics or, much worse, a silkily camouflaged complicity in oppression" by calling for "a strong, explicit, *erotically invested* affirmation of many people's felt desire or need that there be gay people in the immediate world."[18] In chapter 5 I pointed out how many of the clinicians that Sedgwick skillfully took to task for their dangerous antigay therapy practiced upon effeminate boys also saw trans children—in the very same clinic, to be precise. Knowing that the trans child was therefore already a companion of the gay child in her essay, I end with a similar call, routed through B's small but profound archived wish for trans life to grow in the child in the 1950s. There is certainly more than enough advice on "how to bring your kids up trans" today, but it has been confined to a harmful medical narrative that cannot see trans children's growth and flourishing as ends in themselves. For that reason, this book in fact argues precisely against the spirit of the formulation "how to bring your kids up trans." Such a proposal remains wildly insufficient, leaving trans children in the impossible position of living under the sign of a question mark placed on their existence by medicine. If, in the twenty-first century, we adults really desire to learn to care for the many transgender children in our midst, we need to learn first, from B, what it means to wish that there *be* trans children, that to grow trans and live a trans childhood is not merely a possibility but a happy and desirable one. And we need to come into this desire *now*, not in the future.

Acknowledgments

THIS BOOK IS FOR VICKI and the innumerable, unnamable trans children, whose lives have made piercing beauty out of a heavy world inimical to their survival.

This project found its beginning during my time as a graduate student at Rutgers University. I remain grateful for the contributions of the faculty and my fellow graduate students there, especially Fran Bartkowski, Ed Cohen, Jasbir Puar, and Whitney Strub on my dissertation committee. I am also indebted to the Rutgers Institute for Research on Women seminar "Trans Studies: Beyond Hetero and Homo Normativities" and especially to Aren Aizura for shaping my thinking about trans studies.

My colleagues at the University of Pittsburgh, both in the English department and in the Gender, Sexuality, and Women's Studies Program, have been incredibly generous in their support of this work. Immense gratitude goes to my incredible colleagues in Children's Literature, Tyler Bickford and Courtney Weikle-Mills; to Peter Campbell, Paul Johnson, Imani Owens, and Elizabeth Rodriguez Fielder for writing with me; to Todd Reeser, Julie Beaulieu, Natalie Kouri-Towe, and Lisa Brush for being interlocutors in gender studies; and to Don Bialostosky for supporting my research and writing as junior faculty. The students in my graduate seminars "The Body Now" and "Gender and the Child," as well as those in the undergraduate seminar "Literature, Medicine, and Sexology," have left indelible marks on my thinking and on this book. I am thankful to have the privilege of working with brilliant and courageous students from whom I have learned so much, especially Gabby and Brooke. Further thanks also go to Todd for his transformative mentorship and to Julie for teaching me how I could be a queer/trans child *and* a professor at the same time. The archival research for this book and time to write were made possible by a John Money Fellowship from the Kinsey Institute at Indiana University, the Dietrich School of

Arts and Sciences, the Office of the Provost, and a Gender, Sexuality, and Women's Studies Faculty Fellowship.

The labor of many librarians and archivists went into the research for this book, and I am forever in their debt for being patient with my unusual itineraries through archives that had not previously yielded the stories of trans children. At the Kinsey Institute, Liana Zhou and Shawn C. Wilson were instrumental in helping me find the heart of the project, as well as securing permission for the image in this book. Jeanne Vaccaro opened her home to me while I was in Bloomington, providing a wondrous place to dream the project into being. At the LGBT Community Center National History Archive in New York City, the incomparable Rich Wandel generously shared his firsthand knowledge of early trans activism while bringing me boxes. I am particularly indebted to the incredible labor of the staff at the Alan Mason Chesney Medical Archives and the Medical Records Office of the Johns Hopkins Hospital in Baltimore. Marjorie Kehoe and Phoebe Evans Letocha worked with me at every stage of the long process of developing a research protocol and applying to the Privacy Board of the hospital and throughout the exhilarating but meandering research process. I cannot thank them enough. Linda Carson worked tirelessly to welcome me to the already impossibly overtaxed Medical Records Office, not to mention helping me navigate the overwhelming bureaucracy at Hopkins. The staff at the Office were likewise incredibly welcoming when I had to disrupt their day by using the cranky microfilm machine in the middle of their workplace. I also owe thanks to the librarians at the Charles E. Young Special Collections at the University of California, Los Angeles, and to Jennifer Needham at the Special Collections of Hillman Library at the University of Pittsburgh. I further want to thank Laura Wexler for sharing her archival research in Maryland with me.

I owe a debt of gratitude to everyone who read, listened to, and provided feedback on parts of this project at many stages and in many venues. Kadji Amin, Natalia Cecire, Emma Heaney, Meridith Kruse, Brie Owen, and Eliza Steinbock organized important panels and seminars for the growth of this book. Roderick Ferguson's and Lynne Huffer's feedback at our MLA panel, "Foucault and Queer of Color Critique," has been invaluable, as has Rod's support of the project more broadly. The Child Matters Conference hosted by Indiana University Bloomington and organized by Rebekah Sheldon was a profoundly important moment in the development of this book, and I thank Paul Amar, Sarah Chinn, Anna Mae Duane, Clifford Rosky, Kathryn

Bond Stockton, and Mary Zaborskis for two days well spent. The Trans*
Studies conference at the University of Arizona in 2016 was also a watershed moment in showing the true power and ethic of care of trans studies. Toby Beauchamp, Jack Halberstam, Benjy Kahan, Katrina Karkazis,
Tey Meadow, Jennifer Nash, Robert Reid-Pharr, Gabriel Rosenberg, Gayle
Rubin, Gayle Salamon, and Jane Ward all passed through Pitt at decisive
moments in my thinking, generously sharing their time and work. I am
grateful for conversations with Claudia Castañeda, Ann Travers, Elias Vitulli,
and Elizabeth Wilson at similarly key moments that have informed my
thinking. Kyla Schuller has been a true fellow traveler into the strange historical archives of the body and the reader of my dreams. Emma Heaney's
brilliant reading took this book's Conclusion where it needed to go. Kathryn
Bond Stockton is a cherished friend, incomparable mentor, and profoundly
important voice in shaping the ways that the child touches queerness and
transness in this book. For reading the entire book, in more than one form,
and for making me the thinker and writer that I am through a special kind
of friendship, I can never fully convey my gratitude to Rebekah Sheldon
and Jean-Thomas Tremblay, my closest of kin in these pages.

With the University of Minnesota Press I have been the lucky recipient
of Danielle Kasprzak's brilliant editorial vision for this book from day one.
I am ever dazzled by how Dani has seen this book in the moments when
I could not. The anonymous readers provided incredible feedback on the
manuscript, particularly at a critical stage that helped me propel the project into its full form. Any shortcomings in the final version of this book are
very much my own.

There are many, many people whose lives intertwine with mine, in and
outside academia, to whom I am grateful for the ways, quantifiable and
unquantifiable, that they have made the work and life behind this book
possible. I cannot possibly name them all, but I hope they will know, each
in their own way, how much their part in my life matters. Marissa Brostoff,
Summer Kim Lee, Jean-Thomas Tremblay, and Hella Tsaconas knit together
a special kind of cohort that transcends time and institutional form. Erin
English gave me the gift of a vision of what capacious, rigorous, *queer* thinking looks like at just the right moment when I was a baby graduate student,
a baby queer, and a baby New Yorker. There are gorgeous queers all over
this country, but especially in Brooklyn, to whom I owe my voice and confidence. It's hard to express just how profoundly Bryn's genius shared during haircuts means to how I see transness. I think about Mamma often,

wondering how I would translate all this for her, but certain that she would return it with love. I hope this book offers my Mom a special insight into what beautiful things (like a book) can come out of a queer and gender-expansive childhood (mine) lived in the affirmative world that she built for me. There is much I have learned about what it means to grow and give back across the generations from my Dad. I count myself lucky to have the wisdom of a brother who has taught me, by always seeing things more clearly than I do, and long before I ever do, that concepts of age and childhood don't make people. The constant, furry, and cuddly company of B and H while writing this book leaves its imprint in my sheer happiness about the time there spent, as do multiple vegetable gardens now long gone.

And to J, who has fiercely championed my growth and vision, in this book as in all things in our lives, I thank you most of all.

Abbreviations

BK   Bob Kohler Papers, LGBT Center Archive, New York, New York

BUI   Records of the Brady Urological Institute, Alan Chesney Mason Archives, Johns Hopkins Hospital, Baltimore, Maryland

CI   Charles Ihlenfeld Collection, Kinsey Institute, Bloomington, Indiana

EP   Edwards Park Collection, Alan Chesney Mason Archives, Johns Hopkins Hospital, Baltimore, Maryland

HB   Harry Benjamin Collection, Kinsey Institute, Bloomington, Indiana

HHY   Hugh Hampton Young Collection, Alan Chesney Mason Archives, Johns Hopkins Hospital, Baltimore, Maryland

HLH   Records of the Harriet Lane Home, Office of Medical Records, Johns Hopkins Hospital, Baltimore, Maryland

JH   Jeanne Hoff Archive, Kinsey Institute, Bloomington, Indiana

JHH   Records of the Johns Hopkins Hospital, Alan Chesney Mason Archives, Johns Hopkins Hospital, Baltimore, Maryland

JHK   Jeanne Hoff Collection, Kinsey Institute, Bloomington, Indiana

JK   John J. Kearns Papers, LGBT Center Archive, New York, New York

JMH   John Money Collection, Alan Chesney Mason Archives, Johns Hopkins Hospital, Baltimore, Maryland

JMK   John Money Collection, Kinsey Institute, Bloomington, Indiana

LL   Louise Lawrence Collection, Kinsey Institute, Bloomington, Indiana

MJ   Masters and Johnson Collection, Kinsey Institute, Bloomington, Indiana

MRR   Mary Roberts Rinehart Papers, Special Collections Department, University of Pittsburgh

MSA   Maryland State Archives, Court Records for Baltimore City, Annapolis, Maryland

RS   Robert Stoller Papers, Charles E. Young Library Special Collections, University of California, Los Angeles

TC   Thomas Cullen Collection, Alan Chesney Mason Archives, Johns Hopkins Hospital, Baltimore, Maryland

Note: In conformity with federal regulations under the Health Insurance Portability and Accountability Act (HIPAA), certain archival collections consulted during the research for this book are subject to strict privacy conventions concerning the protection of the Personal Health Information (PHI) of individuals described therein. In order to preserve the confidentiality of those records, materials consulted from these collections cannot be cited in standard bibliographical format. In their place, a research code and the collection abbreviation is given in the requisite endnote, providing a coded source for specific documents (e.g., "2001.3, HLH"). Any person wishing to consult the original primary sources corresponding to these codes can apply to the Johns Hopkins Hospital Privacy Board for access. A copy of the code used to conduct research has been deposited at the Alan Chesney Mason Medical Archives, Johns Hopkins Hospital, Baltimore, Maryland.

All names of individuals in this book drawn from such records are pseudonyms invented by the author, unless otherwise stated.

Notes

Introduction

1. James McDonald, "Laverne Cox Declares Transgender State of Emergency," *Out Magazine*, August 20, 2015, https://www.out.com/news-opinion/2015/8/20/laverne-cox-declares-transgender-state-emergency; Janet Mock, *Redefining Realness: My Path to Womanhood, Identity, Love, & So Much More* (New York: Atria Books, 2014); CeCe McDonald, "'Go Beyond Our Natural Selves': The Prison Letters of CeCe McDonald," intr. Omise'eke Natasha Tinsley, *Transgender Studies Quarterly* 4, no. 2 (2017): 243–65; *I Am Jazz*, The Learning Channel, 2015; Moriah Balingit, "Gavin Grimm Just Wanted to Use the Bathroom. He Didn't Think the Nation Would Debate It," *Washington Post*, August 30, 2016, https://www.washingtonpost.com/local/education/gavin-grimm-just-wanted-to-use-the-bathroom-he-didnt-think-the-nation-would-debate-it/. Caitlyn Jenner's late-in-life coming-out and contested attempts to immediately claim a public position of leadership on trans issues also put her into a strange generational relationship with trans children, as well as a frictional relation to black trans women, both of whose public trans visibility and vulnerability long preceded hers. See Julian Gill-Peterson, "Growing Up Trans in the 1960s and 2010s," in *Misfits: An Inquiry into Childhood Belongings*, ed. Markus Bohlmann (Lanham, Md.: Lexington Books), 213–30.

2. For media from the past several years that reflect this figuration, see *I Am Jazz: A Family in Transition*, dir. Jen Stocks, *Oprah Winfrey Network*, November 27, 2011; *PBS Frontline*, Season 34, Episode 1, "Growing Up Trans," PBS, June 29, 2015; Amy Ellis Nutt, *Becoming Nicole: The Transformation of an American Family* (New York: Random House, 2016); "Special Issue: The Gender Revolution," *National Geographic*, January 2017; and 3 *Generations*, dir. Gabby Dellal (Los Angeles: Weinstein Company, 2017). See also Gill-Peterson, "Growing Up Trans in the 1960s and 2010s."

3. C. Riley Snorton and Jin Haritaworn, "Trans Necropolitics: A Transnational Reflection on Violence, Death, and the Trans of Color Afterlife," in *The Transgender Studies Reader 2*, ed. Susan Stryker and Aren Z. Aizura (New York: Routledge, 2013), 66–76.

4. Treva Ellison, Kai M. Green, Matt Richardson, and C. Riley Snorton, "We Got Issues: Toward a Black Trans*/Studies," *Transgender Studies Quarterly* 4, no. 2 (2017): 162–69; Elías Cosenza Krell, "Is Transmisogyny Killing Trans Women of

Color? Black Trans Feminisms and the Exigencies of White Femininity," *Transgender Studies Quarterly* 4, no. 2 (2017): 226–42; Syrus Marcus Ware, "All Power to All People? Black LGBTTI2QQ Activism, Remembrance, and Archiving in Toronto," *Transgender Studies Quarterly* 4, no. 2 (2017): 170–80; and Erin Durban-Albrecht, "Postcolonial Disablement and/as Transition: Trans* Haitian Narratives of Breaking Open and Stitching Together," *Transgender Studies Quarterly* 4, no. 2 (2017): 195–207.

5. Robin Bernstein, *Racial Innocence: Performing American Childhood from Slavery to Civil Rights* (New York: New York University Press, 2011). On the "emptiness" of childhood innocence, see James Kincaid, *Eroticizing Innocence: The Culture of Child Molesting* (Durham, N.C.: Duke University Press, 1998).

6. The high material cost of this figurative separation manifests in one form as the fungibility attached to black trans and trans of color children's lives, a fact illustrated painfully by the case of the murder of Latisha King and the repetition of violence against her during the criminal trial of her killer. See Gayle Salamon, *The Life and Death of Latisha King: A Critical Phenomenology of Transphobia* (New York: New York University Press, 2018).

7. Eva S. Hayward, "Don't Exist," *Transgender Studies Quarterly* 4, no. 2 (2017): 191.

8. The archive of examples here is growing almost daily. For two examples typical of the narrative I am describing, see *PBS Frontline*, "Growing Up Trans," and "The Gender Revolution."

9. On the politics of refusal and racial plasticity, see Sandra Harvey, "The HeLa Bomb and the Science of Unveiling," *Catalyst: Feminism, Theory, Technoscience* 2, no. 2 (2016): 18–20.

10. Theories of trans- or trans* grounded in radical openness or a creative capacity for transformation and mutability, in particular, have gone so far as to equate conceptually trans *with* plasticity. See, for example, Nicholas Chare and Ika Willis, "Trans-: Across/Beyond," *Parallax* 22, no. 3 (2016): 267–89. I follow instead the critical framework of scholars like Zakiyyah Iman Jackson, who shows that plasticity-as-mutability easily underwrites both progressive *and* profoundly dehumanizing projects, particular in the case of slavery, blackness, and the creation of the human. See Jackson, "Losing Manhood: Animality and Plasticity in the (Neo) Slave Narrative," *Qui Parle* 25, no. 1–2 (2016): 95–136. For a historical investigation of the racialization of plasticity in the nineteenth century, the period that precedes this book, see Kyla Schuller, *The Biopolitics of Feeling: Race, Sex, and Science in the Nineteenth Century* (Durham, N.C.: Duke University Press, 2017).

11. To be clear, this is not a criticism of the vital and still emerging scholarship on trans children. This work focuses on the contemporary world not out of any neglect of the past but mostly because of disciplinary convention: it is largely coming out of sociology and ethnographies of the clinic and families with trans

children, rather than from fields that typically engage with archives and extensive history. What I am actually interested in is the generational and historiographical assumptions that have come to suffuse this work in the absence of a historicity to trans children, which I take up later.

12. Tey Meadow, "Child," *Transgender Studies Quarterly* 1, no. 1–2 (2014): 57.

13. This issue frequently turns up in journalistic accounts. See Freda R. Savana, "Looking at Suppressing Puberty for Transgender Kids," *Washington Times*, March 1, 2016, http://www.washingtontimes.com/news/2016/mar/12/looking-at-suppress ing-puberty-for-transgender-kid/. The distinction of reversible/irreversible is also being codified into the standards of care for pediatric trans medicine. See Johanna Olson-Kennedy, Stephen M. Rosenthal, Jennifer Hastings, and Linda Wesp, "Health Considerations for Gender Non-Conforming Children and Transgender Adolescents," *Center of Excellence for Transgender Health*, http://transhealth.ucsf.edu/ trans?page=guidelines-youth.

14. This concern becomes a dramatic plotline for one family with a thirteen-year-old trans child in "Growing Up Trans." I critique the presumptions upon which the entire dispute relies in Gill-Peterson, "Growing Up Trans in the 1960s and 2010s."

15. The most common origin story is that a Dutch clinic developed puberty suppression therapy before it was adopted elsewhere in Europe, the UK, Canada, and the United States. See Peggy T. Cohen-Kettenis and Friedmann Pfäfflin, *Transgenderism and Intersexuality in Childhood and Adolescence: Making Choices* (London: Sage, 2003).

16. Jack Halberstam, "Trans*—Gender Transitivity and New Configurations of Body, History, Memory and Kinship," *Parallax* 22, no. 3 (2016): 367.

17. Meadow, "Child," 58.

18. Halberstam, "Trans*," 367.

19. On the massively unrepresented trans children of color and those without adequate financial or bureaucratic means to access medicine, see Ann Travers, *The Trans Generation: How Trans Kids (and Their Parents) Are Creating a Gender Revolution* (New York: New York University Press, 2018). I return to this issue in the conclusion.

20. I return at more significant length to this problem of generational succession in chapter 5, including by looking at Halberstam's work on the "border wars" between butch lesbians and trans men.

21. See Susan Stryker, Paisley Currah, and Lisa Jean Moore, "Trans-, Trans, or Transgender?," *Women's Studies Quarterly* 36, no. 3–4 (2008): 11–22; Eva Hayward, "More Lessons from a Starfish: Prefixial Flesh and Transspeciated Selves," *Women's Studies Quarterly* 36, no. 3–4 (2008): 64–85; Chare and Willis, "Trans-: Across/Beyond"; and Eliza Steinbock, Marianna Szczygielska, and Anthony Wagner, "Thinking Linking," *Angelaki: Journal of the Theoretical Humanities* 22, no. 2 (2017): 1–10.

22. Susan Stryker, *Transgender History* (Berkeley, Calif.: Seal Press, 2008), 24.

23. Sandy Stone, "The *Empire* Strikes Back: A Posttranssexual Manifesto," 1987, https://sandystone.com/empire-strikes-back.pdf. See also Stone's trenchant reflections on the category in Susan Stryker, "Another Dream of Common Language: An Interview with Sandy Stone," *Transgender Studies Quarterly* 3, no. 1–2 (2016): 303–4.

24. Leslie Feinberg, *Transgender Warriors: Making History from Joan of Arc to Dennis Rodman* (Boston: Beacon Press, 1996), ix, emphasis in original. My thanks to Julie Beaulieu for pointing me toward this passage.

25. Paul Amar, "The Street, the Sponge, and the Ultra: Queer Logics of Children's Rebellion and Political Infantilization," *GLQ: A Journal of Lesbian and Gay Studies* 22, no. 4 (2016): 571.

26. Amar, "The Street," 597.

27. Amar, "The Street," 597.

28. Kathryn Bond Stockton, *The Queer Child, or Growing Sideways in the Twentieth Century* (Durham, N.C.: Duke University Press, 2009).

29. Even in Joanne Meyerowitz's landmark book *How Sex Changed: A History of Transsexuality in the United States* (Cambridge, Mass.: Harvard University Press, 2004), the chapter that covers the era before the 1950s reads like a predicate—an overview of historiographical possibilities, rather than an investigation as detailed as what follows on the midcentury. Although this is in no doubt partly an effect of Meyerowitz being one of the first historians to write in-depth about Christine Jorgensen and 1950s transsexual medicine, it is notable that there are still no book-length studies of the first half of the twentieth century in isolation.

30. Paul B. Preciado, *Testo Junkie: Sex, Drugs, and Biopolitics in the Pharmacopornographic Era*, trans. Bruce Benderson (New York: Feminist Press, 2014). I take up this point in greater detail in chapter 2.

31. Jay Prosser, *Second Skins: The Body Narratives of Transsexuality* (New York: Columbia University Press, 1998), 8; Bernice L. Hausman, *Changing Sex: Transsexualism, Technology, and the Idea of Gender* (Durham, N.C.: Duke University Press, 1995). Preciado's claim in *Testo Junkie* that "the pharmacopornographic business is the *invention of a subject* and then its global reproduction" (36, emphasis in original) reads uncomfortably close to Hausman's that it is "through the analysis of discursive formations that one can trace the conditions of possibility for the emergence of new subjectivities" (viii), which in turn prefaces her argument that "the development of certain medical technologies made the advent of transsexualism possible" (7) and, infamously, that "transsexuals are the dupes of gender" (140).

32. Meyerowitz, *How Sex Changed*, 21.

33. On the challenges of the twentieth-century trans archive, see Laura Peimer, "Trans* Collecting at the Schlesinger Library: Privacy Protection and the Challenges of Description and Access," *Transgender Studies Quarterly* 2, no. 4 (2015):

614–20; Ms. Bob Davis, "Using Archives to Identify the Trans* Women of Casa Susana," *Transgender Studies Quarterly* 2, no. 4 (2015): 621–34; and Chase Joynt and Kristen Schilt, "Anxiety at the Archive," *Transgender Studies Quarterly* 2, no. 4 (2015): 635–44.

34. Meyerowitz, in *How Sex Changed*, and Hausman, in *Changing Sex*, both frame the first half of the twentieth century in this way. On interwar endocrinology, see Alice Dreger, "A History of Intersexuality, from the Age of Gonads to the Age of Consent," *Journal of Clinical Ethics* 9, no. 4 (199): 345–55; and Henry Rubin, *Self-Made Men: Identity and Embodiment among Transsexual Men* (Nashville, Tenn.: Vanderbilt University Press, 2003), 35–59. One noteworthy exception to this framing is Stryker's *Transgender History*. Given that Stryker aims to undermine the dominance of medical discourse in trans history, instead focusing on "the collective political history of transgender social change and activism in the United States" (2), she is able to identify a range of rich sites for investigating the early twentieth century from a trans perspective, as far back as the establishment of the Cercle Hermaphroditos, a trans social club, in New York City in 1895 (41).

35. Meyerowitz, *How Sex Changed*, 21.

36. For a broader reflection on the naming and claiming of trans archives, see K. J. Rawson, "An Inevitably Political Craft," *Transgender Studies Quarterly* 2, no. 4 (2015): 544–52.

37. Ralph Werther, *Autobiography of an Androgyne*, ed. Scott Herring (New Brunswick, N.J.: Rutgers University Press, 2008). Subsequent page references made in-text.

38. Stryker, *Transgender History*, 41.

39. Werther, *Autobiography of an Androgyne*, 21. Subsequent references in-text.

40. Emma Heaney, *The New Woman: Literary Modernism, Queer Theory, and the Trans Feminine Allegory* (Chicago: Northwestern University Press, 2017), 174, emphasis added.

41. Heaney, *The New Woman*, 14.

42. Peter Coviello, *Tomorrow's Parties: Sex and the Untimely in Nineteenth-Century America* (New York: New York University Press, 2013), 20.

43. On the historical shift through which the aspirational model of trans sex produced its difference from cis sex, see Heaney, *The New Woman*, 48.

44. Jennifer Germon, *Gender: A Genealogy of an Idea* (New York: Palgrave Macmillan, 2009); Sharon E. Preves, "Sexing the Intersexed: An Analysis of Sociocultural Responses to Intersexuality," *Signs* 27, no. 2 (2001): 523–56; David A. Rubin, "'An Unnamed Blank That Craved a Name': A Genealogy of Intersex as Gender," *Signs* 37, no. 4 (2012): 883–908; and Jemima Repo, "The Biopolitical Birth of Gender: Social Control, Hermaphroditism, and the New Sexual Apparatus," *Alternatives: Global, Local, Political* 38, no. 3 (2013): 228–44.

45. See Gayle Salamon's important essay "The Meontology of Castration," *Parallax* 22, no. 3 (2016): 312–22.

46. Michael Dillon, *Self: A Study in Endocrinology and Ethics* (London: Heinemann, 1946).

47. Alan L. Hart to Mary Roberts Rinehart, August 3, 1921, Folder 8, Box 21, Series VI, MRR. Hart has also been claimed as a lesbian, notably by Jonathan Ned Katz in *Gay American History: Lesbians and Gay Men in the U.S.A.* (New York: Thomas Y. Crowell, 1992), 390–422. The porosity of the inversion discourse that circulated in this era makes it difficult to disentangle sex from sexuality in the sense of object choice. Nevertheless, in terms of medicine, Hart's interest in hormone therapy, hysterectomy, and gonadectomy certainly makes him an important figure in the history of endocrinology and transsexual medicine before the field came about. For more on identifying trans people from this era, see chapter 2.

48. Louise Lawrence to Harry Benjamin, June 1, 1953, Box 1, Series 1-B, LL.

49. Vicki's letters are discussed in detail in chapter 4.

50. Aaron Devor and Nicholas Matte, "Building a Better World for Transpeople: Reed Erickson and the Erickson Educational Foundation," *International Journal of Transgenderism* 10, no. 1 (2007): 47–68; Aaron Devor and Nicholas Matte, "ONE Inc. and Reed Erickson," *GLQ* 10, no. 2 (2004): 179–209.

51. Abram J. Lewis, "'I Am 64 and Paul McCartney Doesn't Care': The Haunting of the Transgender Archive and the Challenges of Queer History," *Radical History Review* 120 (2014): 22–23.

52. Lewis, "I Am 64," 22.

53. Abram J. Lewis, "Trans Animisms," *Angelaki: Journal of the Theoretical Humanities* 22, no. 2 (2017): 203; Reina Gossett, "Occupy Humor & Grief as Transformative Practices," March 15, 2012, http://www.reinagossett.com/occupy-humor-grief-as-transformative-practices/.

54. For a discussion of this concept in terms of rural trans life, see Jack Halberstam, *In a Queer Time and Place: Transgender Bodies, Subcultural Lives* (New York: New York University Press, 2005), 22–46. On metronormativity in queer theory, where the concept has been explored in greater detail, see Martin F. Manalansan, Chantal Nadeau, Richard T. Rodriguez, and Siobhan B. Somerville, "Queering the Middle: Race, Region and a Queer Midwest," *GLQ: A Journal of Lesbian and Gay Studies* 20, no. 1–2 (2014): 1–12; and Scott Herring, *Another Country: Queer Anti-Urbanism* (New York: New York University Press, 2010).

55. Sylvia Rivera, "Queens in Exile, the Forgotten Ones," in *Street Transvestite Action Revolutionaries: Survival, Revolt, and Queer Antagonist Struggle,* ed. Ehn Nothing (Untorelli Press, 2013), 42.

56. Notes from Martin Duberman Interview with Sylvia Rivera, October 12, 1990, 5–6, Folder 1, JK.

57. Ehn Nothing, "Queers against Society," in *Street Transvestite Action Revolutionaries: Survival, Revolt, and Queer Antagonist Struggle,* ed. Ehn Nothing (Untorelli Press, 2013), 7.

58. Rivera, "Queens in Exile, the Forgotten Ones," 42.

59. Sylvia Rivera and Marsha P. Johnson, "Rapping with a Street Transvestite Revolutionary," in *Street Transvestite Action Revolutionaries: Survival, Revolt, and Queer Antagonist Struggle*, ed. Ehn Nothing (Untorelli Press, 2013), 28.

60. Rivera and Johnson, "Rapping with a Street Transvestite Revolutionary," 29.

61. Notes from Martin Duberman Interview, 7.

62. Some activists have maintained an interest in claiming these street kids as *gay*, rather than trans, although the factual basis for those kinds of distinctions seems rather weak and tends to be part and parcel of political battles over the legacy of the Stonewall riots in the West Village in New York City more than anything else. See David Carter, "Gay Street Youth: The Fire in the Stonewall Riots," *Pride Magazine*, 2003, Folder 18, Box 1, BK.

63. Jessi Gan argues that "Rivera is . . . profoundly important in a Latin@, transgender, and queer historiography where histories of transgender people of color are few and far between." Gan, "'Still at the Back of the Bus': Sylvia Rivera's Struggle," *Centro Journal* 19, no. 1 (2007): 128.

64. While there is an abundant literature about Rivera and Johnson, it tends to repeat the same narratives and vignettes about their lives, presumably because that is all that has been archived or that can be remembered by people who knew them. In addition to the sources mentioned in this introduction, see Martin Duberman, *Stonewall* (New York: Penguin, 1993); Liz Highleyman, "Sylvia Rivera: A Woman before Her Time," in *Smash the Church, Smash the State! The Early Years of Gay Liberation*, ed. Tommi Avicolli Mecca (San Francisco: City Lights Books, 2009), 172–81; Tommi Avicolli Mecca, "Marsha P. Johnson: New York City Legend," in *Smash the Church, Smash the State! The Early Years of Gay Liberation*, ed. Tommi Avicolli Mecca (San Francisco: City Lights Books, 2009), 261–62; Benjamin Shepard, "Sylvia and Sylvia's Children: A Battle for a Queer Public Space," in *That's Revolting! Queer Strategies for Resisting Assimilation*, ed. Mattilda Bernstein Sycamore (New York: Soft Skull Press, 2008); and Leslie Feinberg, "Street Transvestite Action Revolutionaries," *Workers World*, September 24, 2006, http://www.workers.org/2006/us/lavender-red-73/. One nonacademic source of similar narratives comes in the form of obituaries for and remembrances of Rivera. See Michael Bronski, "Sylvia Rivera: 1951–2002," *Z Magazine*, April 1, 2002, https://zcomm.org/zmagazine/sylvia-rivera-1951–2002-by-michael-bronski/; and Riki Wilchins, "A Woman for Her Time," *Village Voice*, February 26, 2002, https://www.villagevoice.com/2002/02/26/a-woman-for-her-time/. Archival holdings on their lives are even more ephemeral, but see BK and JK in particular. Reina Gossett's work in recovering and making Rivera's archive accessible has been instrumental and, far too frequently, uncredited.

65. Stephan Cohen, "An Historical Investigation of School and Community-Based Gay Liberation Youth Groups, New York City, 1969–1975: An Army of Lovers Cannot Fail" (thesis, Harvard University, 2004), 138.

66. Gan, "Still at the Back of the Bus," 133. Shepard concurs in "Sylvia and Sylvia's Children" that even after the dissolution of S.T.A.R., "Rivera played the role of surrogate mother to a community of homeless transgender and queer street kids on the piers" (127).

67. Feinberg, "Street Transvestite Action Revolutionaries."

68. Feinberg, "Street Transvestite Action Revolutionaries."

69. Sylvia Rivera, "Y'all Better Quiet Down," in *Street Transvestite Action Revolutionaries: Survival, Revolt, and Queer Antagonist Struggle,* ed. Ehn Nothing (Untorelli Press, 2013), 30.

70. Dick Leitsch to Bob Kohler, September 12, 1969, Folder 17, Box 1, BK.

71. I also agree that the persistence of transphobic feminist projects within the academy is another area of urgent concern for the field, as Susan Stryker and Talia M. Bettcher point out in "Introduction: Trans/Feminisms," *Transgender Studies Quarterly* 3, no. 1–2 (2016): 5–7. See also Cael M. Keegan's discussion of "compromise" over gender bathroom policies at the National Women Studies Association annual meetings, "On Being the Object of Compromise," *Transgender Studies Quarterly* 3, no. 1–2 (2016): 150–57.

72. Contrast this approach to thinking race and trans together with something like *Trans: Gender and Race in the Age of Unsettled Identities* (Princeton, N.J.: Princeton University Press, 2016), Rogers Brubaker's sociologically driven text that attempts to compare the controversy over Caitlyn Jenner and Rachel Dolezal to think about the incommensurability of transgender and transracial narratives. By taking a highly contemporary, twenty-first-century controversy as his launch point, as if there were no relation between trans and racialized forms of life in the past, and by snubbing trans of color studies scholars who have worked extensively on thinking about race and trans together, Brubaker is able to colonize the subject despite admittedly having *no* expertise in either trans studies or critical race studies (xi). This model also has the effect of entirely flattening the category "race" into an almost meaningless sociological descriptor, which distorts and undermines the position of blackness and the visibility of antiblackness in his analysis. Brubaker's uninterrogated model of subjectivity also reiterates the normative subject of the West as the only intelligible form of gendered and racialized life.

73. Ellison, Green, Richardson, and Snorton, "We Got Issues," 164.

74. Ellison, Green, Richardson, and Snorton, "We Got Issues," 164, emphasis added.

75. Susan Stryker and Aren Z. Aizura, "Transgender Studies 2.0," in *The Transgender Studies Reader 2,* ed. Susan Stryker and Aren Z. Aizura (New York: Routledge, 2013), 10.

76. Snorton and Haritaworn, "Trans Necropolitics," 67.

77. See Alexander G. Weheliye, *Habeas Viscus: Racializing Assemblages, Biopolitics, and Black Feminist Theories of the Human* (Durham, N.C.: Duke University

Press, 2014); and Denise Ferreira da Silva, "Before *Man*: Sylvia Wynter's Rewriting of the Modern Episteme," in *Sylvia Wynter: On Being Human as Praxis*, ed. Katherine McKittrick (Durham, N.C.: Duke University Press, 2015), 90–105.

78. See, for example, Steinbock, Szczygielska, and Wagner, "Thinking Linking." Wynter's concept of "a new science of the word" is also a rich resource for thinking about the undermining and transformation of Western medical science through alternate forms of embodied knowledge previously disqualified by its rationality and coloniality. Sylvia Wynter and Katherine McKittrick, "Unparalleled Catastrophe for Our Species? Or, to Give Humanness a Different Future: Conversations," in *Sylvia Wynter: On Being Human as Praxis*, ed. Katherine McKittrick (Durham, N.C.: Duke University Press, 2015), 14. See also Walter Mignolo's reflections on "*decolonial scientia*" in "Sylvia Wynter: What Does It Mean to Be Human?," in *Sylvia Wynter: On Being Human as Praxis*, ed. Katherine McKittrick (Durham, N.C.: Duke University Press, 2015), 115–18.

79. On the convergences and divergences of trans and indigenous studies, see Scott L. Morgensen, "Conditions of Critique: Responding to Indigenous Resurgence within Gender Studies," *Transgender Studies Quarterly* 3, no. 1–2 (2016): 192–201; and Kale Fajardo, "Queer/Asian Filipinos in Oregon: A Trans*Colonial Approach," lecture given at the University of Pittsburgh, February 29, 2016.

80. Joseli Maria Silva and Marcio Jose Ornat, "Transfeminism and Decolonial Thought: The Contribution of Brazilian *Travestis*," trans. Sean Stroud, *Transgender Studies Quarterly* 3, no. 1–2 (2016): 220.

81. Aren Z. Aizura, Trystan Cotton, Carsten Balzer/Carla LaGata, Marcia Ochoa, and Salvador Vidal-Ortiz, "Introduction," *Transgender Studies Quarterly* 1, no. 3 (2014): 304.

82. Chapter 3, on the invention of gender, takes up this point in greatest detail.

83. C. Riley Snorton, *Black on Both Sides: A Racial History of Trans Identity* (Minneapolis: University of Minnesota Press, 2017), 157.

84. Snorton, *Black on Both Sides*.

85. Susan Stryker, "*We Who Are Sexy*: Christine Jorgensen's Transsexual Whiteness in the Postcolonial Philippines," *Social Semiotics* 19, no. 1 (2009): 79–91.

86. Donna J. Haraway, "Situated Knowledges: The Science Question in Feminism and the Privilege of Partial Perspective," in Haraway, *Simians, Cyborgs, and Women: The Reinvention of Nature* (New York: Routledge, 1991), 193.

87. Haraway, "Situated Knowledges," 190.

88. Haraway, "Situated Knowledges," 190–91.

89. Chela Sandoval, *Methodology of the Oppressed* (Minneapolis: University of Minnesota Press, 2000), 171.

90. Sandoval, *Methodology of the Oppressed*, 175.

91. Cárdenas developed the concept of a "science of the oppressed" as part of collective work with the Electronic Disturbance Theatre. See Leonia Tanczer,

"Hacking the Label: Hacktivism, Race, and Gender," *Ada: A Journal of Gender, New Media, and Technology,* no. 6 (2015): http://adanewmedia.org/2015/01/issue 6-tanczer/. The origin of the term "science of the oppressed," in a very different context from trans of color thought, is actually Monique Wittig's Marxist framework in "One Is Not Born a Woman," in Carole R. McCann and Seung-Kyung Kim, eds., *Feminist Local and Global Theory Perspective Reader,* 3rd ed. (New York: Routledge, 2013), 250. Cárdenas importantly grounds any science of the oppressed in situated practices of knowledge that address contemporary institutions of racist and anti-trans violence, like algorithmic surveillance or everyday street violence. See micha cárdenas, "Trans of Color Poetics: Stitching Bodies, Concepts, and Algorithms," *The Scholar & Feminist Online* 13, no. 3 (2016), http://sfonline.barnard.edu/traversing-technologies/micha-cardenas-trans-of-color-poetics-stitching-bodies-concepts-and-algorithms/; and cárdenas, "Pregnancy: Reproductive Futures in Trans of Color Feminism," *Transgender Studies Quarterly* 3, no. 1–2 (2016): 48–57.

92. Susan Stryker, "De(Subjugated) Knowledges: An Introduction to Transgender Studies," in *The Transgender Studies Reader,* ed. Susan Stryker and Stephen Whittle (New York: Routledge, 2006), 1–18.

93. For several outstanding examples of work that produces situated trans of color knowledges, see Silva and Ornat, "Transfeminism and Decolonial Thought"; Durban-Albrecht, "Postcolonial Disablement and/as Transition"; Dora Silva Santana, "Transitionings and Returnings: Experiments with the Poetics of Transatlantic Water," *Transgender Studies Quarterly* 4, no. 2 (2017): 181–90; Kai M. Green and Treva Ellison, "Tranifest," *Transgender Studies Quarterly* 1, no. 1–2 (2014): 222–25; Kay Gabriel, "Untranslating Gender in Trish Salah's *Lyric Sexology Vol. 1,*" *Transgender Studies Quarterly* 3, no. 3–4 (2016): 524–44; Eliza Steinbock, "Catties and T-Selfies: On the 'I' and the 'We' in Trans-Animal Cute Aesthetics," *Angelaki: Journal of the Theoretical Humanities* 22, no. 2 (2017): 159–78; and Giancarlo Cornejo, "For a Queer Pedagogy of Friendship," *Transgender Studies Quarterly* 1, no. 3 (2014): 352–67. "Response-ability" is from Donna J. Haraway, *Staying with the Trouble: Making Kin in the Chthulucene* (Durham, N.C.: Duke University Press, 2016), 2.

94. Fred Moten, "Blackness and Nothingness (Mysticism in the Flesh)," *South Atlantic Quarterly* 112, no. 4 (2013): 738.

95. Robert Reid-Pharr, *Archives of Flesh: African America, Spain, and Posthumanist Critique* (New York: New York University Press, 2016), 9. References hereafter in-text.

96. This call to recalibrate interpretive practices to *learn* from the lived breaches of humanism encoded in the flesh marks the distinction between Reid-Pharr's posthumanist archival practice and the general "archival turn" that has marked many fields (10)—including transgender studies. Susan Stryker and Paisley Currah, for instance, remark that "perhaps it's no coincidence that 'transgender' as a concept, as an organizing rubric of an emergent social movement, and as an incipient field

of study rose to prominence at the same moment as the archival turn in the early 1990s and signaled similar premillennial and postmodern anxieties regarding the collapse of time and place as did the archival imaginary." "General Editors' Introduction," *Transgender Studies Quarterly* 2, no. 4 (2015): 540.

97. See LaMonda Horton-Stallings's call in *Funk the Erotic: Transaesthetics and Black Sexual Cultures* (Champaign: University of Illinois Press, 2015) for "the intellectual moments in cultural performances and narratives about sex, work, and blackness when black cultural producers' imaginative knowledge challenges the way science and medicine have been the sole influence on what constitutes gender and sexuality" (23–24).

98. Snorton, *Black on Both Sides*, 57.

1. The Racial Plasticity of Gender and the Child

1. Henry Rubin, *Self-Made Men: Identity and Embodiment among Transsexual Men* (Nashville: Vanderbilt University Press, 2003), 35. While work on the era prior to a discourse on transsexuality is comparatively spare, it is notable, for instance, that neither Rubin nor Joanne Meyerowitz, in *How Sex Changed: A History of Transsexuality in the United States* (Cambridge, Mass.: Harvard University Press, 2004), points out the explicitly eugenic context of the leading endocrinologists of the era.

2. Claudia Castañeda, *Figurations: Child, Bodies, Worlds* (Durham, N.C.: Duke University Press, 2002).

3. Indeed, Jeanne Fahnestock claims that metaphor has dominated the study of rhetoric in science, perhaps to the point of granting it *too much* visibility compared to other figures of speech. See *Rhetorical Figures in Science* (Oxford: Oxford University Press, 1999), 4–6. Given the contemporary interest in matter and materiality in feminist, queer, and transgender studies, however, it is an opportune moment to reintroduce the problem of metaphor to the extent that it still incorporates language without deciding in its favor over matter, or vice versa. This chapter suggests that the gulf between the child as a figure and actual living children directs us toward a generative example of the function of metaphor in relation to the living world. For a classic study of metaphor in science, see Mary B. Hesse, *Models and Analogies in Science* (South Bend, Ind.: University of Notre Dame Press, 1966). Hesse relies in particular on the interaction model of metaphor developed by Max Black in *Models and Metaphors: Studies in Language and Philosophy* (Ithaca, N.Y.: Cornell University Press, 1976). Differing conceptions of what counts as metaphor lead into a complex and extended conversation in feminist science studies, beyond the scope of this chapter, over the relation of the experimental apparatus to the world, which is also a question of the relation of matter to meaning-making. In the idiom of Karen Barad's work on "agential realism," metaphor could be read

as one mode of making an agential cut into the real, rather than an external contaminant from human language. See *Meeting the Universe Halfway: Quantum Physics and the Entanglement of Matter and Meaning* (Durham, N.C: Duke University Press, 2007). I follow Donna Haraway's vocabulary for the relation of the natural to the cultural more closely than Barad's in this chapter.

4. For a thorough overview in the case of biology, see Robert J. Richards, *The Romantic Conception of Life: Science and Philosophy in the Age of Goethe* (Chicago: University of Chicago Press, 2002).

5. Gillian Beer, *Darwin's Plots: Evolutionary Narrative in Darwin, George Elliot, and Nineteenth-Century Fiction* (Cambridge: Cambridge University Press, 2000), xxv. Feminist readings of Darwin, notably by Liz Grosz, have evidenced as much. See *Becoming Undone: Darwinian Reflections on Life, Politics, and Art* (Durham, N.C.: Duke University Press, 2011).

6. Donna J. Haraway, *Crystals, Fabrics, and Fields: Metaphors that Shape Embryos* (Berkeley, Calif.: North Atlantic Books, 2004). Subsequent references will be made in-text.

7. Thomas Kuhn, *The Structure of Scientific Revolutions* (Chicago: University of Chicago Press, 1996); Hesse, *Models and Analogies in Science.*

8. See Ernest Starling, *The Croonian Lectures on the Chemical Correlation of the Functions of the Body* (London: Royal College of Physicians, 1905).

9. That being said, there have been many *failed* attempts to isolate plasticity in the living organism as a physical or quasi-physical object, running the spectrum from mechanist, to vitalist, to organicist paradigms. One interesting case is "protoplasm," that enigmatic would-be engine of cell division (and, in that sense, the sort of indeterminacy at the heart of a certain version of the life principle), which was of great interest to biologists at the opening of the twentieth century, in particular. For one prominent reflection from that period, see William Bateson, *Problems of Genetics* (New Haven, Conn.: Yale University Press, 1913), 41. To be clear, this early twentieth-century sense of protoplasm as the material or chemical home of an objective plasticity is rather different from its very specific contemporary meaning in biology as the granular fluid within cell walls.

10. On impressibility and nineteenth-century science, see Kyla Schuller, *The Biopolitics of Feeling: Race, Sex, and Science in the Nineteenth Century* (Durham, N.C.: Duke University Press, 2017).

11. On the emergence of the organismic model in the life sciences, see Haraway, *Crystals, Fabrics, and Fields.*

12. See C. Barker Jørgensen, *John Hunter, A. A. Berthold, and the Origins of Endocrinology* (Odense: Odense University Press, 1971). This model of experiment was also based in the informal observations of livestock farmers for centuries.

13. Arnold Adolph Berthold, "The Transplantation of the Testes," trans. D. P. Quiring, *Bulletin of the History of Medicine* 16 (1944): 400–401, emphasis in original.

14. Charles Darwin, *The Variation of Plants and Animals under Domestication* (New York: Appleton, 1896), 26.

15. Darwin's endorsement was cited as justification of bisexuality's naturalness and sex's plasticity in a range of popular and specialist American scientific periodicals in the late nineteenth century. For a few examples, see C. M. Hollingsworth, "The Theory of Sex and Sexual Genesis," *American Naturalist* 28 (1884): 673–74; Colin A. Scott, "Sex and Art," *American Journal of Psychology* 7, no. 2 (1896): 160; and Thomas A. Reed, *The Sex Cycle of the Germ Plasm: Its Relation to Sex Determination* (Whitefish, Mont.: Kessinger, 2009 [1906]), 18.

16. Starling, *Croonian Lectures*. Across the last several of these lectures in particular, Starling lays out this vision of the endocrine system (which, it should be noted, probably overemphasizes the role of sex).

17. William Bayliss and Ernest Starling, "The Mechanism of Pancreatic Secretion," *Journal of Physiology* 18, no. 5 (1902): 331.

18. Bayliss and Starling, "The Mechanism of Pancreatic Secretion," 339.

19. Starling, *The Croonian Lectures*, 4. Subsequent references will be made in-text.

20. Ernest Starling, "Hormones," *Nature* 112 (1923): 795.

21. Starling, "Hormones," emphasis added.

22. E. Newton Harvey, "Some Physical Properties of Protoplasm," *Journal of Applied Physics* 9 (1938): 68.

23. "Protoplasm," *New Standard Encyclopedia*, vol. 9 (New York: University Society, 1907), no page number; Julius Von Sachs, *History of Botany (1530–1860)*, trans. Henry E. F. Garnsey (Oxford: Clarendon Press, 1890), 327–30.

24. Hans Driesch, "The Potency of the First Two Cleavage Cells in Echinoderm Development: Experimental Production of Partial and Double Formations," in *Foundations of Experimental Embryology*, ed. Benjamin H. Willer and Jane M. Oppenheimer (Englewood Cliffs, N.J.: Prentice Hall, 1964), 39.

25. Ross Granville Harrison, "Observations on the Living Development of Nerve Fiber," *Anatomical Record* 1 (1907): 118.

26. See Jane Maienschein, "The Origins of *Entwicklungsmechanik*," in *A Conceptual History of Endocrinology*, ed. Gilbert F. Scott (New York: Springer, 1991), 43–61.

27. The child study movement was, of course, much broader in scope and reach than just Hall's work, but I focus on him in this chapter for clarity and for his representative thinking. For an introduction to its broader scientific foundations, see Alice Boardman Smutts, *Science in the Service of Children, 1893–1935* (New Haven, Conn.: Yale University Press, 2006).

28. G. Stanley Hall, *Adolescence: Its Psychology and Its Relations to Physiology, Anthropology, Sociology, Sex, Crime, Religion, and Education* (New York: D. Appleton, 1904), xiii. Subsequent references to this book will be made in-text. See also:

"Development is less gradual and more salutatory, suggestive of some ancient period of storm and stress when old moorings were broken and a higher level attained. The annual rate of growth in height, weight, and strength is increased and often doubled, and even more. Important functions previously non-existent arise. Growth of parts and organs loses its former proportions, some permanently and some for a season. Some of these are still growing in old age and others are soon arrested and atrophy" (xiii).

29. For example: "Thus we must conceive growth as due to an impulse which, despite its marvelous predeterminations, is exceedingly plastic to external influences, a few of which can be demonstrated *and more have to be assumed*" (33, emphasis added). Growth is not genetically programmed, nor is plasticity's action representable as such. He then cites an embryo cleavage study similar to Driesch's as evidence (34).

30. See also: "This seems to be nature's provision to expand in all directions its possibilities of the body and soul in this plastic period when without the occasional excess powers would atrophy or suffer arrest for want of use, or larger possibilities would not be realized without this regimen peculiar to nascent periods" (216).

31. Rhythm and periodicity are among his preferred concepts: "There is much to suggest that early adolescence develops in the direction of spurty rather than that of sustained effort, or that the latter comes later. The known changes in circulation, the conjectured modification of the nervous centers, phyletic analogy with the longer than diurnal rhythms of work and rest elsewhere discussed, and common observations as well *as the general concept of plasticity to be shaped by culminative stresses that break out new ways across old ones*—all these suggest this temporary primacy of erethic over plodding increment" (150, emphasis added).

32. As Hall puts it: "The genital tubercle from which the male glans is grown can be seen by the tenth week. Minot finds that the male and female organs have seven parts in common, while there are thirteen homologies which are slowly differentiated as the embryo becomes fully sexed" (413).

33. Hall also recodes "hermaphrodites" in this developmental schema, rather than continuing to categorize them as monstrous creations of nature, different in kind from the rest of the species. In cases of hermaphroditism, he explains, "sexual differentiation which ought to take place in embryonic life *has been incomplete . . .* we now know that the embryological truth of Plato's myth of the bifurcation of an originally bisexual man was a periphrastic adumbration" (413–14, emphasis added). This conversion of hermaphroditism into a developmental sense of intersex is taken up in further detail in chapters 2 and 3.

34. Eugen Steinach, *Sex and Life: Forty Years of Biological and Medical Experiments,* trans. Josef Loebel (New York: Viking Press, 1940), 1. Hereafter cited in-text.

35. D. Schultheiss, J. Denil, and U. Jonas, "Rejuvenation in the Early 20th Century," *Andrologia* 29 (1997): 351–55.

36. Eugen Steinach and Paul Kammerer, "Klima und Mannbarkeit," *Archive fuer Entwicklungsmechanik* 46, no. 2–3 (1920): 391–458.

37. As the original paper has not been translated into English and I do not read German, I am relying here on Cheryl A. Logan's excellent account and analysis, *Hormones, Heredity, and Race: Spectacular Failure in Interwar Failure* (New Brunswick, N.J.: Rutgers University Press, 2013), 65–73.

38. See, for instance, Paul Kammerer, *The Inheritance of Acquired Characteristics*, trans. A. Paul Maeker-Brandon (New York: Koni and Liveright, 1924): "Theoretically, as well as practically, the changeability of living beings is unlimited" (249). For a broader background, see Logan, *Hormones, Heredity, and Race*, 148.

39. Luther Burbank, *The Training of the Human Plant* (New York: Century Co., 1907), 4–5. Hereafter cited in-text.

40. George W. Corner, "Oscar Riddle, 1877–1968, a Biographical Memoir" (Washington, D.C.: National Academy of Sciences, 1974), 435–36.

41. Corner, "Oscar Riddle, 1877–1968," 431, 434.

42. Corner, "Oscar Riddle, 1877–1968," 442.

43. Oscar Riddle, "A Case of Complete Sex-Reversal in the Adult Pigeon," *American Naturalist* 58, no. 655 (1924): 180.

44. Riddle, "A Case of Complete Sex-Reversal," 170.

45. Allen Ezra, "Sex Reversal and the Barrier of Sexuality," *Journal of the American Institute of Homeopathy* 25 (1932): 921.

46. Ezra, "Sex Reversal and the Barrier of Sexuality," 908, emphasis added.

47. Ezra, "Sex Reversal and the Barrier of Sexuality," 908.

48. See Alexandra Stern, *Eugenic Nation: Faults and Frontiers of Better Breeding in Modern America* (Berkeley: University of California Press, 2005); and Gabriel N. Rosenberg, *The 4-H Harvest: Sexuality and the State in Rural America* (Philadelphia: University of Pennsylvania Press, 2015).

49. Carolyn Steedman, *Strange Dislocations: Childhood and the Idea of Human Interiority, 1780–1930* (Cambridge, Mass.: Harvard University Press, 1995), 170, emphasis added.

50. Steedman, *Strange Dislocations*, emphasis in original.

51. Steedman, *Strange Dislocations*, 76.

52. See Jayna Brown, "Being Cellular: Race, the Inhuman, and the Plasticity of Life," *GLQ* 21, 2–3 (2015): 321–41.

53. Steedman, *Strange Dislocations*, 172.

2. Before Transsexuality

1. Joanne Meyerowitz, *How Sex Changed: A History of Transsexuality in the United States* (Cambridge, Mass.: Harvard University Press, 2004), 19. See also

Katie Sutton, "Sexological Cases and the Prehistory of Identity Politics in Inter-war Germany," in *Case Studies and the Dissemination of Knowledge*, ed. Joy Damousi, Brigit Lang, and Katie Sutton (New York: Routledge, 2015), 85–103.

2. "Intersexuality" was a cousin of the theory of bisexuality examined in chapter 1. "Transvestism" encompassed both individuals seeking medical support and those who did not. See Harry Benjamin, *The Transsexual Phenomenon*, electronic edition (Dusseldorf: Symposium, 1999), 16. On the theory of natural bisexuality, see chapter 1.

3. Alan L. Hart to Mary Roberts Rinehart, August 3, 1921, Folder 8, Box 21, Series VI, MRR. Hart's referenced psychiatrist famously published an article on his case in J. Allen Gilbert, "Homosexuality and Its Treatment," *Journal of Nervous and Mental Disease* 52, no. 4 (October 1920): 297–322. Jonathan Ned Katz reads Hart as lesbian in *Gay American History: Lesbians and Gay Men in the U.S.A.* (New York: Plume, 1992), 390–422. The very real porosity of the inversion discourse that circulated in this era makes it difficult to disentangle sex from sexuality in the sense of object choice as would be the custom today. Nevertheless, in terms of medicine, Hart's interest in hysterectomy and gonadectomy certainly makes him an important figure in the history of trans medicine before transsexuality. Katz apparently no longer holds to his reading of Hart as lesbian. See Zagria, "Alan Lucile Hart (1980–1962)," *A Gender Variance Who's Who*, October 20, 2008, https://zagria.blogspot.com/2008/10/alan-lucill-hart-1890–1962-doctor.html.

4. H. M. Coon, "Report to W. B. Campbell," Department of Neuro-Psychiatry, University of Wisconsin–Madison, General Hospital, July 19, 1948, Box 3, Series II-C, HB.

5. Berdeen Frankel Mayer, "Case History and Closing Note," October 2, 1950, Box 3, Series II-C, HB.

6. Coon, "Report."

7. Coon, "Report."

8. Mayer, "Case History."

9. See the extensive correspondence among Val, Kinsey, Benjamin, and Bowman in Box 3, Series II-C, HB.

10. Nonmedical archives, although less available, offer a hint. Figureheads in the American trans community from the 1940s, such as Louise Lawrence in the San Francisco Bay Area, left behind significant correspondence between self-identified "transvestites" throughout the United States, and many of their childhoods would have taken place during the first few decades of the twentieth century. See, for instance, a collection of Lawrence's scrapbooks, containing photos and correspondence from trans people, mostly from the 1940s and 1950s. Folder 7, Box 5, Series III-A, LL.

11. Magnus Hirschfeld, *Transvestites: The Erotic Drive to Cross-Dress*, trans. Michael A. Lombardi Nash (Buffalo, N.Y.: Prometheus Books, 1991). This is the very first English translation of this text.

12. Havelock Ellis, *Studies in the Psychology of Sex*, Vol. II: *Eonism and Other Supplementary Studies* (Philadelphia: F. A. Davis, 1928).

13. Thomas Rennie, a resident psychiatrist at Johns Hopkins, who is discussed in greater detail later in this chapter, represents a good example of an American with a passing familiarity with European sexological concepts who keeps them at arm's length from his clinical determinations.

14. Benjamin, *The Transsexual Phenomenon*, 16.

15. "Profile: Dr. Harry Benjamin, at 95—His Life and Career," *Sexuality Today*, June 9, 1980, 3–4, Box 1, JMK Correspondence. Of course, the fight over the meaning of biology to Freud and to psychoanalysis is one that had a much broader venue during this moment. See Elizabeth Wilson, *Psychosomatic: Feminism and the Neurological Body* (Durham, N.C.: Duke University Press, 2004), 1–3.

16. Benjamin, "Profile," 3.

17. Harry Benjamin to Dr. Steins, September 2, 1922, Box 5, Series II-C, HB. For more on Steinach, see chapter 1.

18. Harry Benjamin to Charles Hamilton, March 18, 1954, Box 5, HB Series. See also Harry Benjamin, "Eugen Steinach, 1861–1944: A Life of Research," *Scientific Monthly* 26 (December 1945): 427–42. Folder 58a, Box 15, Series III-B, HB. For more on Steinach and Kammerer, again, see chapter 1.

19. See various letters between Benjamin, Steinach, and Kammerer, Box 5, Series II-C, HB.

20. Harry Benjamin to Jules S. Bache, November 8, 1925, Box 3, Series II-C, HB. There is an interesting collection of Benjamin's fights with medical journals over publishing pro-Steinach material in the 1920s here. American journals were not as welcoming of Steinach's work, and Benjamin made a point of quarreling with publications that refused his work on that basis. Folder 58b, Box 15, Series II-C, HB.

21. Harry Benjamin, "Reminiscences," *Journal of Sex Research* 6, no. 1 (1970): 4.

22. Benjamin, "Reminiscences," 4.

23. Otto Spengler, "People Just Faint When the Subject Is Broached," in *Gay American History: Lesbian and Gay Men in the U.S.A.*, ed. Jonathan Ned Katz (New York: Plume Press, 1992), 381.

24. Bernard Talmey, "Transvestism: A Contribution to the Study of the Psychology of Sex," *New York Medical Journal* (1915): 298–307; and *Love: A Treatise on the Science of Sex-Attraction, Fourth Edition* (New York: Eugenics, 1919), 297–309.

25. Otto Spengler to Gertrude Atherton, September 10, 1938, Box 3, Series II-C, HB.

26. Harry Benjamin to Gertrude Atherton, September 27, 1938, Box 3, Series II-C, HB.

27. Benjamin, "Profile," 3.

28. Paul Popenoe to Harry Benjamin, November 25, 1936; and Paul Popenoe to Harry Benjamin, May 7, 1935, Box 7, Series II-C, HB.

29. On Riddle and his work at Cold Spring Harbor, see chapter 1.

30. Harry Benjamin to Oscar Riddle, April 1, 1929, Box 7, Series II-C, HB.

31. Oscar Riddle to Harry Benjamin, April 5, 1929, Box 7, Series II-C, HB, 7, emphasis in original.

32. Harry Benjamin to Oscar Riddle, April 22, 1931, Box 7, Series II-C, HB.

33. Oscar Riddle to Harry Benjamin, April 24, 1931, Box 7, Series II-C, HB.

34. Oscar Riddle to Harry Benjamin, January 31, 1930, Box 7, Series II-C, HB.

35. For the broader historical context, see Nancy Ordover, *American Eugenics: Race, Queer Anatomy, and the Science of Nationalism* (Minneapolis: University of Minnesota Press, 2003).

36. Benjamin, "Profile," 4.

37. Young had spent several months in Berlin early in his career, learning from the early inventors of the cystoscope and redesigning the instrument himself many times so as to make it useful for illuminating, visualizing, and recording images of the inside of the body and also affixing appendages to it that could be used for certain surgical procedures, such as removing parts of the prostate or kidney stones. See Hugh Hampton Young, *A Surgeon's Autobiography* (San Diego, Calif.: Harcourt, 1940), 86–91.

38. 1003.1, HHY.

39. Young, *A Surgeon's Autobiography*, 76.

40. See Harriet A. Washington, *Medical Apartheid: The Dark History of Medical Experimentation on African Americans from Colonial Times to the Present* (New York: Harlem Moon Books, 2006), 115–42; and Rebecca Skloot, *The Immortal Life of Henrietta Lacks* (New York: Broadway Paperbacks, 2010), 158–69.

41. 1002.3, HHY.

42. 1002.3, HHY.

43. 1002.4, HHY.

44. For a published overview of the research, teaching, training, and residency dimensions of the Brady Institute, see Young, *A Surgeon's Autobiography*, 235–36.

45. Harriet Lane Home Patient Index Card Series, "Hermaphrodism," EP. The specific cases in question are 2001.2, 2001.3, 2001.7, 2001.9, 2001.10, 2001.11, EP.

46. See Alison Redick, "American History XY: The Medical Treatment of Intersex, 1916–1955 (PhD dissertation, New York University, 2004), 95–96.

47. Young had already seen one intersex patient in his private practice before the opening of the Institute (see 5009.8, BUI), and at least one other physician at Hopkins, Thomas Cullen, had also seen and even published on a case involving a patient diagnosed with hermaphroditism in 1911 (see 3001.1, TC). The published account is Thomas S. Cullen, "A Pseudohermaphrodite," *Surgery, Gynecology, and Obstetrics* (1911): 449–53.

48. Diagnostic Index Card, BUI.

49. Young, *A Surgeon's Autobiography*, 238.

50. Redick argues that this era could therefore be called the "Age of Idiosyncrasy." "American History XY," 18.

51. The model and outline for the ensemble of these surgical techniques is provided at length in Hugh Hampton Young, *Genital Abnormalities, Hermaphroditism, and Related Adrenal Diseases* (Baltimore: Williams & Wilkins, 1937).

52. Redick, "American History XY," 104.

53. To be clear, then, although I did read Stonestreet's medical records as part of researching this chapter, I cannot discuss their contents because of the existing breach of privacy (namely that Young and colleague used Stonestreet's last name and first initial in medical publications discussing the case). Anyone interested in accessing the original documents can apply to the Privacy Board of the Johns Hopkins Hospital and, if granted access, can locate the documents from code for the file, 5007.4, BUI, a copy of which is stored at the Alan Chesney Medical Archives.

54. Young, *A Surgeon's Autobiography*, 204.

55. W. M. C. Quinby, "A Case of Pseudo-Hermaphrodism, with Remarks on Abnormal Function of the Endocrine Glands," *Bulletin of the Johns Hopkins Hospital* 27, no. 300 (1917): 50–53. Hereafter cited in-text.

56. Young, *A Surgeon's Autobiography*, 204.

57. Quinby, "A Case of Pseudohermaphroditism," 53.

58. Young, *A Surgeon's Autobiography*, 205.

59. Young, *A Surgeon's Autobiography*, 205.

60. See, for example, 1006.3 and 1005.6, HHY.

61. See, for example, 5009.11, BUI.

62. See, for example, 1005.1, HHY, from the 1920s; and 1005.2 and 1005.3, HHY, from the 1930s. Because these cases were discussed in *Genital Abnormalities*, with Young's accompanying breach of privacy, I cannot provide any specific details about these individuals.

63. See, for example, 1005.1, HHY.

64. See, for example, 1005.2, HHY.

65. It is not clear what pronouns this child preferred, so I have opted to use plural pronouns. I follow this practice for all intersex and trans children in this book whose gender identities were not archived, but it is most frequent in this chapter and the next.

66. 1005.1, HHY.

67. The procedure is outlined in surgery reports in 5002.1, 5002.2, and 5002.3, BUI.

68. See, for example, the case of a twelve-year-old with a very large adrenal tumor, which required two attempts at surgery, the second of which led to the patient's death. 1006.6, HHY.

69. 5009.11, BUI. Subsequent citations of this code at the end of a paragraph indicate that all quotations and references without notes in that paragraph are from these patient records.

70. Young, *Genital Abnormalities*.

71. 5009.11, BUI. Subsequent citations of this code at the end of a paragraph indicate that all quotations and references without notes in that paragraph are from these patient records.

72. 5009.11, BUI.

73. 5009.11, BUI.

74. For cases of African American intersex children from this era, see 2001.17 and 2001.6, EP. On the long history of antiblackness and nontherapeutic experimentation in American medicine, see Washington, *Medical Apartheid*.

75. Edwards A. Park to Hugh Hampton Young, June 19, 1935, Folder 3, Box 3, Series 1, EP, emphasis added.

76. One place that these strategic adoptions of intersex narratives can be found is in autobiographical texts by public trans figures, for example, Michael Dillon, *Self: A Study in Ethics and Endocrinology* (London: Elsevier Science, 1946); Lilli Elbe, *Man into Woman: An Authentic Record of a Sex Change*, ed. Niels Hoyer (London: Beacon Library, 1933); and Christine Jorgensen, *Christine Jorgensen: A Personal Autobiography* (New York: Bantam Books, 1968).

77. And, as Siobhan Somerville has shown, the sexological framing of inversion was also highly racialized in the United States. See *Queering the Color Line: Race and the Invention of Homosexuality in American Culture* (Durham, N.C.: Duke University Press, 2000).

78. Young, *A Surgeon's Autobiography*, 309–10.

79. Hirschfeld, *Transvestites*, 18.

80. 5014.8, BUI.

81. 5014.1, BUI. Subsequent citations of this code at the end of a paragraph indicate that all quotations and references without notes in that paragraph are from these patient records.

82. 5014.1, BUI.

83. 5014.1, BUI.

84. 5014.1, BUI, emphasis added.

85. See, for example, 5014.12, BUI.

86. 5014.7, BUI.

87. 5014.10, BUI. Subsequent citations of this code at the end of a paragraph indicate that all quotations and references without notes in that paragraph are from these patient records.

88. 5014.10, BUI.

89. Mark Weston was a British athlete and intersex person whose career as a highly successful shot-putter resulted in his transition to living as a man. His surgery

at Charing Cross Hospital in 1936 was intensely covered by the media. "Girl Who Became Man Tells of Metamorphosis," *Reading Eagle,* May 28, 1936, 5.

90. 5014.10, BUI.

91. 5014.10, BUI.

92. 5014.10, BUI.

93. 5014.10, BUI.

94. 5014.10, BUI.

95. Frank R. Lillie, "The Theory of the Free-Martin," *Science* 43 (1916): 611–13.

96. 5014.10, BUI.

97. 5014.10, BUI.

98. 5014.10, BUI, emphasis added.

99. 5014.10, BUI.

100. 5014.11

101. 5014.11, emphasis added.

102. 5014.11.

103. The very idea of a trans child did haunt the Brady Institute because of how the child's exceptional plasticity muddied the distinction between intersex and inversion. For instance, in 1938, around the same time that Bernard and Karen were visiting the Institute, a mother brought in her child, raised a boy, complaining of ostensible "homosexuality." A doctor examined the child and noted that the "mother has been a confidant" about the inversion "and she wrote to Dr. Young following the article in the newspaper regarding 'the changing of boys to girls.'" The mother's connection of her child's potential inversion to Young's sex reassignment of intersex children suggests that outside medical institutions some lay people felt that intersex bodies and inverted bodies, whether homosexual or trans, fell into the same field. The ambiguity of medical discourse, however, is as much an obstacle to interpreting these documents as it is a vital archive. 5014.9, BUI, emphasis added.

104. Records 5016.1, 5016.6, 5016.7, and 5016.8, BUI, all continued into the mid- to late 1960s. Because these records contain material less than fifty years old at the time I was conducting archival research, I was not allowed to read these documents as part of my research protocol.

105. 5016.2, BUI.

106. 5016.4, BUI.

107. 5016.4, BUI.

108. 5016.3, BUI.

109. Emma Heaney, *The New Woman: Literary Modernism, Queer Theory, and the Trans Feminine Allegory* (Chicago: Northwestern University Press, 2017), 175: "This world of trans feminine thriving is more difficult to access in the sexological texts that form a large part of the archive of trans feminine narratives in the period.

The genre of medical writing will always disproportionately contain the words of people who feel (or feel that others feel) that there is a wrong that must be righted, a malady that must be cured. Yet... there is plenty to suggest that many trans women in the period, including those who shared the stories of their lives with sexological researchers, felt likewise 'satisfied." This chapter is in broad agreement with, not to mention indebted to, Heaney's careful parsing of the early twentieth-century trans archive to demonstrate the lived social reality of trans feminine life that sexology and medicine had to willfully misrecognize in order to produce its account of trans experience. Like the trans women whose "satisfying" lives Heaney carefully reads out of the archive, this chapter offers brief glimpses into trans boyhood and girlhood lived in the early twentieth century without reference to medicine in order to show how, even within the medical archive, trans childhood testifies to its social reality and existence, with recognition and satisfaction.

110. Paul B. Preciado, *Testo Junkie: Sex, Drugs, and Biopolitics in the Pharmacophornographic Era*, trans. Bruce Benderson (New York: Feminist Press, 2014), 27–28.

111. Bernice L. Hausman, *Changing Sex, Transsexualism, Technology, and the Idea of Gender* (Durham, N.C.: Duke University Press, 1995). Although, interestingly enough, Hausman does argue for the importance of the early twentieth century in the genealogy of transsexuality (vii).

112. Meyerowitz rejects Hausman's determinist reading of medical technology, suggesting instead that sex reassignment surgery, in particular, took root in Europe before the United States because of local reformist political movements, particularly those associated with Hirschfeld and his interlocutors in Berlin, as well as "a new definition of sex" from the biological sciences that framed it as alterable or changeable. *How Sex Changed*, 21. This chapter is in broad agreement with Meyerowitz, although it offers much more evidence of trans life in the American medical arena because of extensive research in the medical records of the Johns Hopkins Hospital, to which Meyerowitz did not have access.

3. Sex in Crisis

1. The sources on this visit come from Money's published recollections, written almost fifty years later, which are inconsistent about the individual's age, listed once as fifteen and once as seventeen. That inconsistency, the passage of time, and Money's general penchant for renarrating his own career to suit his public image suggest that other details about the case could also be inaccurate. I have also refused to endorse Money's description of this child with a gender marker. See John Money, *Gendermaps: Social Constructionism, Feminism, and Sexosophical History* (New York: Continuum, 1995), 19; and *Biographies of Gender and Hermaphroditism in Paired Comparison* (New York: Elsevier, 1991), 1.

2. Money, *Gendermaps*, 19.

3. Again, *if* we take Money's account at face value.

4. Jennifer Germon, *Gender: A Genealogy of an Idea* (New York: Palgrave Macmillan, 2009), 86.

5. See Germon's chapter, "Stoller's Seductive Dualisms," 63–84, in *Gender,* for a good overview. Stoller's work with transgender children at the University of California, Los Angeles, is discussed in detail in chapters 4 and 5 of this book.

6. Sharon E. Preves, "Sexing the Intersexed: An Analysis of Sociocultural Responses to Intersexuality," *Signs* 27, no. 2 (2001): 523–56; David A. Rubin, "'An Unnamed Blank That Craved a Name': A Genealogy of Intersex as Gender," *Signs* 37, no. 4 (2012): 883–908; Jemima Repo, "The Biopolitical Birth of Gender: Social Control, Hermaphroditism, and the New Sexual Apparatus," *Alternatives: Global, Local, Political* 38, no. 3 (2013): 228–44; and Paul B. Preciado, *Testo Junkie: Sex, Drugs, and Biopolitics in the Pharmacopornographic Era,* trans. Bruce Benderson (New York: Feminist Press, 2014).

7. Germon spends valuable time in *Gender* reconstructing the broader context of Money's doctoral studies, where he very much came to *reflect* hegemonic conceptual contexts in psychology and sexology, rather than overturn them (34).

8. On UNESCO's statements on race, see Sonali Thakkar, "Racial Reformations and the Politics of Plasticity," paper presented at the Modern Languages Association Annual Meeting, Philadelphia, Pa., January 6, 2017.

9. Iain Morland, "Gender, Genitals, and the Meaning of Being Human," in *Fuckology: Critical Essays on John Money's Diagnostic Concepts,* ed. Iain Morland and Nikki Sullivan (Chicago: University of Chicago Press, 2014), 76–77.

10. Morland, "Gender, Genitals, and the Meaning of Being Human," 90.

11. More so than in other chapters of this book, the discussion of the etiology, mechanics, diagnosis, treatment, and pharmacokinetics of CAH and cortisone in this section has been intentionally simplified to reduce some of the quickly overwhelming grain of detail that would address itself better to a specialist audience in medicine. I have made reductions particularly in the complexity of terminology and the modeling of some clinical procedures to condense those specialist concerns in the interest of brevity and the reader's ease in following my argument. If a certain degree of medical accuracy is lost in the process, I believe it to be worth the risk. In any case, the diagnosis and protocols for CAH from this era no longer resemble the current normative medical consensus, so inaccuracy is a highly contextual issue (and this book is hardly invested in the concept of medical accuracy, for that matter). The problem of the entanglement of plasticity, metabolism, and sex that CAH and cortisone signal is the ultimate aim of this section, rather than an exhaustive or finely accurate picture of the condition and its treatment in the late 1940s.

12. Indeed, cases of "female pseudohermaphroditism," of which CAH was probably the most common condition, made up by far the largest single portion of children diagnosed with intersex conditions at the Harriet Lane Home from the 1920s to 1950s, accounting for a little more than 40 percent of total admissions. Pediatric Diagnostic Index Series, "Hermaphrodism," EP.

13. There was also growing speculation, beginning in the 1950s, that the common administration of a synthetic estrogen to prevent miscarriage for women during pregnancy also had virilizing effects on the fetus similar to what occurred in cases of CAH. This may have accounted for some of the sheer volume of admissions to the hospital for these kinds of conditions. Lawson Wilkins, *The Diagnosis and Treatment of Endocrine Disorders in Childhood and Adolescence,* 2nd ed. (Springfield, Ill.: Charles C. Thomas, 1957), 7, 9.

14. One of the other important ways that the medicalization of intersex bodies was justified was through a developmental model in which the study of children might produce insight into the genesis of conditions that were difficult to treat in adults. This was certainly the dominant ethos of the Harriet Lane Home. Whether studying psychiatric conditions, infectious disease, or endocrine disorders, the Home framed its clinical research as producing insights that could not be achieved through work wih adult patients. In the case of a proposed study of heart disease, for instance, Edwards A. Park, the head of the Home, remarked that while "one cannot study effectively rheumatic heart disease in the adult because one there encounters the disease in its already developed form," in children, "particularly in the very young child," by contrast, "one encounters the disease at its very beginning." Edwards A. Park to Hugh Hampton Young, October 19, 1933, Folder 3, Box 3, EP. Park explained the work of the child psychiatrist Leo Kanner to Hugh Hampton Young in similar terms, explaining that its "importance . . . lies, perhaps, not so much in the care of children with behavior disorders as in the study of them, by which he is obtaining an insight into the hitherto greatly neglected subject and information which it is hoped will lead to better understanding of insanity and behavior disturbance in the adult" (Edwards A. Park to Hugh Hampton Young, October 19, 1933, Folder 3, Box 3, EP). For a more thorough overview of the child psychiatry clinic's mandate, see Leo Kanner, "Statement concerning the Psychiatric Clinic of the Harriet Lane Home," 1933, Folder 3, Box 3, EP.

15. Today, CAH is understood to be caused by a genetic mutation. At the time of Wilkins's work, there was no known cause.

16. While this chapter is based on the medical records of the Harriet Lane Home, Wilkins and his colleagues published a series of papers on CAH in the early 1950s that have since become referential texts in postwar pediatric endocrinology. See Lawson Wilkins, R. A. Lewis, R. Klein, and E. Rosenberg, "Suppression of Adrenal Androgen Secretion by Cortisone in a Case of Congenital Adrenal Hyperplasia," *Bulletin of the Johns Hopkins Hospital* 86 (1950): 249–52; Lawson Wilkins,

Lytt I. Gardner, John F. Crigler, Samuel H. Silverman, and Claude J. Migeon, "Further Studies on the Treatment of Congenital Adrenal Hyperplasia with Cortisone: I. Comparison of Oral and Intramuscular Administration of Cortisone, with a Note on the Suppressive Action of Compounds F and B on the Adrenal," *Journal of Clinical Endocrinology and Metabolism* 12, no. 3 (1952): 257–76; and Lawson Wilkins, Lytt I. Gardner, John F. Crigler, Samuel H. Silverman, and Claude J. Migeon, "II. The Effects of Cortisone on Sexual and Somatic Development, with an Hypothesis concerning the Mechanism of Feminization," *Journal of Clinical Endocrinology and Metabolism* 12, no. 3 (1952): 277–95.

17. 2001.15, EP. The rationale for this doctor's refusal of a surgical protocol is not recorded in the archive. Subsequent citations of this code at the end of a paragraph indicate that all quotations and references without notes in that paragraph are from these patient records.

18. 2001.15, EP.

19. 2001.15, EP.

20. 2001.15, EP.

21. Claude Migeon, "Lawson Wilkins and My Life: Part 1," *International Journal of Pediatric Endocrinology,* Supplement 1 (2014): 5–6, 11. Strangely, Wilkins and the Massachusetts researchers apparently reached their conclusion about the ability of cortisone therapy to treat CAH mere days apart.

22. 2001.21, EP.

23. It is extremely difficult to interpret any of this child's self-beliefs on the basis of their records, so I have avoided suggesting what their own gender identity might have been. The doctors at the Home referred to them many times as "a shy and lonely person who is very quiet," with great condescension, attributing very little meaningfulness to their thoughts, behavior, and speech during their stay on the ward.

24. 2001.21, EP.

25. 2001.7, EP. Because it remains unclear from medical records whether or not this child, or any of the other children discussed in this chapter, affirmed the decision to medically reassign their sex as female, I have refrained from using any gendered pronouns to describe them.

26. Wilkins, Gardner, Crigler, Silverman, and Migeon, "Further Studies on the Treatment of Congenital Adrenal Hyperplasia with Cortisone," 279–83.

27. In many cases, however, clitoridectomy had already been performed on the patient as an infant, obviating the question. Wilkins, Gardner, Crigler, Silverman, and Migeon, "Further Studies on the Treatment of Congenital Adrenal Hyperplasia with Cortisone," 283.

28. For an early example of this argument, see Preves, "Sexing the Intersexed," 532–33. For more recent work in intersex studies that covers this argument well, see, for instance, Georgiann Davis, *Contesting Intersex: The Dubious Diagnosis* (New

York: New York University Press, 2015); Morgan Holmes, ed., *Critical Intersex* (New York: Routledge, 2009); and Katrina Karkazis, *Fixing Sex: Intersex, Medical Authority, and Lived Experience* (Durham, N.C.: Duke University Press, 2008).

29. John F. Crigler, Samuel Silverman, and Lawson Wilkins, "Further Studies on the Treatment of Congenital Adrenal Hyperplasia with Cortisone: IV. Effect of Cortisone Compound B in Infants with Disturbed Electrolyte Metabolism," *Pediatrics* 10, no. 4 (1952): 397–413.

30. Migeon, "Lawson Wilkins and My Life," 12.

31. Crigler, Silverman, and Wilkins, "Further Studies . . . IV," 408–11.

32. Crigler, Silverman, and Wilkins, "Further Studies . . . IV," 411. I have narratively minimized the technical role of this second compound for the sake of clarity in this section, although this corticosterone (called "compound B" by Wilkins and his team) also contributed to sodium retention, albeit *without* ameliorating the hyperplasia of the adrenals.

33. Crigler, Silverman, and Wilkins, "Further Studies . . . IV," 397–403.

34. Migeon, "Lawson Wilkins and My Life," 13, emphasis added.

35. Preves, "Sexing the Intersexed," 524, emphasis added.

36. Repo, "The Biopolitical Birth of Gender," 234, emphasis added.

37. Crigler, Silverman, and Wilkins, "Further Studies . . . IV," 411.

38. Hannah Landecker, "The Metabolism of Philosophy in Three Parts," in *Dialectic and Paradox: Configurations of the Third in Modernity*, ed. Bernhard Malkmus and Ian Cooper (Cambridge, Mass.: Harvard University Press, 2013), 193–224.

39. Crigler, Silverman, and Wilkins, "Further Studies . . . IV," 397, 403, 406.

40. The last of these has been given much attention by scholars tracing the genealogy of gender through intersex, but the former two have not. The focus on normalizing surgery in intersex studies has a clear context, given the high material and psychic cost that such coercive procedures incur for infants and children who are either unable to consent or disenfranchised from having any say in the medicalization of their bodies. Stopping the routine practice of genital surgery on infants is an urgent matter. As Davis argues in *Contesting Intersex*, moreover, the constitutive ambiguity between intersex conditions exclusively defined by atypical appearance of the genitals, in contrast to a range of genetic, endocrine, and other metabolic conditions that have sexed and gendered aspects, is why the category itself is unstable and ought to be critically problematized. The recent push to replace the term "intersex" with "Disorders of Sexual Development" (DSD) and the ensuing controversy among medical practitioners and intersex activists is also testament to the instability of the category of knowledge. This chapter draws on these frameworks from intersex studies to argue that the child's growing body and its plasticity in particular point to an even greater material and epistemological inconsistency at the heart of both the categories "intersex" and "gender." The

focus on congenital adrenal hyperplasia (CAH), an intersex condition that involves
the adrenal glands and general metabolism, rather than focusing on the genitals
and gonads exclusively, is in keeping with that destabilizing impulse.

41. John Money, "Hermaphroditism, Gender and Precocity in Hyperadreno-
corticism: Psychologic Findings," *Bulletin of the Johns Hopkins Hospital* 96, no. 6
(1955): 253.

42. Money, "Hermaphroditism, Gender and Precocity," 255. As Repo explains
in "The Biopolitical Birth of Gender," the use of the term "role" here reflects the
influence of one of Money's graduate school mentors at Harvard, the structural
functionalist Talcott Parsons. "Role" described the form of compliance and subjectification embedded in socialization into strict norms (231–31).

43. Money, "Hermaphroditism, Gender, and Precocity," 254.

44. Money, "Hermaphroditism, Gender, and Precocity," 254.

45. For a comprehensive discussion of that paradigm in relation to hermaphroditism specifically, see Alice Dreger, *Hermaphrodites and the Medical Invention of
Sex* (Cambridge, Mass.: Harvard University Press, 1998), 153–55. In his dissertation, Money had reviewed the literature on "hermaphroditism" published in English to undermine the diagnostic criteria set by the German-Swiss pathologist
Edwin Klebs in the 1870s. By Klebs's gonadocentric parameters, "true hermaphroditism" was characterized only by the presence in the body of a mixed "ovotestis"
containing both testicular and ovarian forms of tissue. All other cases were relegated
to two catchall terms: "male pseudohermaphroditism" (where a testis is present
but sex is overall indeterminate) and "female pseudohermaphroditism" (where
an ovary is present but sex is overall indeterminate). The major practical problem
with this tripartite division was its gross inaccuracy. In his dissertation research
Money found essentially zero verifiable cases of "true" intersex conditions, such
that the wide variety of intersex embodiments encountered by doctors were being
relegated to two "pseudo" umbrella categories based on gonads. John Money,
"Hermaphroditism: An Inquiry into the Nature of a Human Paradox" (PhD dissertation, Harvard University, 1951).

46. As Money notes in "Hermaphroditism, Gender and Precocity," 254.

47. "Hermaphroditism, Gender and Precocity," 254.

48. John Money, Joan Hampson, and John Hampson, "Hermaphroditism: Recommendations concerning Assignment of Sex, Change of Sex, and Psychologic
Management," *Johns Hopkins Medical Journal* 97, no. 4 (1955): 285.

49. Money, Hampson, and Hampson, "Hermaphroditism," 285.

50. Money, Hampson, and Hampson, "Hermaphroditism," 285.

51. Money, "Hermaphroditism, Gender and Precocity," 254.

52. Interpreting Money's theory as an extreme form of social constructivism is
more characteristic of the earliest scholarship on intersex and gender. For instance,
Suzanne J. Kessler, in "The Medical Construction of Gender: Case Management

of Intersexed Infants," *Signs* 16, no. 1 (1990): 4, emphasis added, argues that "the process and guidelines by which decisions about gender (re)construction are made *reveal the model for the social construction of gender generally.*" This reading has come under pressure in recent years from scholars in intersex studies, including Rubin, Morland, and Germon. The latter, in particular, takes the time in *Gender* to read in Money's work a more complex argument for the coconstitution of sex and gender as embodied and cultural—to "critically reinvigorate Money's gender" (3). Like Rubin in "An Unnamed Blank That Craved a Name," however, while I find the careful reading of Money imperative, I nonetheless find any reparative impulse in relation to his work decidedly misplaced (887). Money was the direct source of a great deal of inexcusable harm for which he was never held accountable.

53. Money, Hampson, and Hampson, "Hermaphroditism," 289.

54. This has been a site of critique of the medicalization of intersex children since Kessler's work in "The Medical Construction of Gender" in 1990.

55. Money, "Hermaphroditism, Gender and Precocity," 258.

56. Money, "Hermaphroditism, Gender and Precocity," 258. This analogy to the acquisition of language was frequently repeated in their subsequent work on gender, as well as throughout the rest of Money's career.

57. Money, Hampson, and Hampson, "Hermaphroditism," 289.

58. Money, Hampson, and Hampson, "Hermaphroditism," 289.

59. Here lies also the germ of medicine's most gender-normative narrative of transsexuality, whereby sex reassignment and hormones serve to complete the developmental potential of the human, a premise whose many implications for trans children are explored in detail in chapter 4.

60. Money, Hampson, and Hampson, "Hermaphroditism," 291, emphasis added.

61. On the role of metaphor in medical science and Haraway's work, see chapter 1.

62. Preciado, *Testo Junkie*, 113.

63. Preciado, *Testo Junkie*.

64. Preciado, *Testo Junkie*, 348, 351, 385.

65. Preciado, *Testo Junkie*, 385, emphasis in original.

66. See 2001.9, 2001.15, and 2001.23, EP.

67. Money, Hampson, and Hampson, "Hermaphroditism," 297.

68. Money, Hampson, and Hampson, "Hermaphroditism."

69. Money, Hampson, and Hampson, "Hermaphroditism."

70. Money, Hampson, and Hampson, "Hermaphroditism," 298, emphasis added.

71. Money, Hampson, and Hampson, "Hermaphroditism," emphasis added.

72. Money, Hampson, and Hampson, "Hermaphroditism," 299.

73. See chapter 2.

4. From Johns Hopkins to the Midwest

1. John Money and Florence Schwartz, "Public Opinion and Social Issues in Transsexualism: A Case Study in Medical Sociology," in *Transsexualism and Sex Reassignment,* ed. Richard Green and John Money (Baltimore: Johns Hopkins University Press, 1969), 255–56.

2. Joanne Meyerowitz, *How Sex Changed: A History of Transsexuality in the United States* (Durham, N.C.: Duke University Press, 2002), 220

3. Money and Schwartz, "Public Opinion," 256.

4. John Hopkins University, Office of Public Relations, "Statement of the Establishment of a Clinic for Transsexuals at the John Hopkins Medical Institutions," November 21, 1966, Folder 3, Bio Files Box, JMH.

5. John Money to Ram. W. Rapoport, August 2, 1973, Box 7, JMK. This letter outlines Money's approach to diagnosis and treatment in the 1960s and early 1970s.

6. John Money to Burton H. Wolfe, March 28, 1969, Box 9, JMK.

7. Frederick P. McGehan, "20 Sex-Change Operations Done at Hopkins since 1966," *Baltimore Sun,* February 16, 1969, 15.

8. Here I am thinking of the three books that address this time period: Meyerowitz, *How Sex Changed;* Susan Stryker, *Transgender History* (Berkeley, Calif.: Seal Press, 2008); and Bernice Hausman, *Changing Sex: Transsexualism, Technology, and the Idea of Gender* (Durham, N.C.: Duke University Press, 1995).

9. *State of Maryland v. [G.L.],* Indictment #1531 Y, January 5, 1965, MSA.

10. I use plural pronouns to refer to G.L. to avoid assigning any gender to them, given that their identity is completely suppressed in the archive.

11. Money and Schwartz, "Public Opinion," 255.

12. On the Compton's Cafeteria Riot, see Stryker, *Transgender History,* 72–73.

13. I am drawing here on Kathryn Bond Stockton's concept of sideways growth, to which I return later in this chapter in greater detail. *The Queer Child, or Growing Sideways in the Twentieth Century* (Durham, N.C.: Duke University Press, 2009).

14. Because the medical records of individuals from less than fifty years ago were not accessible under the HIPAA regulations governing my research protocol, I was not able to read those documents.

15. I also discuss Lane's childhood briefly in chapter 2.

16. 5016.3, BUI. Subsequent citations of this code at the end of a paragraph indicate that all quotations and references without notes in that paragraph are from these patient records.

17. 5016.3, BUI.

18. 5016.3, BUI.

19. 5016.3, BUI. Another major example is Louise Lawrence, who worked with Harry Benjamin during his summer trips to San Francisco, Alfred Kinsey, and Karl Bowman of the Langley Porter Psychiatric Clinic. See chapter 2.

20. 5016.2, BUI. Subsequent citations of this code at the end of a paragraph indicate that all quotations and references without notes in that paragraph are from these patient records.

21. 5016.2, BUI.

22. 5016.2, BUI.

23. 5016.2, BUI.

24. Harry Benjamin, "Operated Transsexuals (Male), Charts," no date (circa 1970), Folder 25, Box 28, HB.

25. Elmer Belt to Harry Benjamin, August 24, 1959, Box 3, Series II-C, HB. His approach to trans medicine, interestingly, was based in a gonadal theory reminiscent of interwar endocrinology: Belt felt very strongly that the "testes" of trans women should be implanted in the abdomen during surgery, not removed. Outlining his rationale to an interested colleague, he explained: "It is not necessary to disturb the patient's endocrine balance to maintain his condition as a trans-sexual since the faulty tissues lay within the substance of the testis in the first place." While this was a fairly circular notion of hormones for the 1950s, Belt's conviction underscores the omnipresence and impact of the endocrine body for the emergence of transsexual medicine in the postwar period. Elmer Belt to Robert P. McDonald, June 2, 1958, Box 3, Series II-C, HB. While Belt's correspondence from the late 1950s refers variously to "these boys" or "this young man" among his patients, he did not officially take on any children as candidates for surgery. "H.S." to Elmer Belt, no date (c. 1958), Box 3, Series II-C, HB; Elmer Belt to Carroll C. Carlson, May 20, 1958, Box 3, Series II-C, HB. In a letter to his friend and colleague Benjamin, Belt explained in 1958 that he had just seen an eighteen-year-old "who is trans-sexual and earnestly desires an operative procedure for the change of his sex"; however, Belt turned them away for being under the age of medical consent. Elmer Belt to Harry Benjamin, September 11, 1958, Box 3, Series II-C, HB.

26. Harry Benjamin to Elmer Belt, July 12, 1960, Box 3, Series II-C, HB.

27. See Hausman, *Changing Sex*, 1–6.

28. Harry Benjamin to Elmer Belt, October 29, 1965, Box 3, Series II-C, HB. See R. A. Gorski and J. W. Wagner, "Gonadal Activity and Sexual Differentiation of the Hypothalamus," *Endocrinology* 76, no. 2 (February 1965): 226–39. This body of research can be read in relation to Eugen Steinach and Oscar Riddle's earlier work on the sexed body and brain in animals from chapter 1. See also Roger A. Gorski, "Modification of Ovulatory Mechanisms by Postnatal Administration of Estrogen to the Rat," *American Journal of Physiology* 205, no. 5 (November 1963): 842–44.

29. David O. Cauldwell, "Psychopathia Transsexualis," *Sexology* 16 (1949): 274–80.

30. Louise Lawrence to Harry Benjamin, October 18, 1953, Folder 1, Box 1, Series 1B, LL.

31. Meyerowitz, *How Sex Changed*, 102.

32. See Louise Lawrence's letters to Alfred Kinsey and Harry Benjamin in Folder 1, Box 1, Series 1B, LL.

33. Harry Benjamin, "Transvestism and Transsexualism," *International Journal of Sexology* 7, no. 1 (August 1953): 12–13, emphasis added. For more on Steinach, see chapter 1.

34. Aaron Devor and Nicholas Matte, "Building a Better World for Transpeople: Reed Erickson and the Erickson Educational Foundation," *International Journal of Transgenderism* 10, no. 1 (2007): 47–68.

35. Harry Benjamin Foundation for Research in Gender Role Orientation, Promotional Flyer, 1966, Folder 1, Box 23, HB.

36. Harry Benjamin Foundation, Trustees Meeting Minutes, September 29, 1967, Folder 1, Box 23, HB.

37. Harry Benjamin, "Male Transsexuals: Ages When First Seen," December 31, 1965, Folder 24, Box 28, HB.

38. Harry Benjamin, "Male Transsexuals: First Evidence of T.S.ism (for book)," Folder 24, Box 28, HB.

39. Harry Benjamin, *The Transsexual Phenomenon*, electronic edition (Dusseldorf: Symposium Publishing, 1999), 6.

40. Benjamin, *The Transsexual Phenomenon*, 7.

41. Benjamin, *The Transsexual Phenomenon*, 8, emphasis in original.

42. Gayle Rubin, "Thinking Sex: Notes for a Radical Theory of the Politics of Sexuality," in *Deviations: A Gayle Rubin Reader* (Durham, N.C.: Duke University Press, 2011), 154.

43. Benjamin, *The Transsexual Phenomenon*, 9.

44. Benjamin, *The Transsexual Phenomenon*, 11.

45. Benjamin, *The Transsexual Phenomenon*, 11.

46. Louise Lawrence to Alfred Kinsey, June 20, 1952, Folder 1, Box 1, Series 1B, LL.

47. Benjamin, *The Transsexual Phenomenon*, 16.

48. Benjamin, *The Transsexual Phenomenon*, 16.

49. Benjamin, *The Transsexual Phenomenon*, 17.

50. Benjamin, *The Transsexual Phenomenon*, 23.

51. Patrick Healy and Geoff Quinn, "Gender Program Rapped," *UCLA Daily Bruin*, Friday, February 7, 1975, no page number, Box 8, RS.

52. Department of Psychiatry, University of California, Los Angeles, undated typed memo (c. 1963), Box 16, RS.

53. Robert Stoller, *Sex and Gender, Vol. II: The Transsexual Experiment* (New York: Jason Aronson, 1975), 11, emphasis in original.

54. Stoller, *Sex and Gender, Vol. II: The Transsexual Experiment*, 2.

55. Stoller, *Sex and Gender, Vol. II: The Transsexual Experiment*, 81.

56. Stoller, *Sex and Gender, Vol. II: The Transsexual Experiment*, 107.

57. Stoller, *Sex and Gender, Vol. II: The Transsexual Experiment*, 101.

58. Richard Green, "Sissy Boy [name redacted]," April 29, 1969, typed interview transcript, Box 8, RS.

59. Eve Kosofsky Sedgwick, "How to Bring Your Kids Up Gay," *Social Text* 29 (1991): 18–27.

60. For several examples suggesting the range of answers to this question, see E. M. Litin, M. E. Giffin, and A. E. Johnson, "Parental Influence in Unusual Sexual Behavior in Children," *Psychoanalytic Quarterly* 25 (1956): 37–55; R. Euguene Holemon and George Winokur, "Effeminate Homosexuality: A Disease of Childhood," *American Journal of Orthopsychiatry* 35 (1965): 48–56; Bernard Zuger, "The Role of Familial Factors in Persistent Effeminate Behavior in Boys," *American Journal of Psychiatry* 126, no. 8 (February 1970): 151–54; Richard Green and John Money, "Stage-Acting, Role-Taking and Effeminate Impersonation during Boyhood," *Archives of General Psychiatry* 15 (November 1966): 535–38; and George A. Rekers, O. Ivar Lovaas, and Benson Low, "The Behavioral Treatment of a 'Transsexual' Preadolescent Boy," *Journal of Abnormal Child Psychology* 2, no. 2 (June 1974): 99–116.

61. Alan S. Ruttenberg, "A Case Study of a Five-Year-Old Transsexual Boy," conference paper, location of presentation not given, February 21, 1967, Box 8, RS.

62. Ruttenberg, "A Case Study of a Five-Year-Old Transsexual Boy," 2.

63. Lawrence E. Newman, "Transsexualism in Adolescence: Problems in Evaluation and Treatment," typed manuscript, 3, no date, Box 9, RS.

64. Newman, "Transsexualism in Adolescence," 12–13, emphasis added.

65. Newman, "Transsexualism in Adolescence," 16–19.

66. Robert Stoller, Memorandum "RE: Research Meeting," November 12, 1963; and Robert Stoller, Memorandum, March 31, 1964, Box 16, RS.

67. Richard Green, Memorandum, May 25, 1970; Richard Green, Memorandum, March 20, 1970; Richard Green, Memorandum, October 8, 1969; and Richard Green, Memorandum, April 1, 1969, Box 16, RS.

68. Robert Stoller, typed manuscript, November 19, 1963, Box 16, RS.

69. For instance, see "TY" to Mr. Nelson, no date (1966), Box 6, Series II-C, HB. This letter was written to the author of an article about transsexuality in the *Evansville Courier* and was forwarded upon receipt to Benjamin.

70. At least two of the children who wrote to Benjamin's practice referenced each other in their letters, suggesting they had traded his address. They are discussed later.

71. See Mrs. Morton Phillips (Dear Abby) to Harry Benjamin, various letters, Box 6, Series II-C, HB.

72. See, for example, "WL" to Harry Benjamin, January 20, 1969, Box 4, Series II-C, HB.

73. "HU" to Harry Benjamin, no date (c.1969), Box 4, Series II-C, HB.

74. "MK" to Harry Benjamin, November 28, 1969, 2, Box 4, Series II-C, HB.

75. "WL" to Harry Benjamin, January 20, 1969, Box 4, Series II-C, HB, 3, emphasis added.

76. "GV" to Harry Benjamin, no date (c. March 1971), 1, Box 5, Series II-C, HB, emphasis added.

77. "MK" to Harry Benjamin, November 28, 1969, 1–2, Box 4, Series II-C, HB.

78. Harry Benjamin to "Vicki," March 20, 1970, Box 7, Series II-C, HB.

79. "PF" to Harry Benjamin, May 20, 1970, Box 5, Series II-C, HB.

80. "GV" to Harry Benjamin, no date (c. March 1971), 2, Box 5, Series II-C, HB.

81. "GV" to Harry Benjamin, no date (c. 1971), Box 5, Series II-C, HB, emphasis added.

82. "YC" to Leo Wollman, December 1968, Box 6, Series II-C, HB.

83. To preserve confidentiality, I use a different pseudonym from the one that she used in her letters.

84. "Vicki" to Leo Wollman, November 28, 1968, Box 7, Series II-C, HB.

85. Virginia Allen to "Vicki," December 24, 1968, Box 7, Series II-C, HB.

86. "Vicki" to Leo Wollman, no date (c. December 1968); "Vicki" to Leo Wollman, no date (January 1969); "Vicki" to Leo Wollman, no date (February 1969); and "Vicki" to Harry Benjamin, May 14, 1969, Box 7, Series II-C, HB.

87. "Vicki" to Leo Wollman, no date (c. February 1969); and Virginia Allen to "Vicki," February 20, 1969, Box 7, Series II-C, HB.

88. "Vicki" to Leo Wollman, March 30, 1969, Box 7, Series II-C, HB.

89. "Vicki" to Harry Benjamin, no date (c. 1969), Box 7, Series II-C, HB.

90. Kathryn Bond Stockton, "The Queer Child Now and Its Paradoxical Global Effects," *GLQ: A Journal of Lesbian and Gay Studies* 22, no. 4 (2016): 506.

91. Stockton, *The Queer Child*, 11.

92. Stockton, *The Queer Child*, 3–4.

93. Stockton, *The Queer Child*, 13.

94. Stockton, *The Queer Child*, 13.

95. "Vicki" to Leo Wollman, November 28, 1968.

96. Photographs in "Vicki" to Leo Wollman, November 28, 1968.

97. Virginia Allen to "Vicki," December 24, 1968, Box 7, Series II-C, HB.

98. "Vicki" to Leo Wollman, no date (c. December 1968), Box 7, Series II-C, HB.

99. "Vicki" to Leo Wollman, February 1969, Box 7, Series II-C, HB.

100. "Vicki" to Leo Wollman, February 1969, emphasis added, Box 7, Series II-C, HB.

101. "Vicki" to Leo Wollman, March 30, 1969, Box 7, Series II-C, HB.

102. "Vicki" to Leo Wollman, May 14, 1969, Box 7, Series II-C, HB.

103. Harry Benjamin to "Vicki," May 22, 1969, Box 7, Series II-C, HB.

104. "Vicki" to Harry Benjamin, June 15, 1970, Box 7, Series II-C, HB.

105. Eugene Hoff, Summary of Interview with "NB," July 24, 1978, Folder 43, Box 2, JH.

106. See Robin Bernstein, *Racial Innocence: Performing American Childhood from Slavery to Civil Rights* (New York: New York University Press, 2011).

5. Transgender Boyhood, Race, and Puberty in the 1970s

1. Ram W. Rapoport to John Money, July 27, 1973, Box 7, JMK.

2. John Money to Ram W. Rapoport, August 2, 1973, 1, Box 7, JMK.

3. John Money to Ram W. Rapoport, August 2, 1973, 1, Box 7, JMK, 2.

4. John Money to Ram W. Rapoport, August 2, 1973, 1, Box 7, JMK, 2.

5. John Money to Ram W. Rapoport, August 2, 1973, 1, Box 7, JMK, 3. This is odd because Hopkins most certainly would not have approved surgery for a seventeen-year-old during the 1970s. Money may have disagreed with that policy, but he also lacked the ability to change it.

6. Joanne Meyerowitz, *How Sex Changed: A History of Transsexuality in the United States* (Cambridge, Mass.: Harvard University Press), 222. The timeline and model of the Stanford Program reflected the emergent norms of the field, but perhaps in one of its most rigid forms. An initial consultation, followed by psychiatric evaluation, an endocrine exam, a "grooming clinic" run by "a postoperative transsexual patient and a professional model regarding electrolysis, proper clothing, with proper emphasis on womanly counseling," a meeting with an employment counselor, and a consultation with a lawyer were involved. After each of these hurdles had been cleared, the clinic's committee would meet to decide on "final clearance" before approving surgery. Clients were also required to live in their gender identity for a year, on hormones, before surgery. Follow-up appointments after surgery were meant to take place annually for five years. The estimated cost (excluding follow-ups) of the full program was approximately $3,000 to $4,000 in 1972. Erickson Educational Foundation, Enclosure to John Money, June 27, 1972, Box 2, JMK.

7. John Money and Richard Green, eds. *Transsexualism and Sex Reassignment* (Baltimore: Johns Hopkins University Press, 1969).

8. See Meyerowitz, *How Sex Changed*, 271–74.

9. One of the earliest evaluations of the historicity of trans masculine experience is [Aaron] Devor's *FTM: Female-to-Male Transsexuals in Society* (Bloomington: Indiana University Press, 1997), 3–36. Conspicuously, Devor's historical chronology ends in the 1960s and so does not comment on the border wars that were contemporary with the publication of the book. By contrast, Leslie Feinberg's

Transgender Warriors: Making History from Joan of Arc to Dennis Rodman (Boston: Beacon Press, 1996) makes much more general claims about the potential reclamation of historical trans masculine figures. For a recent review of the disproportionate visibility of trans women in relation to that of trans men in transgender studies, see Matthew Heinz, *Entering Transmasculinity: The Inevitability of Discourse* (Bristol, England: Intellect Press, 2016), 13–14.

10. As Meyerowitz explores in *How Sex Changed,* 271–74, these private clinics did not close down in the 1980s by any means. The point is rather that their approach to access to surgeries was dealt an inevitable blow with the incorporation of transsexual diagnosis into the *DSM.*

11. For instance, when the New Jersey Medical School in Newark began seeing trans clients in 1972, Blue Cross Blue Shield would generally cover medical procedures *after* an individual had been at the clinic for one year. The medical school also reported: "We have been instrumental in having the State of New Jersey Medicaid program pay for sex reassignment procedures in 15 cases. This is the first time that a state medical agency has considered transsexualism to be a medical disorder requiring surgical correction." See Richard M. Samuels, Harish K. Malhotra, and Mona M. Devanesan, "A Gender Dysphoria Program in New Jersey," *Journal of the Medical Society of New Jersey* 74, no. 1 (January 1977): 37. In a 1975 issue of the Erickson Educational Foundation publication, Ira Dushoff reported "that more than 15 carriers of national repute have paid for sex reassignment surgery such as reconstructive in nature." See "Insurance Information," *Erickson Educational Foundation Newsletter* 8, 1 (Spring 1975), 3, Digital Transgender Archive, https://archive.org/details/newslettervol8eric.

12. David Valentine, *Imagining Transgender: An Ethnography of a Category* (Durham, N.C.: Duke University Press, 2007), 55, emphasis in original.

13. As chapter 4 details, for endocrinologists like Harry Benjamin who bridged both epistemological traditions, the unruly relationship between homosexuality and transsexuality proved impossible to reconcile.

14. Valentine, *Imagining Transgender,* 59.

15. Eve Kosofsky Sedgwick, "How to Bring Your Kids Up Gay," *Social Text* 29 (1991): 21, emphasis in original.

16. Sedgwick, "How to Bring Your Kids Up Gay," 21.

17. Sedgwick, "How to Bring Your Kids Up Gay," 20.

18. See, for one of the earliest examples, Patricia Leigh Brown, "Supporting Boys or Girls When the Line Isn't Clear," *New York Times,* December 2, 2006, http://www.nytimes.com/2006/12/02/us/02child.html.

19. Including in the 1960s, in the case of the University of California, Los Angeles. See chapter 4.

20. Jack Halberstam, *Female Masculinity* (Durham, N.C.: Duke University Press, 1998), 144, emphasis added.

21. Radclyffe Hall, *The Well of Loneliness* (London: Wordsworth Classics, 2005). On the early twentieth century, see Elizabeth Lapovsky Kennedy and Madeline D. Davis, *Boots of Leather, Slippers of Gold: The History of a Lesbian Community* (New York: Routledge, 2014).

22. See the introduction to this book for more on Hart and Dillon. See chapter 2 for more on Bernard.

23. Halberstam, *Female Masculinity*, 142.

24. At the same time, it is worth pointing out that some of the impetus for taking up the border war in this moment was the murder of Brandon Teena in 1993 and the subsequent litigation over naming and identity. See C. Jacob Hale, "Consuming the Living, Dis(re)membering the Dead in the Butch/FTM Borderlands," *GLQ* 4, no. 2 (1998): 311–48. Interestingly, in *Self-Made Men: Identity and Embodiment among Transsexual Men* (Nashville, Tenn.: Vanderbilt University Press, 2003), Henry Rubin located the emergence of trans masculine identity and community in the 1970s, much earlier than Halberstam (although he was relying there on data from medical professionals, who reported an apparent uptick in trans men seeking surgery that we should probably regard with a high degree of scrutiny as the basis of an argument about identity and demography). In any case, however, Rubin's explanation for that emergence also repeated the narrative of sequence and precedence: "The rise in the number of FTMs in the 1970s is the unintended consequence of identity work in the lesbian community" (64). I should add that I do not mean to pin this problem on Halberstam or Rubin; these two books are incredibly important for taking trans masculinity seriously as an object of analysis. I am also not trying to argue that lesbian feminism or butch lesbian politics were irrelevant to trans masculinity or transgender boyhood. The specific problem I see is the generational presumption of temporal sequence from lesbian to transgender. I do not see that succession holding up, even in the loosest sense, in the 1970s or even earlier in the twentieth century (see especially chapter 2 of this book). Since that narrative of succession has worked in tandem with the contemporary discourse that makes trans children products of the present and future, rather than subjects bearing a past, this chapter aims to overturn that dimension of the border wars narrative in particular. The related point to make here is that there simply *is not* much of an explicit generational narrative around the relationship between trans masculinity and butch masculinity. Rather, the narrative has been left *implicit* by a lack of detailed historical analysis—and that is precisely the problem this chapter seeks to remedy. One noteworthy exception to this historical assumption of succession and competition comes from Jeanne Córdova. See Talia M. Bettcher, "A Conversation with Jeanne Córdova," *Transgender Studies Quarterly* 3, no. 1–2 (2016): 285–93.

25. Meyerowitz, *How Sex Changed*, 253.

26. The clinic had been far from prolific in its actual work, moreover. At the time of its closing, only one hundred clients had been granted access to surgery. Joann Rodgers, "Hopkins Ceases Sex-Change Operations," *News American*, August 12, 1979, no page, Folder 3, JMH. See also Mark Bowden, "Power Struggle Erupted into New Hopkins Policy on Sex-Change Surgery," *Baltimore Sun*, April 7, 1980, no page, Folder 3, JM.

27. Harry Benjamin to Elmer Belt, July 28, 1958; Harry Benjamin to Elmer Belt, March 6, 1960; and Elmer Belt to Harry Benjamin, February 22, 1960, Box 3, Series II-C, HB.

28. See Gayle Salamon, "The Meontology of Masculinity: Notes on Castration Elation," *Parallax* 22, no. 3 (2016): 312–22.

29. "D.N." to Charles Ihlenfeld, no date, 1975, Box 3, Series II-C, HB.

30. Charles Ihlenfeld to "D.N.," June 19, 1975, Box 3, Series II-C, HB.

31. "N.Y. Academy of Medicine," *Erickson Educational Foundation Newsletter* 6, no. 1 (Spring 1973): 1, Digital Transgender Archive, https://archive.org/details/newslettervol6eric_u6k9.

32. For example, see Jeanne Hoff, [patient name and record number redacted], February 1976, Folder 46, Box 3, JH. This seventeen-year-old trans child managed to arrange to fly from New Hampshire to New York City and back in one day in order to take an appointment in Benjamin's practice. However, they did not have permission from their parents to do so. "We consult with and advice [sic] under-age patients without parental consent, but have not, to our knowledge, treated such patients," explained Virginia Allen to this patient in a letter dated September 22, 1975, Folder 36, Box 3, JH Box 3.

33. "D.U." to Charles Ihlenfeld, July 2, 1976, Box 3, Series II-C, HB.

34. Virginia Allen to "D.U.," July 9, 1976, Box 3, Series II-C, HB

35. Agnes C. Nagy, [patient record name redacted], [date redacted], 1976, Folder 52, Box 5, JH.

36. See, for example, Elaine Ferranti to John Money, August 27, 1974, Box 2, JMK, writing for advice on opening a gender clinic.

37. Frank Knight to John Money, October 11, 1977, Box 4, JMK.

38. Raymond Lemberg to John Money, March 27, 1979, Box 4, JMK.

39. Roy N. Killingworth to John Money, October 4, 1971, Box 4, JMK.

40. John K. Meyer to Roy N. Killingworth, November 2, 1971, Box 4, JMK.

41. Dorothy Baker to Social Service Department Director, Johns Hopkins Hospital, April 10, 1969, Box 1, JMK.

42. John Money to Dorothy Baker, April 30, 1969, Box 1, JMK.

43. Still, having carefully considered the document in its entirety, I do not doubt the source enough to cast it as fictitious.

44. [Name illegible due to damage to document] to John Money, January 5, 1976, Box 1, JMK.

45. For example, Granato also performed surgery for a sixteen-year-old trans girl in 1975. Jeanne Hoff, [case notes], May 31, 1977, Folder 27, Box 2, JH.

46. See, for instance, Howard Grotsky to Johns Hopkins University Chairman, Department of Psychiatry, July 21, 1975, Box 3, JMK, for an example of a clinician looking for a way to arrange surgery for a sixteen-year-old trans girl with parental support and consent. Because Hopkins had a strict policy not to accept for surgery candidates under the age of twenty-one, Grotsky's inquiry was rejected. Mark F. Schwartz to Howard Grotsky, July 28, 1975, Box 3, JMK.

47. S. Otto Hesterly to Richard Green and John Money, August 1, 1971, Box 3, JMK. Again, this person was turned away because of Hopkins's age requirement in the reply to the letter. John K. Meyer to Otto Hesterly, August 20, 1971, Box 3, JMK.

48. Charles Ihlenfeld, "The Transexual," unpublished manuscript with handwritten revisions, *Sexuality*, August 4, 1971, Box 7, Series II-C, HB, 1–4.

49. Ihlenfeld, "The Transexual," 4.

50. Ihlenfeld, "The Transexual," 5.

51. Ihlenfeld, "The Transexual," 7.

52. Robert Stoller, *Sex and Gender, Vol. II: The Transsexual Experiment* (New York: Jason Aronson, 1975), 81.

53. Harry Benjamin to John P. Curran, January 5, 1971, Box 4, Series II-C, HB.

54. Garrett Oppenheim, "Ihlenfeld Cautions on Hormones," *Transition* 8 (January/February 1979): 1, 3, 15, emphasis added, Folder 4, Series I, CI.

55. Oppenheim, "Ihlenfeld Cautions on Hormones," 15, emphasis added. That "difficulty" is likely a reference to the way that the symptomatology for transsexuality in childhood differed only slightly from the symptomatology for homosexuality as established by the psychogenic theories on hand.

56. Anonymous, "Letter: Hormones at Age 17," *Transition* 8 (January/February 1979): 7, Folder 4, Series I, CI.

57. Anonymous, "Letter: Hormones at Age 17."

58. The possible implication is that if a child could succeed with a claim of legal emancipation before age eighteen, they would be empowered to make their own health-care decisions. Even if this was a buried implication of Levidow's printed response, I have come across no discussion elsewhere, speculative or concrete, of that possibility for trans children in this era.

59. Lawrence Newman, "Transsexualism: A Disorder of Sexual Identity," *Medical Insight* (November 1970): 37, Folder 50, Box 28, MJ.

60. Newman, "Transsexualism," 37.

61. Newman, "Transsexualism," 39, emphasis added.

62. Newman, "Transsexualism," 39, emphasis added.

63. W. A. Marshall and J. M. Tanner, "Variations in Pattern of Pubertal Changes in Girls," *Archives of Disease in Childhood* 44, no. 235 (1969): 291–303; and "Variations

in the Pattern of Pubertal Changes in Boys," *Archives of Disease in Childhood* 45, no. 239 (1970): 23–33.

64. I take up this point in a broader context of thinking race and trans together in Julian Gill-Peterson, "The Technical Capacities of the Body: Assembling Race, Technology, and Transgender," *Transgender Studies Quarterly* 1, no. 3 (2014): 413.

65. Joseph L. Rauh to John Money, September 29, 1970, Box 7, JMK.

66. Ronald A. Rabin, Psychiatric Consultation Adolescent Service, [patient name redacted], 1970, Box 7, JMK, 1.

67. Ronald A. Rabin, Psychiatric Consultation Adolescent Service, [patient name redacted], 1970, Box 7, JMK, 1.

68. Ronald A. Rabin, Psychiatric Consultation Adolescent Service, [patient name redacted], 1970, Box 7, JMK, 3.

69. Ronald A. Rabin, Psychiatric Consultation Adolescent Service, [patient name redacted], 1970, Box 7, JMK, 4.

70. John Money to Joseph L. Rauh, October 5, 1970, Box 7, JMK, 1, emphasis added.

71. John Money to Joseph L. Rauh, October 5, 1970, Box 7, JMK, 2, emphasis added.

72. For an example of an inquiry from a juvenile parole officer, in this case about a trans girl incarcerated in juvenile homes for boys since age eight because she had run away from home, see Richard S. Peterson to John Money, September 10, 1974, Box 8, JMK.

73. Gary L. Nitz to Alejandro Rodriguez, October 19, 1971, Box 6, JMK.

74. T. Kerby Neill to John Money, October 26, 1978, Box 7, JMK.

75. T. Kerby Neill to John Money, October 26, 1978, Box 7, JMK, 3.

76. Kathryn Bond Stockton, "The Queer Child Now and Its Paradoxical Global Effects," *GLQ* 22, no. 4 (2016): 531–32, n.8, emphasis in original.

77. Claudia Castañeda, "Developing Gender: The Medical Treatment of Transgender Young People," *Social Science and Medicine* 143 (November 2014): 262–70.

78. Although a few formal counseling programs for and by trans people had opened in San Francisco earlier in the decade. See Meyerowtiz, *How Sex Changed,* 234–35.

79. Jeanne Hoff, [case notes], June 17, 1977, Folder 3, Box 2, JH.

80. Jeanne Hoff, [case notes, medical record number redacted], September 7, 1977, Folder 34, Box 1, JH, emphasis added.

81. Jeanne Hoff, [case notes, medical record number redacted], September 4, 1976, Box 1, JH.

82. Jeanne Hoff, [case notes, medical record number redacted], November 2, 1976, Box 1, JH.

83. Leah C. Schaefer to Agnes C. Nagy, September 18, 1976, Box 1, JH.

84. Jeanne Hoff, [case notes, medical record number redacted], April 15, 1980, Folder 3, Box 3, JH.

85. [Name redacted] to Jeanne Hoff, July 4, 1999, Folder 3, Box 3, JH.

Conclusion

1. Ryan Gados, "Trump Administration Working on New Transgender Bathroom Directive," *Fox News*, February 22, 2017, http://www.foxnews.com/poli tics/2017/02/22/trump-administration-working-on-new-transgender-bath room-directive.html. For several examples of media coverage from the past few years that labels trans children's access to bathrooms as a "new issue," see "CBS News Poll: Transgender Kids and School Bathrooms," *CBS News*, June 8, 2014, http://www.cbsnews.com/news/cbs-news-poll-transgender-kids-and-school -bathrooms; David Lightman and Lesley Clark, "Will the Transgender Bathroom Issue Split the Republican Party?" *Charlotte Observer*, May 13, 2016, http://www .charlotteobserver.com/news/politics-government/article77530152.html; and Beth Walton, "Discovering Emma: A Kindergartner's Transgender Journey," *Citizen Times*, May 20, 2017, http://www.citizen-times.com/story/news/local/2017/05/ 20/discovering-emma-kindergartners-transgender-journey/99975676/.

2. Sheryl Gay Stolberg, "Bathroom Case Puts Transgender Student on National Stage," *New York Times*, February 23, 2017, https://www.nytimes.com/2017/02/23/ us/gavin-grimm-transgender-rights-bathroom.html.

3. Ariane de Vogue, "Meet Gavin Grimm, the Transgender Students at the Center of Bathroom Debate," *CNN*, September 8, 2016, http://www.cnn.com/ 2016/09/08/politics/transgender-bathroom-issues-gavin-grimm/index.html, emphasis added.

4. H. M. Coon, Report to W. B. Campbell, Department of Neuro-Psychiatry, University of Wisconsin–Madison, General Hospital, July 19, 1948, Box 3, Series II-C, HB.

5. Claudia Castañeda, "Developing Gender: The Medical Treatment of Transgender Young People," *Social Science & Medicine* 143 (2015): 267–68.

6. Sahar Sadjadi, "The Endocrinologist's Office—Puberty Suppression: Saving Children from a Natural Disaster?" *Journal of Medical Humanities* 34, no. 2 (2013): 255–60; Tey Meadow, *Trans Kids: Being Gendered in the Twenty-First Century* (Berkeley: University of California Press, 2018).

7. Ann Travers, *The Trans Generation: How Trans Kids (and Their Parents) Are Creating a Gender Revolution* (New York: New York University Press, 2018).

8. Dean Spade, "Mutilating Gender," in *The Transgender Studies Reader*, ed. Susan Stryker and Stephen Whittle (New York: Routledge, 2006), 315–32; Eric A. Stanley, "Gender Self-Determination," *Transgender Studies Quarterly* 1, no. 1–2

(2014): 89–91; Paisley Currah, "Transgender Rights without a Theory of Gender?" *Tulsa Law Review* 52, no. 3 (2017): 441–51.

9. On the flexible child as a biological body under neoliberalism, see Julian Gill-Peterson, "The Value of the Future: The Child as Human Capital and the Neoliberal Labor of Race," *Women's Studies Quarterly* 43, no. 1–2 (2015): 181–96, and "Neurofeminism: An Eco-pharmacology of Childhood ADHD," in *Mattering: Feminism, Science and Materialism,* ed. Victoria Pitts-Taylor (New York: New York University Press), 188–203.

10. Paul B. Preciado, *Testo Junkie: Sex, Drugs, and Biopolitics in the Pharmacopornographic Era,* trans. Bruce Benderson (New York: Feminist Press, 2014), 385. I take up this critique of Preciado in detail in chapter 3.

11. Rebekah Sheldon, *The Child to Come: Life after the Human Catastrophe* (Minneapolis: University of Minnesota Press), 151.

12. Sheldon, *The Child to Come,* 151.

13. Sheldon, *The Child to Come,* 180.

14. My thanks to Claudia Castañeda for discussing this question with me.

15. See Folder 7, Box 5, Series III A, LL.

16. Lawrence herself seems to have maintained an interest in these histories of childhood public cross-dressing, collecting clippings of newspaper articles about children who, after participating in Mummer and Ragamuffin parades, ran away from home dressed in the clothes of the opposite sex. See "Boys Will Be Girls" and "She's a He," *Inside Detective,* July 1941, Folder 2, Box 4, Series III A, LL.

17. Louise Lawrence, Scrapbook, no date (circa 1950s), Folder 7, Box 5, Series III A, LL.

18. Eve Kosofsky Sedgwick, "How to Bring Your Kids Up Gay," *Social Text* 29 (1991): 26, emphasis in original.

Index

"Agnes," 123–24, 137–38, 144
Aizura, Aren, 25
Alabama, 21, 84–89
Allan, Virginia, 152, 154
Amar, Paul, 10
American Psychiatric Association, 167
antiblackness, 2, 4, 25, 79–80, 185–90, 201. *See also* psychiatry; racialized gender; transsexuality
anti-trans: medicine, 80–90, 135–37, 144–48, 159–60, 185–86; narratives questioning children's transness, vii, 10, 155 (*see also* childhood: trans as etiology for gender); politics, vii–ix, 1, 195–96; violence, ix–x, 1–2, 23–24
archive: of medicine, 12, 26, 90–91, 175, 177, 187; of this book, 20–21, 23, 31–32, 59–60, 62, 203; of trans history, 11–21, 31, 59–62, 90, 95, 160, 191–92
Arizona, 174
Arkansas, 178

Baltimore, 63, 69, 74, 76–77, 81, 84, 89–91, 104, 107, 129–30, 135
bathroom bills, 2, 195–96
Belt, Elmer, 137, 171–72, 244n25
Benjamin, Harry, 19, 21, 33, 61, 64–68, 91, 94, 129–30, 137–60, 167, 171–74, 178–80, 192, 201

Berlin, 13, 53, 66, 232n37, 236n112
"Bernard," 84–89
binary. *See* gender; sex; transition
biopolitics, 9, 16, 26, 94, 112, 198, 202. *See also* Foucault, Michel
bisexuality, as theory of sex. *See* plasticity; sex
blackness, 25, 30–32, 186–87, 225n97
Boston, 106
Bowman, Karl, 61

California, 52, 104–5, 151
Canada, 217n15
cárdenas, micha, 29
Castañeda, Claudia, 36, 191, 197
Chicago, 165
child: definition and use of term, 9–10; as eugenic concept, 52–53; as figure, viii, 2–3, 36, 56–57
child development: as explanation for gender variance, 47–49, 76–78, 88–89, 119, 141–42; as justification for anti-trans medicine, 145–46. *See also* Hall, G. Stanley
childhood: trans as etiology for gender, viii, 4, 8, 118, 144, 198, 202–3
children, oppression of, 8, 10, 196–98
cisgender, vii, 6, 15, 23, 27, 141, 181, 199, 202–3, 219n43
Cold War, 94
Colorado, 187

· 257 ·

Haritaworn, Jin, 26
Harry Benjamin Foundation, 139–40
Hart, Alan, 18, 60–62, 90, 170
Hausman, Bernice, 12, 94
Hayward, Eva, 2
Heaney, Emma, 15, 93
hermaphroditism. *See* intersex
Herring, Scott, 13–15, 220n54
heterosexuality, 71, 88
Hirschfeld, Magnus, 59, 64–65, 68, 81, 138, 142
Hoff, Jeanne, 160, 171–74, 192–93
homosexuality: distinction from trans identity, 167–68, 176; as misrecognition of trans people, 4, 13, 29, 186–88; overlap with trans identity, 13–14, 60–61, 80–81, 84–90, 135–36, 142, 144, 151–52; psychiatric medicalization of, 83–90, 135; use of term, 9
hormones: cortisone, 106–14; "discovery" of in science, 41–44; early medical therapies, 79, 83; trans children's access to, 149, 151, 153–54, 157–58, 173, 178–79, 193. *See also* endocrinology
Houston, 137

identity. *See* homosexuality: overlap with trans identity; intersex: relation to trans identity; multiple trans childhoods; transvestism and transvestite: as trans identity
identity politics, vii, 14, 16, 22, 190
Ihlenfeld, Charles, 171–74, 178–83
intersex: field of intersex studies, 240–41n40, 241–42n52; as indicative of plasticity, 112–13; medicalization of children, 68–70, 75–80, 103–14, 120, 124–26; relation to trans

identity, 15, 62–63, 80–90, 92–93, 99, 137–38, 140–41, 144; use of term, 9
inversion. *See* homosexuality
Italy, 137

Jennings, Jazz, 1
Johns Hopkins Hospital, 13, 17, 19, 21, 22, 27, 46, 63–64, 68–72, 75, 79–105, 115, 121, 124, 130, 137, 165, 171, 175–78, 187; Brady Urological Institute, 68–76, 79–83, 87, 89, 91, 99, 104, 133–36; Gender Identity Clinic, 129–30, 133; Harriet Lane Home for Children, 70, 78–80, 88, 100, 103–13, 124
Johnson, Marsha P., 21–25
Jorgensen, Christine, 11, 22, 91, 94, 137–39, 142, 150–51
June, Jennie, 13–16

Kammerer, Paul, 51–52, 57, 65, 67
Kanner, Leo, 70, 107, 238n14
"Karen," 89–90
Katz, Jonathan Ned, 60, 230n3
Kentucky, 187
Kinsey, Alfred, 18, 61, 68
Krafft-Ebing, Richard von, 13
Krell, Elías Cosenza, 1

"Lane," 133–35, 243n15
Lawrence, Louise, 18, 138–39, 142, 151, 203–4, 206
lesbian–trans masculine border wars, 170–71, 188, 190–91, 250n24
letters of trans children to doctors, 151–79, 172–74
Lewis, Abram J., 19–20
Lillie, Frank R., 87
London, 42, 172
Los Angeles, 20–21, 149, 171–72

JULIAN GILL-PETERSON is assistant professor of English at the
University of Pittsburgh.

Printed and bound by CPI Group (UK) Ltd, Croydon, CR0 4YY

09/06/2025

14685650-0001